The Consumer
Health Information
Source Book

CONSUMER INFORMATION SERIES

The Consumer Health Information Source Book
   by Alan M. Rees and Blanche A. Young
The Travel Book: A Guide to the Travel Guides
   by Jon O. Heise

The Consumer Health Information Source Book

Alan M. Rees
and Blanche A. Young

R. R. Bowker Company
New York & London, 1981

To June Marguerite Rees, M.D.

Published by R. R. Bowker Company
1180 Avenue of the Americas, New York, NY 10036
Copyright © 1981 by Xerox Corporation
All rights reserved
Printed and bound in the United States of America

Library of Congress Cataloging in Publication Data

Rees, Alan M
    The consumer health information source book.

    (Consumer information series)
    Includes indexes.
    1. Health—Bibliography.   2. Medicine, Popular—
Bibliography.   3. Health—Information services—United
States—Directories.   4. Medicine—Information services
—United States—Directories.   5. Health education—
Audio-visual aids-Catalogs.   I. Young, Blanche A., joint
author.   II. Title.   III. Series: Consumer information
series (New York)   [DNLM: 1. Bibliography of medi-
cine.   2. Medicine—Directories—Bibliography.
3. Medicine—Popular works.   ZWB 130 R328c]
Z6673.R43   [RA776]   016.613   80-28793
ISBN 0-8352-1336-6   AACR1

Contents

Foreword

The individual is the key decision-maker in health practice and medicine. It is the individual who must decide when to seek medical help, where to go, who to see, what information to give, what demands to make, and what advice to accept. These decisions determine whether the individual benefits or suffers from medical care, and whether the American public's multimillion dollar annual expenditure on medical care represents a wise investment or a misguided attempt to buy health. Important as these decisions are, they are secondary to another set of decisions—whether to exercise, control weight, drink moderately, reduce stress, stop smoking, and prevent accidents. These decisions are the true determinants of health. The rise of the self-care movement and the new emphasis on health promotion all attest to the acknowledgment of the critical importance of these decisions. Within the medical care system, the recognition of the individual's responsibility for health and the physician's responsibility to advise and assist in the individual's decision-making has resulted in the most significant change in the doctor-patient relationship in the last century, perhaps ever.

Intelligent decision-making is impossible, however, without relevant, up-to-date, and usable information on a wide range of topics. The individual needs information on the benefits, risks, and costs of medical care; selection of a physician; surgical procedures; second opinions; signs and symptoms; how and when to utilize medical services; exercise; smoking; nutrition; stress; and more. Despite this enormous need for information, the individual in search of help may find that too much rather than too little health information is the problem. Every day greets new medical advances and theories, new information sources, new media. Much of the health information currently available is good, but more of it is mediocre or misleading. When first confronted, the wealth of health information materials may seem to be a hopeless morass of conflicting information in a bewildering variety of formats.

Yet, relevant and reliable health information is available on almost every subject—*if you know where to look!* This is the importance of this book. In *The Consumer Health Information Source Book,* Alan Rees and Blanche Young have provided organized access to an excellent selection of materials and information sources, both print and nonprint. The simple, straightforward approach of this book transcends the enormous variety of information presented. The *Source Book* is the first of its kind in assembling a vast array of sources of consumer health information. Whoever searches for health information—consumers, physicians, health care practitioners, health educators, librarians—will find this book an invaluable guide.

Donald M. Vickery, M.D.
President, Center for Consumer
   Health Education
Vienna, Virginia

Preface

This book assembles, describes, and evaluates the principal sources of health information for the layperson. It is both an annotated bibliography of current literature and a guide to organizations that provide health information. *The Consumer Health Information Source Book* is a title in Bowker's Consumer Information Series.

Consumer health information is the term commonly used to describe information on health and medical topics for the general public. It encompasses information on wellness, physical fitness, preventive medicine, and self-health care, which are all primarily concerned with health maintenance and the promotion of good health practices. Consumer health information also includes patient education information, which generally focuses on the management of illness within the hospital setting. It is hoped that this book will prove valuable both to consumers and to professionals who must respond to the health information needs of the public. Such professionals include physicians, nurses, patient and health educators, and librarians in public, medical, and health sciences libraries.

Better access to consumer information is necessary to permit effective decision-making by the public. Today, the burgeoning demand for consumer information and consumer health information stems from the public's recent claim to high-quality services and products in all sectors of the economy. The extension of consumerism to the health care market place attests to the public's recognition of the importance of good health to improving the quality of life in America.

In addition, recent developments in medical research, technology, and health care services have placed more pressure on the individual to keep informed of the relative benefits, risks, and costs of care and treatment in order to make responsible decisions. The modern medical consumer requires the knowledge to choose among an often bewildering variety of medical and health care alternatives. And, more than ever before, the patient recognizes that consent to care and treatment can and should be "informed consent."

Thus, the average layperson is now not only more concerned about health, but realizes that he or she must assume individual responsibility and become an active partner in the doctor-patient relationship. Passive dependence upon professional medical opinion is no longer sufficient. "Consumers (sometimes known as patients) . . . are insisting, with considerable success, that they deserve not just a piece of the action, but a piece of the knowledge. The passive role of the patient is passé," states Robert Hardy in *SICK: How People Feel about Being Sick and What They Think of Those Who Care for Them* (Chicago: Teach'em, 1978). Interviewed in the Summer 1980 issue of *Medical Self-Care* magazine, Sidney M. Wolfe, M.D., director of the Public Citizen Health Research Group, a consumer advocacy organization, points to "the erosion of the traditional view that the doctor knows everything and the patient knows nothing."

That the individual can now in large measure influence his or her own health through improvement of health practices and life-style is the basis of the self-health care movement. As Donald M. Vickery, M.D., explains in *LifePlan for Your Health* (Reading, MA: Addison-Wesley, 1979): "Doctors cannot manage your health even if they are so inclined. *You* decide when to go to the doctor, what health facilities to use, whether to take the doctor's advice." Vickery also explodes a number of common fallacies, such as "health depends most on good medical care; doctors and only doctors can tell you if you're healthy; and that medicine has a cure for every disease." Health care cannot be equated with medical care.

Unfortunately, the consumer in the past has not been equipped with the information necessary to judge the effectiveness and efficiency of health care services or to accept responsibility for managing his or her own health. There is no shortage of consumer health information, yet coordinated delivery at local, state, regional, and federal levels does not exist at the present time. The situation is in marked contrast to the organized access to, and delivery of, the professional literature of the health sciences provided by libraries utilizing MEDLINE and other data bases. Resource sharing and interlibrary loan make this literature readily available.

It is hoped that *The Consumer Health Information Source Book* will contribute toward a better informed consumer by providing, for the first time, organized subject access to the vast amount of consumer health information currently available. A concerted effort has been made to bring together the most important, up-to-date, and useful materials and sources on the most significant topics of health care concern.

Book titles were selected and evaluated by the authors according to defined criteria: currency (publication date of 1975 of later); qualifications and/or institutional affiliation of author; significance and validity of content (accuracy, comprehensiveness, documentation, objectivity); quality of writing (style and readability); organization and ease of use (indexes, illustrations, and special features are noted); reference value in locating additional sources of information (bibliographies, lists of resource organizations); physical aspects (quality of print, paper, and binding; aesthetic appeal); and consumer orientation or usefulness in making judicious decisions about one's health and appropriate use of health care services. Works considered especially valuable are indicated as such in the text by the terms recommended and highly recommended. Expert opinion was sought from the medical staff of University Hospitals of Cleveland and the faculty of the School of Medicine at Case Western Reserve University in the formulation and application of these criteria. It should be noted that on many topics there is a lack of consensus in the medical community.

Users of this book are advised to read the Guide to Use section, following the Acknowledgments, for a detailed description of the contents of the *Source Book* and information on further research and materials acquisition.

The publication of this book is the first attempt at organizing the bibliography and literature of consumer health information. A subsequent title in the Consumer Information Series, a handbook tentatively entitled *Developing Consumer Health Information Services,* is currently in preparation. This latter book will describe the design, implementation, and operation of health information services and programs in various library settings.

Acknowledgments

It is most pleasing to acknowledge the assistance of a number of persons in the preparation of this book. Our thanks to Robert G. Cheshier, Majorie Saunders, and Margaret Henning of the Cleveland Health Sciences Library for assistance and encouragement; to Eleanor Goodchild, architect of the Consumer Health Information Program and Services (CHIPS) project, for helpful suggestions and for supplying many items of information; to Ellen Gartenfeld, project director of the Community Health Information Network (CHIN), for bringing the importance of consumer health information to our attention in 1978; to William Fissinger, vice-president for development of University Hospitals of Cleveland, and to Scott Inkley, M.D., chief of staff of University Hospitals and professor of medicine, Case Western Reserve University, for making many of the splendid resources of University Hospitals available; to Robert Botti, M.D., Jerome Paulson, M.D., Robert Kellermeyer, M.D., and A. Brian Little, M.D., professors of medicine, for recognizing the significance of consumer health information; to friend and colleague Susan Crawford of the American Medical Association for continuing advice and for the gift of materials; to Rita Book, special assistant to the dean, School of Library Science, Case Western Reserve University, for assistance in organizing education programs for librarians in consumer health information; to Cari Tobias Gross, Lucille Lang, and John Lonsak of the Cuyahoga County Public Library System for supplying book materials; to Robin Gallagher for perseverance in the typing of a difficult manuscript; and finally, to the Cleveland Foundation for their perception of the need for consumer health information services in Cleveland through their grant support.

Guide to Use

The Consumer Health Information Source Book is divided into three parts. Part I (Chapters 1–2) describes in narrative the health information needs of the public in light of changing social trends, such as medical consumerism and health promotion, and discusses current efforts to respond to these information requirements. It includes, in Chapter 2, an annotated bibliography of the seminal, landmark publications relating to the consumer health information movement.

Part II (Chapters 3–7) is a guide to Reference and Research Aids. Chapters 3 and 4 are "bibliographies of bibliographies" of print and audiovisual materials: Chapter 3 discusses bibliographies that relate to general consumer health information materials, patient education materials, Spanish-language materials, and government publications; while Chapter 4 examines bibliographies on 12 major health topics, such as alcoholism and diet and nutrition. Chapters 5, 6, and 7 include consumer health magazines, journals, and newsletters; professional medical literature suitable for supplementing popular consumer health collections; and profiles of the federal health information clearinghouses.

Part III (Chapters 8–17) comprises the main body of the book, providing in-depth descriptions of the primary sources of health information for the consumer—books, pamphlets, audiovisual producers and distributors, and resource organizations. Each chapter is devoted to a major focus of health concern, such as wellness, physical fitness, and self-health care, the focus of Chapter 8. Subsequent chapters discuss the health concerns of special groups—women, children, and the elderly—and health problems, such as heart disease and stroke, cancer, diabetes, mental health, alcoholism, and drug abuse.

Each chapter in Part III is divided into four sections: books, pamphlets, audiovisual producers and distributors, and resource organizations.

1. *Books.* The first section of each chapter is an annotated bibliography of books. Titles are arranged under subject areas and then alphabetically by author within major subcategories. For example, Children's Health is the sub-

ject of Chapter 9; subcategories include Infant and Preschool Care; Nutrition and Physical Fitness, Dental Care, and so forth. Entries contain full bibliographic information: author, title, city of publication, publisher, date, number of pages, and price; city, publisher, and price for paperback edition, if any; and a descriptive, evaluative annotation. British publisher and price are also cited for titles available in the United Kingdom. Out-of-print titles are designated "OP." Publication data is based upon *Books in Print 1979–1980* and *British Books in Print 1979.* All books included (more than 700) were published between 1975 and early 1980.

2. *Pamphlets.* Following the book annotations are lists of the major publishers and distributors of pamphlets and booklet materials. Entries are arranged alphabetically by name of organization and provide ordering addresses and lists of selected titles. Because of the diversity of pricing policies for such materials, prices are only cited for pamphlet and booklet materials known to cost $3 or more, either individually or as a series package. Many organizations supply pamphlets at no cost or minimum cost if they are requested in limited quantities. However, either payment may be required for large numbers of copies or an assurance that copies will be used for specific purposes. Requests for bulk orders should be accompanied by a statement noting target population, mode of distribution, and intended usage. As a rule, commercial producers charge for their pamphlets and booklets.

The significance of pamphlets and booklets in satisfying consumer health information needs should be stressed. Most pamphlets are simple, short, succinct, and endorsed by reputable health-related organizations. Pamphlets can be readily utilized for distribution to those requiring minimal explanation in easily comprehensible language. Moreover, they can be most helpful in relation to many medical topics where book literature for the lay reader is scant or nonexistent, for example, cystic fibrosis, Parkinson's disease, or epilepsy.

3. *Audiovisual Producers and Distributors.* Following the Pamphlets section is an alphabetically arranged directory of audiovisual producers and distributors, providing addresses and relevant subject coverage for each organization.

4. *Resource Organizations.* Concluding each chapter is an alphabetical list of information and referral sources, with addresses, that may be contacted to satisfy information requests relating to the subject coverage of the particular chapter. Such sources include voluntary health organizations, self-health care groups, parents groups, information centers, health education and counseling agencies, government agencies, public health groups, research centers, professional associations, consumer advocacy groups, and others. Both local and national organizations are listed. Many national health-related organizations, such as the American Cancer Society, maintain regional offices or affiliates to which national centers refer local information requests and inquiries, and which can most efficiently be contacted directly. Users of this book are urged to consider the lists of resource organizations as a core directory on which to build their own community-based information and referral source lists.

Many of the organizations in Part III of *The Consumer Health Information Source Book* provide a variety of materials and services and are thus listed in all three sections—pamphlets, audiovisual producers and distributors, and resource organizations. For further aid in reference, Appendix 1 and Appendix 2 are composite lists of the names and addresses of pamphlet suppliers and audiovisual producers and distributors included in Part III. These lists should prove especially useful for individuals who wish to request catalogs and publication lists from a large number of organizations. Appendix 1, the Organizational Guide to Pamphlets Suppliers, lists all pamphlet publishers and distributors alphabetically within six groups, delineating the major types of pamphlet-producing organizations: commercial firms, government agencies and clearinghouses, insurance companies, pharmaceutical companies, professional associations and societies, and voluntary health organizations. Appendix 2, the Directory of Audiovisual Producers and Distributors, incorporates all audiovisual suppliers in one alphabetical listing.

Names and addresses of American and British book publishers are provided in Appendix 3. This Directory of Publishers also includes publishers of bibliographies and other publications whose addresses are not included in the bibliographic information of the text entries.

Cross-references are used in the text to refer readers to other relevant chapters and sections. To further facilitate access, author, title, and subject indexes are included. The importance of consulting the indexes in using this book should be noted.

Part I

Consumer Health Information

Chapter 1

The Needs of Consumers for Health Information

HEALTH CARE AND THE AMERICAN PUBLIC

The United States spent 8.8 percent of its Gross National Product on health in 1977, involving an expenditure of more than $163 billion. Americans visited their doctors more than one billion times in that year. In 1980, the health care industry will account for 9 percent of the GNP or some $200 billion.[1] Dollars spent on health care, which amounted to $43 billion, or $217 per capita, in 1965 reached $192 billion, or $863 per capita in 1978.[2] Health care costs increase at the rate of $1 million per hour. The money spent in one day on health care in the United States exceeds the GNP of most nations in the world. Almost 5 percent of the total U.S. work force is employed in the health care industry, which includes more than 400,000 physicians, 100,000 dentists, and over 800,000 registered nurses affiliated with 7,200 hospitals, 20,100 nursing homes, and 6,200 other inpatient facilities.[3] A high social and economic priority is given in the United States to health care delivery, education, and research.

The quality of health care enjoyed by the populace has never been higher. Great progress has been made in increasing life expectancy and in reducing infant mortality. However, much disillusionment pervades the health care system in that public expectations far exceed the return from the enormous financial investment. The funding of additional health care resources and services appears to have little effect on most indicators of health status. The great emphasis upon medical technology appears to produce diminishing returns, and many question the cost effectiveness of specific medical procedures and services. The United States does not rank among the top ten nations with respect to most health indicators.

3

Health Promotion

The limits of medical intervention in the management of illness and disability are increasingly apparent. More sophisticated instrumentation and expensive health facilities do not ensure good health. As Joseph Califano, former Secretary of the Department of Health, Education and Welfare, has noted, "the road to better health in the nation's future cannot be paved only with the gold bricks of medication and expensive technology. The next dramatic breakthrough in the health of our people should be in prevention and promotion." [4] In this connection, *Healthy People: The Surgeon General's Report on Health Promotion and Disease Prevention* concludes that "health promotion is an idea whose time has come." [5]

Health promotion represents a hope for the future and serves as a rallying point for new efforts in health care. "Health promotion," a recent report of the National Chamber Foundation points out, "is a social movement of major proportions. It is gaining in popularity due to rapidly rising health care costs and concern that health status in general is not improving even though an increasing number of dollars is being spent on health care." [6] It is now realized that prevention is preferable to cure; that it is less expensive to keep people healthy than to treat sickness; that deficiencies in life-style account for more than one half of all mortality; and that changes in personal habits, and control of health hazards in the environment, will do most to improve the nation's health. Marc Lalonde, former Minister of National Health and Welfare of Canada, argues that "the traditional view of equating the level of health in Canada with the availability of physicians and hospitals is inadequate . . . There is little doubt that future improvements in the level of health of Canadians lies mainly in improving the environment, moderating self-imposed risks, and adding to our knowledge of human biology." [7] He adds that "for these environmental and behavioral threats to health, the organized health care system can do little more than serve as a catchment net for the victims." [8]

It is not surprising that great emphasis is currently placed upon self-care programs, health activation systems, health behavior modification, smoking cessation, hypertension screening, stress management utilizing yoga, transcendental and other forms of meditation, holistic medicine, health hazard appraisal, and alternative healing methods. Attention is increasingly focused upon the role of the individual in maintaining his or her own wellness. Many writers and educators speak of "patient power" and stress the need for persons to take primary responsibility for their health. "It is a time for the patient to stop feeling ignorant of his body and of his health; to stop blindly accepting whatever he is told. It is a time for him to ask questions, to read, to understand . . . It is a time for the patient to make the final decision concerning his own body." [9] Keith Sehnert, M.D., one of the founding fathers of the self-health care movement and author of the landmark book *How to Be Your Own Doctor—Sometimes,* [10] asserts that it is possible to be your own or your family's own doctor a great deal more than doctor-dependent people realize.

The public is vitally concerned with health and its preservation. *The Perrier Study: Fitness in America* reveals that more than 90 million American adults participate in some form of physical activity on a regular basis.[11] *The General Mills American Family Report, 1978–1979: Family Health in an Era of Stress,* a comprehensive study of the health needs, beliefs, and practices of Americans, demonstrates that health and staying healthy has become a major priority of the American public. Seventy percent of the adults interviewed for the survey by Yankelovich, Skelly, and White believe that Americans are more conscious about their health than they were a few years ago, and only 12 percent feel that they are less concerned.[12] Great interest is focused upon self-health care, physical fitness, exercise, drug abuse, hypertension, alcoholism, teenage pregnancy, sexual dysfunction, pregnancy and childbirth, mental disorders, nutrition, immunization, abortion, smoking, the handicapped, suicide, cancer, nursing homes, death and dying, hospices, medication, health insurance, the increasing cost of health care, and many other health-related topics.

"As people learn more about the relationships between lifestyles, health risk factors and disease," notes an American Hospital Association health information survey, "they are becoming increasingly conscious of their own health." [13] Indeed, the popularity of "doctor shows" on television, syndicated medical news columns, health articles in *Family Circle, Vogue, Redbook,* and other popular magazines, and the annual publication of more than a thousand health-related books by some eighty publishing houses all attest to the rapidly growing demand for health information. Companies such as General Mills, Xerox, Exxon, and Kimberly Clark have initiated health promotion programs to help employees and their families achieve and maintain their health, increase productivity by reducing disability and absenteeism, and thereby lower health insurance costs. Bonuses, vacations, and other incentives toward health are further awarded.

Medical Consumerism

Public interest in health is also manifested in the form of medical consumerism. The basic assumptions of this movement are that health care systems are overutilized often to the detriment of health, and that medical providers tend to generate unnecessary demand for their services. Better-informed consumers can make more intelligent and economical use of the health care system. Organizations such as the Public Citizen Health Research Group in Washington and the Center for Medical Consumers and Health Care Information in New York City are concerned with self-care initiatives, health promotion, and containment of costs.

Consumers are supported by the *Patient's Bill of Rights* of the American Hospital Association in insisting that the public has the right to obtain complete, current information concerning diagnosis, treatment, and prognosis in terms they can understand. Informed consent means that patients should play an active and intelligent role in the decision-making process concerning the risks and alternatives involved in their treatment.[14] The medical profession is now more responsive to the need to educate the public and to place more responsibility on individuals for their own health. A more sophisticated public would, it is believed, improve the doctor-patient relationship, promote health, and reduce health care costs by encouraging more prudent use of medical services. Anne Somers, professor of community medicine and family medicine at Rutgers University, expresses the belief that "it is not possible to sustain financially an adequate health care system in a country like the United States, unless accompanied by an effective program of consumer health education." [15]

Contrary to popular belief, the traditional medical establishment is supportive of health promotion and lay health initiative. The House of Delegates of the American Medical Association recommended in 1978 that "Consumers and patients should be encouraged and assisted to become more active and knowledgeable participants in making health care utilization decisions by developing health and patient education programs that inform consumers and patients about the costs and benefits associated with potential and alternative courses of treatment and emphasizing self-help programs directed at well and worried-well individuals." [16]

The American Hospital Association established in 1978 its Center for Health Promotion to coordinate and expand the association's activities and programs in patient education, community health education, and employee health. The center has produced a number of patient education teaching manuals and has organized several conferences. In addition to the American Medical Association and the American Hospital Association, other organizations such as the American Dental Association, the American Academy of Pediatrics, and the American College of Obstetricians and Gynecologists are also active in health promotion.

Public Demand for Health Information

Healthy People: The Surgeon General's Report on Health Promotion and Disease Prevention stresses that Americans have a deep interest in improving their health. *The General Mills American Family Report, 1978–1979: Family Health in an Era of Stress* confirms this conclusion and points out that despite the importance attached to health a majority of Americans feel that they are not well informed about good medical care, mental illness, nutrition, and diet. Fewer than three out of ten felt that they were well informed. The level of knowledge varies by demographic group. Eighty percent of those who consider themselves well informed are in the middle to upper socioeconomic groups. The least informed are to be found among the poorer socioeconomic groups and minorities.

Doctors and dentists are the most common sources of health information, followed by television programs, news stories, and popular magazines and newspapers. A Louis Harris survey, conducted in 1978 for the Pacific Mutual

Life Insurance Company, entitled *Health Maintenance,* reveals that there are still substantial minorities, and in some cases majorities, who are completely unaware of the health risks they are taking. The Harris survey revealed that Americans would like to learn more about how to perform self-examination for hypertension, breast cancer, and heart irregularities; what can be done to reduce the chances of heart attack; the effects of various drugs; the influence of fat and food additives on diet; the nutritional value of different foods; general information on how to stay healthy; and how to cope with stress and anxiety.[17]

The National Health Council's report, *Promoting Health: A Source Book,* which describes the major health promotion programs currently underway, emphasizes the need to supply this information: "If we are going to turn the health care system towards prevention and health promotion, we must expect and allow the citizen and consumer to play a larger role, ask him or her to take on larger responsibilities for health, both personally or socially." [18]

However, the provision of accurate, timely, and relevant information is a formidable task. The challenge to satisfy the health information needs of the American public can be met only if the multitude of information resources can be assembled and exploited in an effective and efficient manner, a task that will involve coordinated and concerted effort on a national basis.

Furthermore, it is generally agreed that the mere supply of health information does not, in itself, ensure behavioral change leading to improved health status. A recent Kellogg Foundation report notes that "the adoption of healthy life styles may result either by chance (health information), by informed decision (health education), or by design (health promotion)." [19] Within this context, health information in the form of printed or audiovisual materials must be viewed as a primary ingredient in the overall process of improving health knowledge and producing positive health changes in the populace.

Role of the Federal Government

The viewpoint of the medical consumer has been built into a number of legislative programs. These include the Health Maintenance Organization Act of 1973, the Comprehensive School Health Act of 1974, and the National Health Planning and Resources Development Act of 1974. The last act provides for a majority of consumers to serve on the planning boards of health systems agencies and statewide coordinating councils.

The National Health Education and Disease Prevention Act of 1975 was followed by the National Consumer Health Information and Health Promotion Act of 1976. The 1976 legislation provided for the establishment of the Office of Health Information and Health Promotion (OHIHP)* in the Office of the Assistant Secretary of Health, Department of Health, Education, and Welfare (now the Department of Health and Human Services—HHS). This

---

*Subsequently expanded in title to the Office of Health Information, Health Promotion, Physical Fitness and Sports Medicine.

office is charged with the coordination of all Public Health Service (PHS) and HHS departmental activities in health education, physical fitness, sports medicine, preventive services, and education. OHIHP fosters the appropriate use of health care facilities and resources that contribute to health promotion and is responsible for facilitating access to health information by the public. The office has sponsored a series of eight Regional Health Promotion Forums to stimulate health promotion activities throughout the country and has been active in the areas of smoking and health, nutrition, and school health.

A number of federal clearinghouses, such as the National Clearinghouse for Family Planning Information, the National Clearinghouse for Mental Health Information, the Cancer Information Clearinghouse, and the Alcohol Information Clearinghouse, exist to provide information services in specific health areas (see chapter 7 for a description of clearinghouse services and publications). At present, however, the network of federal information clearinghouses relating to human services is under scrutiny as a result of numerous complaints regarding inadequate announcement of the availability of informational materials, the unresponsiveness of the clearinghouses to consumer requests, and the lack of an efficient document delivery system. With a few exceptions, most of the federal health information clearinghouses lack clear objectives and do not provide prompt, efficient service. After much delay, a National Clearinghouse for Health Information has been funded to serve as a "referral center, providing a focal point for access to consumer health information sources within the federal establishment. While it is a worthy objective to strive for such coordination, there still remains the problem of the organization of federally produced materials.

Availability of Health Information

In terms of quantity, much consumer-oriented health information exists. In addition to the 1,000 books published annually, an amount increasing at about 10 percent per year, a massive body of pamphlet and booklet literature emanates from community health organizations such as the American Cancer Society and the Arthritis Foundation. Approximately 100 such organizations produce health-related pamphlets for the public. Both pharmaceutical and insurance companies also generate and distribute pamphlets. Furthermore, the federal health-related clearinghouses produce as well as disseminate pamphlets, booklets, and other materials. Federal agencies, particularly the National Cancer Institute and the National Heart, Lung and Blood Institute, have invested large sums of money in the production of consumer-oriented pamphlets and booklets.

In addition, several thousand consumer health/patient education audiovisuals are available from some 50 major producers and distributors. Most of these are designed for patient education purposes, mainly in the hospital setting.

Unfortunately, the massive amount of book, pamphlet, and audiovisual materials available does not reach the public in any effective or systematic manner. Consumer health information services, both in the hospital and in community settings, have been developed with little coordination. To rationalize the system at this time is extremely difficult and complex. Several major problems exist: lack of bibliographic control and announcement mechanisms; lack of any formal mechanism for evaluating quality; the related lack of a professional consensus on many issues such as breast surgery and nutrition; and the existence of a very inadequate distribution system, which is unresponsive to the demands of the public.

The identification, selection, and acquisition of information materials is time-consuming and expensive and requires both specialized knowledge of health topics and relevant information sources. Few libraries or hospitals have the personnel or resources to acquire these specialized print and nonprint materials in any thorough or systematic manner. It is frustrating and costly to assemble comprehensive pamphlet collections on popular health topics. It is even more expensive to purchase audiovisuals for patient education. Few directories or bibliographies exist. No general mechanism for the announcement and review of pamphlet and audiovisual resources is available. The existing reviews of books and audiovisuals are essentially nonevaluative in nature and do not take into account criteria such as comprehensiveness, accuracy, reading level, authority, target audience, and so on. Public libraries have endeavored to meet the health information needs of lay people by purchasing books with little or no guidance as to quality. Likewise, hospitals tend to purchase expensive audiovisuals utilizing locally produced evaluation protocols.

If the problems of evaluation, bibliographical control, announcement, and dissemination can be solved, vast resources of consumer health information can be assembled and utilized. Librarians, patients educators, and community health educators share the common objective of creating a better-informed public with respect to health. It is hoped that the sources of consumer health information materials listed in this book will furnish some assistance in meeting this challenge.

HEALTH INFORMATION IN THE COMMUNITY

As discussed above, a number of recent surveys and research studies reveal that Americans are not well informed on factors affecting their health. Few Americans understand the essentials of physical fitness and health maintenance. Widespread confusion exists on what is, and what is not, good for one's health. Very few persons know exactly when, and when not, to seek professional medical advice. Widespread ignorance exists on how to select a physician. Most people are not equipped to make prudent and economical use of the health care delivery system. Less than one in four Americans is well informed on basic health problems and the poor, who perhaps need health information most, have least access to it.

The Physician and the Consumer

Despite the claims of some militant consumer groups, no conspiracy exists to deny the individual's right to obtain accurate and understandable information relevant to his or her physical condition. The old attitude to the effect that "the less the patient knows, the better" is rapidly disappearing from the medical scene.

Lynn Baker expresses a typical physician's opinion:

> Ideally, after making a diagnosis a physician should sit down with the patient and family members and give a crash course in the problem. This might be followed by an audiovisual presentation the family could refer to later, again and again, if necessary. Also helpful would be printed information on the disease as well as typewritten instruction sheets detailing therapy . . . the physician would always be available to answer questions and bring the patient up to date on therapeutic advances . . . But all of this is a pipe dream, of course. If each of us did all these things we would see no more than a few patients a day.[20]

The constraints of time and the economics of medical practice militate against such extensive patient education activity. One health educator believes that "it is a mirage to expect doctors to be disseminators of health information. The physician is not well prepared, doesn't have access to information, and—pardon my cynicism—lacks the financial incentive for providing it." [21]

Many writers recognize that patient dissatisfaction is most often related to insufficient, contradictory, and confusing information in which many questions remain unanswered. Barbara Nowak, writing in the *Journal of the American Medical Association,* considers that "consumers think that they are not receiving the encouragement and reassurance that are a part of the total care package, and this is attributable to poor communication." [22] The quality of the doctor-patient relationship is very closely correlated with the adequacy of the communication that takes place.[23] Alice O'Donnell considers that health education is "as much a part of the internists' and family physicians' responsibility as it is of the pediatricians'."[24] Another physician gives a prescription to his colleagues on how to make the most of their time with patients: "avoid jargon, ask if patient has a question, address the patient and note the decision, monitor compliance carefully, make sure the patient understands the reasons for his specific regimen, use clearly written literature to supplement face-to-face instructions and take advantage of the patient education expertise of others." [25] Yet another physician stresses that "consumers have a right to as much information about their medical situation as they can comprehend and assimilate without undue stress." [26]

Patients share these attitudes and increasingly insist on a parity relationship in which medical decisions are made jointly following informed discussion of the various options available to them. Consumers are becoming much more aggressive in shopping for medical services in a competitive market place in which physicians seek patients and hospitals endeavor to fill empty beds. Health services are increasingly scrutinized and evaluated by consumers who demand courteous and frank disclosure of the procedures prescribed.

In physicians' offices it is now not uncommon to find health pamphlets, books, and magazines on a wide variety of topics. Health articles are often posted on bulletin boards while "no smoking" posters are prominently displayed. Many physicians utilize models, diagrams, and charts to explain health problems to patients. Some obstetricians, gynecologists, and surgeons employ audiovisual programs to explain childbirth and surgical procedures. Use of such audiovisual materials improves the physician-patient relationship, stimulates more meaningful dialogue, and reduces the level of anxiety.

The Hospital and the Consumer

Some form of patient education now exists in more than 3,000 hospitals. This is carried out by physicians, nurses, dietitians, pharmacists, physical therapists, and social workers. A number of hospitals employ full-time patient education coordinators. Individualized instruction is often supplemented by audiovisual programs relating to topics such as presurgical preparation, childbirth, diabetes management, hypertension, and health maintenance. Nursing staff are often used to coordinate and conduct patient education.[27] Closed-circuit television is increasingly used to bring programs to patients in their beds. The Greater Cleveland Hospital Association, for example, uses microwave transmission to bring patient education programming to patients in some 19 hospitals in northeast Ohio.

A more structured educational program has been implemented in some hospitals. This involves a referral of a patient by a physician to the health education center for the purpose of viewing audiovisual programs calculated to lead to a better comprehension of the nature and management of specific health problems. The physician writes a prescription for a specific health education program, which is then filled by the health education center. Compliance with the educational prescription is monitored and assessed by the center staff and subsequently recorded on the patient's chart, so that the physician can determine whether the patient has viewed and understood the program prescribed. Patient education of this type exists at the Kaiser-Permanente Medical Center in Oakland, California,[28] the Cleveland Clinic, and elsewhere. Judith Topper has reviewed the various types of patient education activities in hospitals.[29]

Hospitals are also involved in community health education programs by providing lectures for the general public. Others sponsor radio talks, television programs, and newspaper columns in which problems are discussed and questions answered on popular health topics. A few hospitals have launched ambitious community health education programs. Notably, Mount Auburn Hospital in Cambridge, Massachusetts, and the Swedish Medical Center in Englewood, Colorado, have developed innovative and successful health education programs for the community at large.

In Manhattan, Lenox Hill Hospital's storefront Health Education Center provides interested persons with accurate health information without charge.[30] Among the services offered are health screening, taped health messages, audiovisual programming, pamphlets, and flyers. Other storefront education centers are being developed by hospitals in various parts of the United States. Although regarded by some as a public relations gimmick, these consumer health information services are obviously popular and well received.

Blue Cross–Blue Shield has established health education programs in several parts of the United States. The Center for Health Education in Manhattan operated by Blue Cross–Blue Shield of Greater New York offers access to displays, exhibits, videotapes, medical age appraisal, and a number of relevant publications. Seminars, workshops, and lectures are held for the public on topics such as food and nutrition, physical fitness, stress relaxation techniques, smoking cessation, and alcoholism.

Many communities have health fairs to disseminate health information to the public.[31] These fairs typically involve the cooperation of local media (television, radio, and newspapers), medical societies, health maintenance organizations, academic institutions, hospitals, nursing homes, voluntary health organizations such as the American Heart Association, and self-health care groups. Screening services for hypertension and oral health are often provided together with workshops on topics such as nutrition, diet, stress reduction, and family planning.

Tel-Med is offered in many communities. This is a telephone library providing taped recordings, lasting from three to five minutes, on more than 100 topics. These programs are informative and accurate, covering specific topics in categories such as birth control, cancer, common medical problems, dental health, diabetes, diet and nutrition, digestive diseases, first aid, heart and circulatory diseases, human sexuality, kidney ailments, mental health, respiratory diseases, allergies, skin, smoking, venereal disease, vision and hearing, and health concerns of women. The most popular programs are, not surprisingly, related to human sexuality. Tel-Med is sponsored in some communities by hospitals and in others by the local medical society, health maintenance organization, or other institution. One disadvantage of Tel-Med is that it is restricted to the local telephone calling area, so that in large communities such as Los Angeles, only partial coverage can be attained by any one Tel-Med operation.

Libraries and Health Information

The health sciences library has as its central mission the delivery of information services to health sciences personnel in various settings. Some 2,900 libraries located in medical schools, dental schools, hospitals, health maintenance organizations, health systems agencies, and other health-related organizations exist to provide informational support to those engaged in patient care, education, research, and health planning.[32] However, these health sciences libraries exist primarily for the delivery of information to professionals. Access to the libraries of medical schools, for example, is necessarily restricted and often denied to the general public. The layperson has been forced to turn to local public libraries or to hospital libraries.

Most public librarians are aware of the great lay interest in health topics. Information requests have proliferated on subjects such as alcoholism, drug abuse, mental health, teenage pregnancy, abortion, medication, cancer, hypertension, stress, nutrition, human sexuality, diabetes, arthritis, and so on. On the basis of a public and medical library survey, three Houston librarians have classified such requests into four categories relating to disease information, medical procedures, and drugs; directory information; questions about specific books and holdings; and other factual information.[33] Likewise, patients and their families request books and pamphlets from hospital libraries to explain and clarify medical problems. Many professionals in the hospital setting also turn to the hospital librarian for assistance in identifying materials suitable for use by their patients.

In public libraries, a number of innovative consumer health information programs have been established. CHIPS (Consumer Health Information Program and Services/Salud y Bienestar) has as its major goal the formation of a health information network to serve the consumer, the public library client, and the hospital patient. Initially funded by an LSCA Title I grant for three years from 1976 to 1979, this bilingual project coordinates efforts of the Carson Regional Library of the Los Angeles County Public Library and the Harbor General Hospital—UCLA Medical Center Libraries. The populace served is over 2 million people of multiethnic backgrounds. The cooperative endeavor, linking the resources of a large public library system with a backup hospital library, has resulted in the successful build-up of health information materials, greater accessibility of these materials, strengthened interlibrary loan arrangements, establishment of contact with some 40 health-related organizations in the community, and installation of Tel-Med as a health information line. Eleanor Goodchild, project director and architect of the CHIPS program, notes that "libraries of all types, it would seem, need to become active participants in the CHE (Consumer Health Education) movement. To do so will require more emphasis on cooperative efforts between different types of libraries, health agencies, hospitals and consumers."[34]

Another innovative project is CHIN (Community Health Information Network) coordinated at Mount Auburn Hospital in Cambridge, Massachusetts. CHIN has created a cooperative network involving the public libraries of Arlington, Belmont, Cambridge, Lexington, Somerville, and Watertown. Emphasis has been placed upon the development of an efficient interlibrary loan system to improve the public libraries' access to health sciences library resources, the creation of basic collections of reference books, texts and journals in public libraries, the provision of backup reference services by the network office, and the planning of a series of health education programs for presentation in public libraries. CHIN coordinator Ellen Gartenfeld states that the growth of the project is viewed as "a validation of our belief that such a health information network is necessary and that this type of public/health sciences library cooperation is a viable solution to the demands created by the growing consumer health education movement."[35] She adds succinctly: "What we are talking about is not 'do-it-yourself medicine' but the development of knowledgeable consumers of health care."

In Cleveland, the School of Library Science at Case Western Reserve University has been engaged in the development of public library-based, consumer health information services. In 1979, a project funded by the Cleveland Foundation accomplished two objectives: identification of sources of health-related information and creation of lists of recommended materials for public library usage; and design and conduct of a series of educational programs to improve the knowledge and skills of public library personnel in responding to the health information requests of library patrons.[36] With the assistance of the medical staff of University Hospitals of Cleveland, four programs were held—Cancer, Heart Disease and Hypertension, Health Problems of Children, and Health Concerns of Women. Each program included a lecture by a medical school faculty member, creation of a bibliography of book, pamphlet, and audiovisual resources, and a workshop to discuss the informational materials. Pamphlet collections in the four areas were also assembled and made available. A quarterly newsletter, *Healthline Cleveland,* was initiated to identify and describe the wide range of informational resources available in the health field relevant and appropriate for public library usage.

The next phase of this activity, initiated in September 1980 under LSCA Title I funding, is an operational one, involving collection development to strengthen and extend the health-related information services of ten public library systems in northeast Ohio and the linkage of two public libraries to the Health Education Television Network of the Greater Cleveland Hospital Association. Through this link-up, public library patrons will have access to the same 12 hours of health education programming viewed daily by patients in participating northeast Ohio hospitals.

Health information services are being created in a number of other public library systems. Kelly Jennings of the Tulsa (Oklahoma) City-County Library System has produced a number of resource lists and has established successful liaison with community health agencies. In addition, she recently completed a consumer health information training manual for public library staff.[37] In Pennsylvania, the Philipsburg State General Hospital in cooperation with the Centre County and Clearfield Library Systems, with LSCA Title I funding, is engaged in collection development, networking, and sponsoring educational programs for library personnel. Similar activity has been reported in New Mexico, Maryland, and New York.

Some hospital libraries have also been active in providing health information to patients and their families. In particular, the libraries at the Veterans Administration Hospitals in San Francisco and Minneapolis have planned and executed innovative services to patients involving the use of books, pamphlets, audiovisuals, posters, and games. The Minneapolis VA Library is actively involved in patient education programs. Annette Swezey and Anita Kaufman have described the use of a library cart service to provide information to arthritic patients in a clinic milieu.[38] Joanne Marshall and John Hamilton have designed and carried out a project in which clinical librarians, as members of the health care team, provide information to gastroenterology patients to assist them in participating knowledgeably in their own health care.[39] Separately, Marshall describes the preparation of "patient education packages" for use in the clinic and the ward.[40] She concludes that patients and their families appreciate the increased accessibility of information resources that the clinical librarian provides.

The Role of the Library

Somers has defined consumer health education as "a process that informs, motivates and helps people to adopt and maintain healthy practices and life-styles, advocates environmental changes as needed to facilitate this goal, and conducts professional training and research to the same end." [41] Elsewhere, Somers considers that the essential goal is "to provide people with enough information and motivation to help them understand the factors that promote health and those that threaten health, and so be in a position to make informed choices or 'tradeoffs' in their own lives." [42]

Two writers illustrate the debate over the role of health information in health education. Lawrence Green, director of the Office of Health Information, Health Promotion, Physical Fitness and Sports Medicine, considers that health information is often neither a necessary nor a sufficient component of effective health education, which refers to strategies or learning experiences designed to effect voluntary adjustment of behavior conducive to health.[43] Donald M. Vickery, coauthor of *Take Care of Yourself: A Consumer's Guide to Medical Care,* argues against the conventional belief that information does not mean education and education does not ensure behavioral change. He notes that of the 33 million Americans who have ceased smoking since 1964, 95 percent of them did so without benefit of any specific educational intervention beyond information. He poses a rhetorical question: "When does repetition of information become educational? The dividing line between information and education is far from clear."[44] Certainly, it is difficult to conceive of educational activity without some form of information base.

Neither the hospital librarian nor the public librarian is a health educator, however. The essential role of the librarian involves the identifying, assembling, cataloging, and disseminating information materials. Health sciences librarians are constantly called upon to utilize their skills to identify, acquire, and make available books, journals, and audiovisuals in support of patient care, research, and educational activities of health sciences professionals. In particular, the health sciences librarian plays a very important role in medical schools and teaching hospitals in relation to intern and residency training programs. The extension of these library-related skills to the identification, acquisition, and organization of patient education materials, both print and audiovisual, is entirely logical. As one librarian notes, "The hospital librarian is the most knowledgable member of the hospital organization with regard to the selection, evaluation, organization and storage of information. It is logical that the hospital librarian should contribute his skills to patient education." [45]

Hospital librarian Britain Roth is in agreement with this point of view, yet stresses that control of patient education must remain in the hands of physicians and nurses, who would review audiovisual programs for intellectual content and audience level in relation to patient education objectives.[46] Caren Quay of the Kaiser-Permanente Medical Center library states that she does not offer patients materials not explicitly approved for use in the library. She points out that "if the information exists (i.e., in language understood by people who are not medical professionals) but has been rejected by the medical staff, I consider the reasons for its rejection. If it is a decision based on content I must respect that choice, for it is a choice of materials consistent with a particular medical practice." [47]

There is little doubt that the hospital librarian can be most helpful in deploying professional skills for the purpose of identifying, acquiring, and organizing patient education materials. Most health professionals have neither the time nor the specialized knowledge to seek out and obtain relevant book, pamphlet, and audiovisual materials. The principal point of dispute would appear to be related to the evaluation and selection of materials for specific patient populations. Many physicians and nursing personnel wish to reserve for themselves the judgment whether a pamphlet or audiovisual contains accurate, relevant, and appropriate information that would be supportive rather than threatening to a patient's well-being.

The librarian need have no qualms about yielding this judgment. In fact, the librarian can be most helpful in identifying and obtaining appropriate evaluation protocols that may be adapted by patient educators for their use. Also, the librarian can assist in organizing meetings of the patient education committee and arranging for the screening of candidate programs for preview. Furthermore, the librarian can serve as a liaison with audiovisual producers and distributors and bring new programs to the attention of patient education personnel. In short, the hospital librarian can function best as a health information expert with specialized knowledge of health information resources designed for both professional and lay audiences.

Within the public library setting, the librarian can play a similar role. In this context, the librarian can be a most effective agent in providing authoritative and relevant health information to the community. It is to be noted that under no circumstances can the librarian give medical advice, since this is the prerogative of licensed health professionals. Medical information is not to be equated with medical advice. Lynn Foster and Phyllis Self note that it is often difficult to decide whether answering a particular question involves giving advice. They consider medical advice to consist of the following: recommending a method, procedure, or treatment to follow; recommending alternate drugs; assisting the patient in self-diagnosis; and interpreting medical information to the patron. Their message can be succinctly stated—stay away from diagnosis and treatment.[48] Marilyn Vent and Patricia Weaver-Myers concur and warn: "Do not slip into the advice syndrome."[49]

It is, however, encouraging to note that many medical practitioners are most hopeful that the library, as a social agency, can play a far more active role in disseminating health information. Gartenfeld points out, with respect to the CHIN experience, that "we have not encountered any opposition from providers of health services, and we do not believe that this is accidental." [50]

The notion that the public library should not provide medical information is a phantom issue. The fear of lawsuits does not appear to have any justification. There can be no real dispute that the community has a right to have free and unimpeded access to relevant and authoritative health information. The obstacle to providing consumer health information services in the public library is one of priority. Confronted with scarce and limited financial resources to meet the multiple information needs of the community, it is necessary to assess the social importance of health to the community. Public librarians should not find this assessment difficult when they consider the dominant position held by health in the mass media and in printed publications.

The Interfacing of Public and Health Sciences Libraries

The major library response to the health information needs of the community must necessarily come from the public library. Traditionally, public libraries have been highly sensitive to the information needs of the communities they serve, yet as a group public librarians have little more understanding of health problems than the public they serve. Also, their knowledge of the wide range of specialized informational materials available is limited. On the other hand, health sciences librarians have little experience in providing library services to the general public. In this connection, health sciences librarians "are presently inexperienced in, and their libraries ill-suited for, extensive service to the non-medical public." [51]

Effective consumer health information services will necessitate multitype library cooperation involving public, hospital, and academic health sciences libraries. The public library should be able to draw upon the specialized publications and materials contained in health sciences libraries. Of even greater importance is the specialized knowledge of health and information resources possessed by the health sciences librarian. This fact suggests that health sciences librarians can best serve as consultants, educators, and reference specialists in order to assist the public library to discharge its responsibility to provide information to the community.

The library has the potential of being a vital force in creating an informed populace and in promoting health in the community. In addition to network linkages between types of libraries, it will be necessary to create community-wide networks, on perhaps a state or regional basis, to link libraries with voluntary health organizations, government agencies, health systems agencies, medical schools, medical societies, and schools of public health.

To satisfy the health information needs of the American public in sickness and health, a concerted and coordinated effort is necessary involving physicians, nurses, pharmacists, dietitians, patient educators, and librarians. The role of both public and health sciences librarians is to provide health information to members of the community and to supply informational support to the educational activity undertaken by health professionals to promote the health of the American populace.

NOTES

1. *Health: United States.* Office of the Assistant Secretary for Health, Public Health Service, 1978. DHEW Pubn. No. (PHS) 78-1232. p. 3.
2. Alain C. Enthoven. *Health Plan: The Only Practical Solution to the Soaring Cost of Medical Care.* (Reading, MA: Addison-Wesley, 1980), p. xvi.
3. *Health: United States,* p. 25.
4. *Promoting Health: Issues and Strategies.* Office of Health Information and Health Promotion, Office of the Assistant Secretary for Health, January, 1979, p. 1.
5. *Healthy People: The Surgeon General's Report on Health Promotion and Disease Prevention.* Office of the Assistant Secretary for Health, Public Health Service, 1979. DHEW Pubn. No. (PHS) 79-55071. See also *Healthy People: The Surgeon General's Report on Health Promotion and Disease Prevention. Background Papers,* 1979. DHEW Pubn. No. (PHS) 77-55071A.
6. *A National Health Care Strategy.* A Series of Five Reports on Business Involvement With Health. (Washington, D.C.: National Chamber Foundation, 1979).
7. Marc Lalonde. *A New Perspective on the Health Care of Canadians.* (Quebec: Information Canada, 1974), p. 18.
8. Lalonde, p. 5.
9. Shirley Linde. *The Whole Health Catalog: How to Stay Well Cheaper.* (New York: Rawson, 1977), p. 3.
10. Keith Sehnert. *How to Be Your Own Doctor—Sometimes.* (New York: Grossett, 1977).
11. *The Perrier Study: Fitness in America.* Conducted by Louis Harris and Associates. (New York: Perrier-Great Waters of France, 1979).
12. *The General Mills Family Report 1978–1979: Family Health in an Era of Stress.* (Minneapolis: General Mills, 1979).
13. *Health: What They Know, What They Do, What They Want: A National Survey of Consumers and Businesses.* (Chicago: American Hospital Association, 1978).
14. James E. Ludlam. *Informed Consent.* (Chicago: American Hospital Association, 1978), p. 5.
15. Anne R. Somers. "Consumer Health Education: How Are We? Where Are We Going?" *Canadian Journal of Public Health* 68 (Sept./Oct. 1977): p. 364.
16. *Proceedings of the House of Delegates.* (Chicago: American Medical Association, 1978).
17. *Health Maintenance.* Survey conducted by Louis Harris and Associates. (Newport Beach, CA.: Pacific Mutual Life Insurance Company, 1978).
18. *Promoting Health: A Source Book.* Regional Forums on Community Health Promotion. (New York: National Health Council, 1979), p. 11.
19. *Viewpoint: Toward a Healthier America.* A Summary Report on Health Issues and Related Programming of the Kellogg Foundation. (Battle Creek, MI: Kellogg Foundation, 1979), pp. 9-10.
20. Lynn Baker. "Rx for Physicians: Education While We Medicate." *Medical World News* 20 (April 30, 1979): p. 75.

21. "Information: Key to Health." *The General Mills Family Forum. A Digest of the Proceedings.* (Held in Chicago, Oct. 18, 1979). (Minneapolis: General Mills, 1980), p. 19.

22. Barbara Nowak. "Marketing Medicine to Today's Consumer." *Journal of the American Medical Association* 242 (November 30, 1979): p. 2403.

23. Betty Mathews and others. "Hospital Based Health Education: For Patients, Staff and the Community." *Health Values* 3 (Jan.–Feb. 1979): p. 33.

24. Alice Anne O'Donnell. "Outlook 1979/Patient Education: Selecting Patient Education Materials." *Patient Care* 13 (Jan. 15, 1979): p. 167.

25. "Patient Education—What It Can Do." *Internist* 18 (Oct. 1977): p. 12.

26. Bruce Cume and John H. Renner. "Patient Education: Developing a Health Care Partnership." *Postgraduate Medicine* 65 (Jan. 1979): p. 178.

27. Lois Fuhrer and Ronni Bernstein. "Making Patient Education a Part of Patient Care." *American Journal of Nursing* (Nov. 1976): pp. 1798–1799.

28. Bobbie F. Collen and Kriker Soghikian. "A Health Education Library for Patients." *Health Services Reports* 89 (May–June 1974): pp. 236–243.

29. Judith Topper. "Hospitals as Centers for Consumer Health Information." *Bulletin of the American Society for Information Science* 4 (April 1978): pp. 13–14.

30. "Storefront Education at Lenox Hill." *Health Care Education* 7 (April 1978): pp. 23–27.

31. Tom Ferguson. "A Health Fair for Your Community." *Medical Self-Care* 6 (Fall 1979): pp. 3–8.

32. Alan M. Rees and others. *Directory of Health Sciences Libraries in the United States, 1979.* (Cleveland, OH: Case Western Reserve University, 1980).

33. Dottie Eakin and others. "Consumer Health Information: Libraries as Partners." *Bulletin of the Medical Library Association* 68 (April 1980): p. 221.

34. Eleanor Goodchild and others. "The CHIPS Project: A Health Information Network to Serve the Consumer." *Bulletin of the Medical Library Association* 66 (Oct. 1978): pp. 432–436.

35. Ellen Gartenfeld. "The Community Health Information Network: A Model for Hospital and Public Library Cooperation." *Library Journal* 169 (Oct. 1, 1978): pp. 1911–1914.

36. Alan M. Rees. "The Informed Medical Consumer—In Sickness and Health." Paper presented at the 80th Annual Meeting of the Medical Library Association, Washington, D.C., June 14, 1980.

37. Kelly Jennings. *Consumer Health Information: The Public Librarian's Role* (Tulsa, OK: Tulsa City-County Library System, 1980). 34 pp. (Manual).

38. Annette Swezey and Anita Kaufman. "Library Cart Service Provides Information for Clinic Patients." *Hospitals* 51 (Sept. 1, 1977): pp. 65–67.

39. Joanne Marshall and John Hamilton. "The Clinical Librarian and the Patient: Report of a Project at McMaster University Medical Center." *Bulletin of the Medical Library Association* 66 (Oct. 1978): pp. 420–425.

40. Joanne Marshall. "Clinical Librarians Join Health Care Teams to Provide Information Directly." *Canadian Library Journal* 36 (Feb.–April 1979): pp. 27–28.

41. Anne R. Somers. *Promoting Health: Consumer Education and National Policy* (Germantown, MD: Aspen Systems, 1976), p. 42.

42. Anne R. Somers. "Consumer Health Education: Where Are We? Where Are We Going?" p. 366.

43. Lawrence W. Green. "Health Information and Health Education: There's a Big Difference Between Them." *Bulletin of the American Society for Information Science* 4 (April 1978): p. 15.

44. Donald M. Vickery. "Is It a Change for the Better?" *Hospitals* 53 (Oct. 1, 1979): p. 89.

45. Cheryl Lynn Harris. "Hospital-Based Patient Education Programs and the Role of the Hospital Librarian." *Bulletin of the Medical Library Association* 66 (April 1978): p. 213.

46. Britain G. Roth. "Health Information for Patients: The Hospital Library's Role." *Bulletin of the Medical Library Association* 66 (Jan. 1978): pp. 14–18.

47. Caren Quay. "The Role of the Librarian in Patient Education Efforts." Paper presented at the Second Annual National Symposium on Patient Education, Oct. 21, 1978, San Francisco.

48. Lynn Foster and Phyllis Self. "Legal and Medical Reference: A Dilemma for Public Libraries." *Illinois Libraries* 60 (March 1978): p. 244.

49. Marilyn Vent and Patricia Weaver-Myers. "Health Information Sources and Services for the Small Public Library." *Oklahoma Librarian* 28 (Jan. 1978): p. 17.

50. Ellen Gartenfeld. "The Community Health Information Network," p. 1914.

51. Dottie Eakin. "Consumer Health Information: Libraries as Partners," p. 227.

Chapter 2

Readings on the Consumer Health Information Movement

A number of seminal books, conference papers, proceedings and articles have been published on the general subject of health information for the layperson. This chapter contains a representative selection of significant publications. The listing is divided into three sections: Health Promotion and Medical Consumerism; Libraries and Consumer Health Information Services; and Patient Education Theory and Practice. Many of the works cited here are discussed in context in the preceding chapter.

HEALTH PROMOTION AND MEDICAL CONSUMERISM

Consumerism and Health Care. Publication No. 52-1727. New York: Natl. League for Nursing, 1978. 58 pp. $3.95.
A collection of provocative papers that discuss the consumer's role in health care; the impact of consumerism on health professionals; the consumer and the health care professionals ("contented marriage or shotgun wedding"); and implications of the American Hospital Association's *Patient's Bill of Rights* on the health care system. Although written from the point of view of the nursing profession, this is an important summary of enlightened thinking. It deserves to be updated, since the bibliography, in particular, is outdated.

The General Mills Family Report, 1978–1979: Family Health in an Era of Stress. Minneapolis: General Mills, 1979. 192 pp.
A survey conducted by Yankelovich, Skelly, and White revealed that health and staying healthy has become a major priority of the American public. Yet despite the high level of interest in and the importance they attach to health, fewer than one third of the U.S. population can be called really well informed.

According to the report, "The health information most desired by the American public is where to go for help when needed (i.e., government health agencies, health organizations, etc.). This type of information is followed by how to teach children better health and eating habits, how to manage the family's health better, how to cope with stress, the most important signals of physical and health problems, effective diets and exercises for weight control, information on nutrition, reliable remedies for minor health problems, how best to exercise and keep physically fit, how to communicate with teenagers about sex, drinking and drugs, how to cope with serious illness in the family and how to prevent and care for childhood diseases."

Health: What They Know, What They Do, What They Want: A National Survey of Consumers and Businesses. Chicago: Amer. Hospital Assn., 1978. 32 pp.
The need to provide the American public with more information about preventing illness and staying healthy is evident. This conclusion is based on a nationwide survey in ten cities, which explored health practices in the United States and evaluated the level of consumer awareness about health information and educational programs. Survey findings indicate that there is a demand to make health information more readily available and that many persons are unaware of the information and education services currently offered. Stress reduction, home safety, balanced diet, weight control, and how the health care system functions are the topics most often requested by the layperson.

Health Maintenance: A Nationwide Survey of the Barriers toward Better Health and Ways of Overcoming Them, Conducted among Representative Samples of the American Public, Business, and Labor Leaders. Conducted by Louis Harris and Associates. Newport Beach, CA: Pacific Mutual Life Insurance, 1978. 88 pp.
The objectives of the survey were to identify the numbers and types of people who are putting themselves at risk, to measure the knowledge of each of these groups, and to determine the potential for changing their behavior by health education and giving them knowledge that they do not currently have. It is concluded that a landslide majority of 92–95 percent agree that "if we Americans lived healthier lives, ate more nutritious food, smoked less, maintained our proper weight and exercised regularly, it would do more to improve our health than anything doctors and medicine could do for us." Of particular interest is a tabulation of health topics that people would like to learn most about and a listing of information sources used to obtain health care information, such as advice from doctors, public service messages, advice from pharmacists, and so forth.

Healthy People: The Surgeon General's Report on Health Promotion and Disease Prevention. Office of the Assistant Secretary for Health, Public Health Service, 1979. DHEW Pubn. No. (PHS) 79-55071. 177 pp.
This report notes the emerging consensus among scientists and the health community that the nation's health strategy must be dramatically recast to

emphasize the prevention of disease. The individual can do more to ensure his own health and well-being than any doctor, any hospital and drug, or any exotic medical device. The report stresses that the health of Americans can be most significantly improved through actions individuals can take for themselves, such as elimination of cigarette smoking; reduction of alcohol misuse; adoption of dietary changes to reduce intake of excess calories, fat, salt and sugar; employment of exercise and periodic screening for high blood pressure; and adherence to speed laws and use of seat belts. Finally, *Healthy People* outlines a strategy for implementing defined health goals relating to infants, children, adolescents, adults, and the elderly. The respective roles of individuals, families, health professionals, health institutions, schools, business and labor, and communities are defined.

Information Needs of Californians: A Survey Commissioned by the State Library of California for the Govenor's Conference on Libraries and Information Services. Sacramento, CA: California State Lib., March 1979. 10 pp.

Information Needs of Californians: Introductory Materials for the Survey Report Prepared for the Governor's Conference on Libraries and Information Services. Sacramento, CA: California State Lib., March 1979. 8 pp.

The first title *Information Needs of Californians: A Survey* summarizes the major findings of a statewide survey of California citizens undertaken to identify their needs for information, the ways they seek to satisfy these needs, and how well these needs are met. The random sample used consisted of about 1,000 households, drawn from 50 large geographic areas in California. Interviews were obtained from 646 persons, 14 years of age or older, and 3,869 information-seeking situations were identified. The greatest number related to money matters, consumer issues, housing or home care, and health. Data are analyzed by racial group, age and urban/rural variables. *Introductory Materials* discusses the implications of the survey and notes that while 21 percent of people surveyed often turn to libraries, only 7 percent resort to libraries to resolve specific everyday problems. It suggests that libraries, to be more responsive, should perhaps emphasize subject areas most often cited in everyday situations: money matters, consumer issues, home care, job-related issues, and health.

Lalonde, Marc. *A New Perspective on the Health of Canadians: A Working Document.* Quebec: Information Canada, 1974. 76 pp.

A landmark document produced by the then minister of National Health and Welfare of Canada. Lalonde outlines a new strategy for improving the health of Canadians based upon health promotion and preventive medicine. "The evidence uncovered by the analysis of sickness and death now indicates that improvement in the environment and an abatement in the level of risks imposed upon themselves by individuals, taken together, constitute the most promising ways by which further advances can be made." Lalonde concludes that faced with environmental and behavioral threats to health, "the organized health care system can do little more than serve as a catchment net for the victims."

Lazes, Peter, ed. *The Handbook of Health Education.* Germantown, MD: Aspen
  Systems, 1979. 430 pp. $25.
A comprehensive description of a wide variety of community health education
programs in schools, hospitals, health maintenance organizations, and other
settings. Case histories illustrate the effective use of media such as brochures,
pamphlets, recorded telephone messages, cable television, public service spot
announcements, closed-circuit television, and portable bedside teaching carts.
Self-health care and the consumer viewpoint are also included. An appendix,
listing health education resources such as government agencies, organizations, associations, publications, magazines, and newsletters, is incomplete
and is lacking in descriptive detail. This publication will interest those concerned with patient education and the promotion of health in the community.

Marshall, Carter. *Toward an Educated Health Consumer: Mass Communication and
  Quality in Medical Care.* Report of Conferences Sponsored by John E.
  Fogarty Intl. Center for Advanced Study in the Health Sciences. Natl.
  Insts. of Health. DHEW Pubn. No. (NIH) 77-881. 63 pp.
Describes the growth of the consumer movement and the technological advances that have occurred in the communication field in relation to the
adoption of preventive measures for maintenance of lifetime well-being. An
excellent review of health education and the feasibility of modifying health
behavior by mass communication techniques.

Meyer, Linn. "Consumers Must Become Partners in Their Own Care."
  Hospitals 51 (April 1, 1977): 79–82.
Argues that self-health care is a lay movement that has the right of certain
experimentation. A new social contract must evolve between professionals
and lay persons. Education can significantly achieve a modification of life-
style. "More than money is needed to stop the public from smoking, drinking,
eating too much, and driving too fast; although our national resources are
finite, there is no limit to the amount of money that could be spent on health;
there is not now, nor will there ever be, a medical Utopia." Stresses the
importance of an informed public.

A National Health Care Strategy. A Series of Five Reports on Business Involvement with Health. Washington, DC: Natl. Chamber Foundation, 1979. $15.
Analyzes the necessity for the involvement of industry in health promotion
activity, especially in relation to physical fitness, smoking cessation, alcohol
abuse, nutrition and weight control, screening programs such as for hypertension, medical self-care, and stress management. Emphasizes the need for
educational programs supported by good information resources.

The Perrier Study: Fitness in America. New York: Perrier—Great Waters of
  France, 1979. 59 pp. $5.
This study was conducted by Louis Harris and Associates for Great Waters of
France, the U.S. distributor of Perrier Water. The study provides insight into

the attitudes, knowledge, and behavior¯of Americans regarding physical fitness and exercise. It indicates that a truly national commitment to physical fitness has begun to emerge. More than 90 million adults now participate in some form of physical activity on a regular basis.

Preventive Medicine USA: Health Promotion and Consumer Health Education. A Task Force Sponsored by John E. Fogarty Intl. Center for Advanced Study in the Health Sciences, Natl. Insts. of Health, and Amer. College of Preventive Medicine. New York: Prodist, 1976. 851 pp. $29.95.
Emphasizes the relation of health status to life-style and its current challenge to consumer health education. Summarizes and analyzes programs, practices, and problems of health education. Recommends that the nation's basic health policy should be health promotion.

Schoolman, Harold. "Health Education for the Public." Unpublished paper. Natl. Lib. of Medicine, Bethesda, MD, 1979. 6 pp.
Dr. Schoolman is Deputy Director for Research and Education at the National Library of Medicine. He discusses the proliferation of health education techniques including telephone, teletype, and Braille teletype dial-access systems, closed circuit television, videocassettes and computer-assisted instruction. Regarding the pamphlet literature emanating from the federal clearinghouses, other government agencies and from the private sector, Schoolman notes that this literature lacks minimal quality assurance and has little bibliographic control. No adequate announcement and distribution system presently exists, which is a problem that needs to be solved. Since medical libraries do not provide access to the general public, Schoolman concludes that "only the public library has any real contact with the vast majority of potential users" of this literature.

Somers, Anne R. "Consumer Health Education: Where Are We? Where Are We Going?" *Canadian Journal of Public Health* 68 (September/October 1977): 362–368.
Somers, Anne R. *Promoting Health: Consumer Education and National Policy.* Germantown, MD: Aspen Systems, 1976. $12.95.
Dr. Somers is professor of community medicine and family medicine at Rutgers University and is a leading theorist and exponent of health promotion. She believes that it is not possible to sustain financially an adequate national health care system in the United States unless it is accompanied by an effective program of consumer health education. The single overriding goal of health education should be "to provide people with enough information and motivation to help them understand the factors that promote health and those that threaten health, and so to be in a position to make informed choices or 'tradeoffs' in their own lives."

Taylor, Flora. "When You and Your Partner the Doctor Talk about Diagnosis." *FDA Consumer* 13 (November 1979): 13–15.
Stresses the need for the patient to assume a positive role by asking the doctor

for all information that will enable the patient to work with the doctor and make his or her own contribution in treating the illness. Taylor advises the patient to request the doctor to explain the diagnosis, to indicate which body systems are involved, the disease process at work, whether it is contagious, what the course of the illness will be, what forms of treatment are available, the risks and benefits of each, and the pros and cons of the treatment alternatives. Good communication will result in a true partnership between patient and physician and better medical care.

Vickery, Donald M. "Is It a Change for the Better?" *Hospitals* 53 (October 1, 1979): 87–90.
Points out that decision makers within the hospitals must consider whether their primary mission is the improvement of the community's health or the management of a growing inpatient service. Dr. Vickery considers that it is inevitable that hospitals will move further into consumer health education (that is, patient education, health information, health promotion, and health education). Emphasis should be placed on health promotion rather than disease detection. Available evidence points to the efficacy of consumer health education rather than screening. The author notes that health information can be an effective catalyst for behavioral change toward a healthier life-style.

Viewpoint: Toward a Healthier America. A Summary Report on Health Issues and Related Programming of the Kellogg Foundation. Battle Creek, MI: Kellogg Foundation, 1980. 30 pp.
A most lucid and informative analysis of health promotion, this report discusses the differences between health information, health education, and health promotion. It concludes that "While a combination of three might prove most useful, there seems to be the greatest opportunity for improving health status . . . by placing highest priority on health promotion." The discussion of national activity is followed by a summary of Kellogg Foundation initiatives in health promotion and disease prevention. These projects are described in a number of areas: health education–educational setting; health education–community agencies; health promotion/life-style–educational setting; health promotion/life-style–health providers; health promotion/life-style–community agencies; health promotion/life-style–work site; health promotion/self-care–community agencies. An excellent state-of-the-art review.

LIBRARIES AND CONSUMER HEALTH INFORMATION SERVICES

Allen, Luella, and Manning, Martha. "Women's Health Information: A Role for Health Sciences Libraries." Paper delivered at the 80th Annual Meeting of the Medical Lib. Assn., Washington, DC, June 18, 1980. 10 pp.
Describes how two health sciences librarians at the University of Buffalo provided library service at Women's Place, a referral and counseling service in

Buffalo, New York. The operation of a health information hotline was aimed at disseminating "timely, authoritative, unambiguous and understandable" information to the layperson. Unfortunately, the service was suspended because of a fire that destroyed the office.

Davies, Nicholas E. "Bringing Order to the Literature of Health Education." *New England Journal of Medicine* 302 (June 26, 1980): 1476–1478.
Argues that the literature of health education for the public is jumbled, confused, and untidy.Much of the material is impossible to classify, catalog, store, and retrieve. Amid this chaos, the public turns to the publications of cultists, faddists, and opportunists. Davies believes that the simplest method for making improvements is the construction of a "Brandon List" (a core list of essential publications) for the literature of health education and calls for the funding of an impartial group, sophisticated in health care, to produce such a library list of recommended publications.

Eakin, Dottie, Jackson, Sara, and Hannigan, Gale. "Consumer Health Information: Libraries as Partners." *Bulletin of the Medical Library Association* 68 (April 1980): 220–229.
Discusses the results of a survey conducted at the Houston Public Library and the Houston Academy of Medicine-Texas Medical Center Library to determine the numbers and types of questions asked by the public. The authors relate their experience to the broader issues of the respective roles of public, academic, and hospital libraries and consider that librarians must become partners with health professionals, health organizations, and educators.

Foster, Eloise. "Patient/Health Education in the Context of the Consumer Education Movement." In *Patient/Health Education: The Librarian's Role.* Detroit: Wayne State Univ., Div. of Library Science, 1979.
The author is director of the Library of the American Hospital Association and presented this paper at an Office of Education institute on "Patient/Health Education: The Librarian's Role" held at Wayne State University, February 5–9, 1979. Ms. Foster argues that an essential component of consumer health education is to "inform people about health, illness, disability, and ways in which they can improve and protect their own health, including more efficient use of the delivery system." The role of the librarian is reviewed within this context. Edited by M. T. Larson, the institute proceedings are annotated below.

Foster, Lynn, and Self, Phyllis. "Legal and Medical Reference: A Dilemma for Public Libraries." *Illinois Libraries* 60 (March 1978): 243–248.
Militant consumerism is generating a demand on the part of the layperson for medical and legal information. This constitutes a challenge for the public librarian, who is confronted with the problem of what constitutes medical/legal advice. The authors consider that advice would be recommending treatment procedures; advising alternate drugs that may produce the

same results as those presently taken; assisting patients to diagnose themselves; and interpreting medical information to the layperson. Unfortunately, they concede, it is difficult to determine where the boundary between advice and information falls. A list of recommended medical and legal books is appended.

Gartenfeld, Ellen. "The Community Health Information Network." *Library Journal* 103 (October 1, 1978): 1911–1914.
Describes CHIN (Community Health Information Network), a cooperative library network established with LSCA funding, linking Mount Auburn Hospital, Cambridge, Massachusetts, with the six public library systems of its catchment area. Emphasis has been placed on collection development, improvement of the interlibrary loan system, and education of public library staff.

Goodchild, Eleanor, and others. "The CHIPS Project. A Health Information Network to Serve the Consumer." *Bulletin of the Medical Library Association* 66 (October 1978): 432–436.
CHIPS (Consumer Health Information Program and Services/Salud y Bienestar) is an LSCA Title I funded project that has as its major goal the formation of a health information network to serve the consumer, the public library client, and the hospital patient. Funded for three years, 1976–1979, in the amount of $230,000, this bilingual project coordinates efforts of the Carson Regional Library of the Los Angeles County Public Library and Harbor General Hospital-UCLA Medical Center Library to provide health information resources and services to the public. The target population is over 2 million people of diverse ethnic backgrounds.

Green, Lawrence W. "Health Information and Health Education: There's a Big Difference Between Them." *Bulletin of the American Society for Information Science* 4 (April 1978): 15–16.
According to Green, *health education* is the term used more broadly and frequently to refer to strategies or learning experiences designed to bring about voluntary adjustment of behavior conducive to health. *Health information* is often neither a necessary nor a sufficient component of effective health education. Information may be one element of a strategy, but most behavioral changes require more than health information. Green argues that health information specialists can play a vital role in making esoteric or centralized sources more accessible, comprehensible, and credible for local consumption.

Harris, Cheryl Lynn. "Hospital-Based Patient Education Programs and the Role of the Hospital Librarian." *Bulletin of the Medical Library Association* 66 (April 1978): 210–217.

An examination of current advances in hospital-based patient education and a delineation of an expanded role for the hospital librarian in this context. Describes the patient education programs at Kaiser-Permanente Medical Center in Oakland, California, and at the Veterans Administration Hospital Library in Minneapolis, Minnesota. The role of the hospital librarian is defined as an informed intermediary between the health practitioner and the information sources required for conducting patient education.

Jennings, Kelly. *Consumer Health Information: The Public Librarian's Role.* Manual. Tulsa, OK: Tulsa City-County Library System, 1980. 34 pp.
An 11-part manual that discusses why and how to develop and utilize consumer health information collections in public libraries. Topics covered include: evaluation and selection of health materials, sources of health information, the public librarian and medical reference work, developing reference guidelines, legal aspects of medical reference, and building community support.

Larson, M. T., ed. *Patient/Health Education: The Librarian's Role.* Proceedings of an Invitational Institute held February 5–9, 1979 at Wayne State Univ. Detroit: Wayne State Univ., Div. of Lib. Science, 1979.
Contains a number of papers presented on consumer health information services and patient education, including Eloise Foster's paper, annotated above. Concludes that public libraries have a major responsibility for providing health information to the layperson and that health sciences libraries should share in this responsibility. Coordination should be maintained between local and regional libraries and health agencies.

Marshall, Joanne Gard. "Clinical Librarians Join Health Care Team to Provide Information Directly." *Canadian Library Journal* 36 (February/April 1979): 23–28.
Describes a project at McMaster University to explore and evaluate the role of the clinical librarian in providing information to patients in a gastroenterology program. Based upon questions asked by patients, a core of patient education materials was assembled, including pamphlets, journal articles, and audiovisuals. A series of "patient resource guides" was prepared in cooperation with the Hamilton (Ontario) Public Library. Many patients comment that they feel more comfortable asking a librarian for information than they do asking their physician.

Marshall, Joanne Gard. "Patient Use of Health Sciences Libraries." *Ontario Library Review* 64 (March 1980): 35–37.
A questionnaire administered to patients at the McMaster University Medical Center indicated that a significant number of patients listed medical libraries or medical books as useful sources of information. They consider that reading

about a treatment and its alternatives can serve as a "second medical opinion" and provides reassurance that they are receiving quality medical care. Concludes that although it is not always possible to give patients access to medical libraries, special attention should be given to serving the public by alternate means.

Marshall, Joanne Gard, and Hamilton, John D. "The Clinical Librarian and the Patient: Report of a Project at McMaster University Medical Center." *Bulletin of the Medical Library Association* 66 (October 1978): 420–425.
Summarizes a research project designed to assist patients in participating more knowledgeably in their own health care and to assist health professionals in applying the latest information from the biomedical literature to patient care and education.

Roth, Britain G. "Health Information for Patients: The Hospital Library's Role." *Bulletin of the Medical Library Association* 66 (January 1978): 14–18.
Roth proposes that hospital libraries should collaborate with health professionals in supplying health information to patients, in addition to their more traditional role of providing recreational reading for patients and serving the informational needs of the physicians and medical staff. Materials for patients should include topics such as diet, family adjustments to illness, home care, sexual activity, future complications, pre- and postoperative procedures, and normal health conditions.

Vent, Marilyn, and Weaver-Meyers, Patricia. "Health Information Sources and Services for the Small Public Library." *Oklahoma Librarian* 28 (January 1978): 17–21.
Argues that librarians can provide health information to the lay public "if they do not slip into the advice syndrome." The authors consider that basic reference books, popular works, and medical library services can, in all probability, provide the answers to any information request. A list of recommended reference works is supplied together with a description of local health information sources available in Oklahoma City.

Weck, Egan. "Look Who's Reading the *PDR* Now!" *FDA Consumer* 13 (November 1979): 16–20.
The *PDR* (*Physicians' Desk Reference*) is one of the "hottest" volumes kept at the reference desk in libraries. Also, the *PDR* is a best-seller in bookstores; its annual sales now exceed 150,000 copies. With the growth of the consumer movement, there has been an ever-increasing public demand for information about prescription drugs. Despite the technical language of the *PDR* the essential content is comprehensible to most laymen. Of particular use are the product identification pictures and listings by manufacturers, brand names, generic names, and classification by type of product such as analgesics, diuretics, and so forth. Formerly unavailable to the public, this book is now a widely used source for consumer health information concerning drugs.

PATIENT EDUCATION THEORY AND PRACTICE

Baker, Lynn. "Rx for Physicians: Educate While We Medicate." *Medical World News* 20 (April 30, 1979): 75.
Most patients have immense curiosity about their medical problems. Physicians "should start recognizing that when it comes to patient care a good article in a popular magazine is every bit as important to a patient as a good article in a prestigious medical journal is to a physician." Underlines the necessity for patient education in which the physician is totally committed.

Bryan, Thornton, and others. "Selecting Patient Education Materials." *Patient Care* 13 (January 15, 1979): 167–177.
Underlines the necessity to make patient education a basic part of every contact with patients. "One of the big problems," states Dr. Huffman, "remains the profusion of patient education aids." Unless we can catalog this mass of material and make it more generally available, practicing physicians will not be able to give patient education the importance it deserves in everyday practice.

Currie, Bruce, and Renner, John. "Patient Education: Developing a Health Care Partnership." *Postgraduate Medicine* 65 (January 1979): 177–182.
Increasingly, patients are insisting on becoming partners in their own health care. Physicians who welcome such involvement should try to determine the medical IQ and knowledge-base of the patient and then provide an appropriate educational experience. An atmosphere encouraging genuine dialogue is essential to a successful doctor-patient relationship.

Fuhrer, Lois, and Bernstein, Ronni. "Making Patient Education a Part of Patient Care." *American Journal of Nursing* 76 (November 1976): 1798–1799.
Description of a patient education program in a 535 bed hospital utilizing nursing personnel to teach patients with conditions including diabetes, coronary disease, gynecological disease, hypertension, and ostomies.

Hospital Inpatient Education: Survey Findings and Analysis. Chicago: Amer. Hospital Assn., 1979.
A summary of what the nation's hospitals are doing in patient education, including information about topics, focus of program, budget, use of video in patient teaching, and so forth.

The Hospital's Responsibility for Health Promotion. Statement. Chicago: Amer. Hospital Assn., 1979.
Asserts that hospitals have a responsibility to take a leadership role in helping ensure the good health of their communities. In addition to the primary

mission of providing health care and related education to the sick and injured the hospital has a responsibility to work with others in the community to assess the health status of the community; identify target areas and population groups for hospital-based and cooperative health promotion programs; develop programs to help upgrade the health in those target areas; ensure that persons who are apparently healthy have access to information about how to stay well and prevent disease; provide appropriate health education programs to aid those persons who choose to alter their personal health behavior or develop a more healthful lifestyle; and establish the hospital as an institution in the community that is concerned about good health in addition to one concerned about treating illness.

Implementing Patient Education in the Hospital. Chicago: Amer. Hospital Assn., 1979. 293 pp. $34.25.
Provides patient education coordinators with the materials and information needed to assess, plan, implement, and evaluate their hospital's programs. Contains highly practical, action-oriented information. Also contains a comprehensive bibliography covering benefits and evaluation of patient education programs; evaluative research; financing patient education; health beliefs and attitudes; implementing patient education in different settings; innovative patient education media and methods; interviewing; patient-provider communication and compliance; patient teaching; and special education techniques.

McCormick, Rose-Marie Duda, and Gilson-Parkevich, Tamar. *Patient and Family Education: Tools, Techniques and Theory.* New York: Wiley, 1979. 327 pp. $14.95.
A practical working handbook of useful guidelines based upon actual experience at Children's Hospital in Columbus, Ohio. Outlines how to apply patient education theory in specific settings; how to develop a system for creating teaching aids; how to evaluate the effectiveness of patient instruction. Features 79 "Helping Hands," step-by-step model instruction sheets on a variety of health topics.

National Patient Education Symposium. Atlanta, GA: Center for Disease Control, Bureau of Health Educ., 1978. 119 pp.
Proceedings of a 1977 national conference that focused attention on the theory, methodology, economics, and evaluation of patient education activities. Contains the transcript of presentations by leading health educators Lowell Levin, Elizabeth Lee, Lawrence Green, and William Carlyon, among others. A valuable state-of-the-art review.

Patient Education: The Concept; Selected Reading References; Organizational Resources. New York: Metropolitan Life Insurance, 1978. 6 pp.
A short bibliography of journal articles and books on the theory and im-

plementation of patient education programs. Also contains a listing of several dozen voluntary and professional health organizations that supply free or inexpensive patient education materials.

Patient Education 1973–1978. Natl. Lib. of Medicine Literature Search No. 78. Bethesda, MD: Natl. Lib. of Medicine, Reference Services Div.
Contains 295 citations of English-language literature derived from the MED-LINE data base.

A Patient's Bill of Rights. Statement. Chicago: Amer. Hospital Assn., 1975.
Six of the twelve sections refer to the patient's right to obtain specific information from the hospital or physician. The sections include information concerning diagnosis, treatment and prognosis, necessary procedures, and the patient's requirements for continuing health care following discharge. The *Bill of Rights* has served to stimulate the demand for accurate, relevant medical information as an established right of the consumer. Defines the notion of informed consent.

Proceedings, National Symposium on Patients' Rights in Health Care. May 17–18, 1976. Health Services Admin. DHEW Pubn. No. (HSA) 76-7002. 91 pp.
An analysis of patients' rights within the general context of consumer responsibilities and involvement. Emphasizes the need for consumer health education, consumer advocacy, more effective regulatory activities, and broad community involvement in health care.

Selected References on Patient Education. Health Resources Admin., Div. of Facilities Development, 1974. DHEW Pubn. No. (DFD) E-2. 10 pp.
Short descriptive annotations on some 50 journal articles and monographs relating to the theory, methodology, and evaluation of patient and health education programs.

Simmons, Jeanette. *Patient Education: An Annotated Bibliography.* Bureau of Health Educ., Center for Disease Control. Atlanta: Center for Disease Control, 1975. 13 pp.
An annotated bibliography with the primary focus on the objectives methodology, organization, and evaluation of patient education programs.

Part II

Reference and Research Aids

Chapter 3

Bibliographies and Selection Guides

The publications listed in this chapter are bibliographies, indexes, and guides to general consumer health information materials, including books, pamphlets, and audiovisuals. Entries are arranged in four sections: General Materials; Patient Education Materials; Spanish-Language Materials; and Government Publications. Many of the bibliographies were developed for use in connection with specific consumer health or patient education projects and thus emphasize materials available or accessible locally. Bibliographies relating to specific health topics are annotated in Chapter 4.

GENERAL MATERIALS

Alexander, Carole Klein. *Health Care for the Layman: A Basic Book Collection for the Education Center.* New York: New York Univ. Medical Center, Patient Educ. Center, 1979. 12 pp.
A selected guide to books relating to basic topics such as aging, arthritis, diabetes, gastrointestinal system, oncology, plastic surgery, stress, gynecology, heart disease, and urology. Contains very short descriptions of each item. A good selection of basic books on a variety of topics.

Available Catalogs or Listings of Sources for Health Education Materials. New York: New York Metropolitan Reference and Research Lib. Agency (METRO), n.d. 3 pp.
A selection of some ten directories and catalogs of consumer health/patient education materials. Contains address and ordering information.

Bennet, Steven J., and Parker, Richard A., eds. *Health Source 1979: A Popular Index to Books about Nutrition, Lifestyle, Health Care.* Cambridge, MA: Bennett and Parker Pubns., 1979. 65 pp.

Lists over 700 popular books published since 1975 with a cost of less than $10. Most of the books selected "attempt to demystify medical knowledge and practices by translating medical concepts into everyday language, and by promoting the idea that self-help leads to self-health." Major topics covered are nutrition (vegetarian and natural foods cookery, vitamins, salt, fiber, weight loss); life-style and well-being (stress, staying in shape, kicking the smoking habit); holistic healing arts (acupuncture, Shiatsu, massage, homeopathy, naturopathy); childbirth; body and soul (yoga, biofeedback, oriental exercise and meditation). Contains lists of publishers and distributors and author and subject indexes. Lacks annotations, but useful as a guide to the self-health care literature.

Bibliography Series. Cambridge, MA: Community Health Information Network (CHIN), Mount Auburn Hospital, 1979–.

A number of bibliographies have been compiled for the CHIN In-Service Training Program. Some of the bibliographies have annotations. Titles of the bibliographies compiled since September 1979 are:

> *Books for Children and Young Adults on Selected Health-Related Topics*
> *Breast Cancer*
> *Consumer Health Information*
> *Government Agencies Which Produce Materials on Health for the Consumer*
> *Growing Older*
> *The Informed Health Care Consumer*
> *Physical Fitness*
> *Preventive Medicine—A Selected Bibliography*
> *Professional Reading List on Health Information*
> *Selected List of Reference Books for the Core Collection*
> *Sources of Free or Inexpensive Materials*
> *Stress*

Bolce, Frederica S. *Medical Books for the Non-Medical Library.* Cleveland, OH: Cleveland Area Metropolitan Lib. System (CAMLS), November 1978. 10 pp.

Lists 44 principal works in the major medical specialties. Very useful for identifying major textbooks in specialties such as gastroenterology, pediatrics, or psychiatry. Also has a selected list of journals such as the *Journal of the American Medical Association* and *New England Journal of Medicine.* The 108 works listed are reference materials rather than books likely to be read by the lay public.

Bunting, Allison, and others. *Selected List of Medical Reference Works for Public Libraries.* Los Angeles: Pacific Southwest Regional Medical Lib. Service, January 1979. 14 pp.

An excellent evaluative list of bibliographies, selection aids, dictionaries, directories, encyclopedias, handbooks, and textbooks. Very useful comparative discussion of the major sources of information on drugs and poisoning. Highly valuable for the building of a core collection. Compiled by the staffs of UCLA Biomedical Library and the Consumer Health Information Program and Services (CHIPS) libraries.

Calebretta, Nancy, comp. *Medical Library Materials for Non-Medical Libraries.* New York: New York Metropolitan Reference and Research Lib. Agency (METRO), 1978. 30 pp.
A ten-page annotated guide that includes selection aids; list of publishers with addresses; and primary reference sources, such as dictionaries, handbooks, and textbooks. Largely duplicates the listing contained in Bunting et al.'s *Selected List . . . ,* described above.

Catalog: Health and Safety Educational Materials. New York: Metropolitan Life Insurance, Health and Safety Educ. Div., 1978. 7 pp.
Identifies booklets on topics such as health maintenance organizations, stress and health, immunization, heart attacks, and so forth, available from Metropolitan. Also lists films available on loan.

Consumer Health Education: A Directory, 1975. Amer. Public Health Assn. and Health Resources Admin., 1976. DHEW Pubn. No. (HRA) 76-607. 47 pp.
A listing, produced by the American Public Health Association, of the objectives and programs of some 50 major voluntary health organizations in the United States, such as the American Cancer Society, American Heart Association, La Leche League, Epilepsy Foundation of America, Mental Health Materials Center, and Sex Information and Education Council of the United States (SIECUS). In each instance, available books, pamphlets, audiovisuals, and other information materials are noted. A subject index is provided. Unfortunately, the list is somewhat out of date.

Consumer Health Information: Print and Audiovisual Resources. Chicago: Amer. Hospital Assn., Center for Health Promotion, 1978. 5 pp.
Names and addresses of suppliers of health information and education materials relating to arthritis, cancer, diabetes, heart disease, hypertension, and nutrition. Each entry indicates the availability of pamphlets, films and slides, catalogs, and Spanish-language materials. A good selection.

Consumers Index. Ann Arbor, MI: Pierian. Qtrly. $59.50/yr.
One of the feature sections of this quarterly publication is devoted to health and personal care. Popular articles are listed from some 100 periodicals. Topics covered include aging, breast feeding, health problems of children, headaches, hypertension, pregnancy, breast cancer, stress, and so forth. This publication provides good access to the large number of popular health articles now appearing in *Ladies Home Journal, Mademoiselle, Family Circle, Good*

Housekeeping, Consumer Reports, Parents Magazine, McCall's, Woman's Day, Vogue, Changing Times, and other such magazines.

Freedom Booklist. Phoenix, AZ: Samaritan Health Service, Health Educ. Resource Center, 1980. 8 pp.
Seven book lists on fitness; reduction of environmental and personal risks; emotional well-being; educated eating; drug decisions; occupational satisfaction; and management of stress. A good selection but lacks annotations or evaluation.

Hamilton, Patricia, comp. *Sources of Free and Low Cost Health Education Materials for Consumers.* New York: New York Metropolitan Reference and Research Lib. Agency (METRO), 1978. 12 pp.
Lists agencies, organizations, societies, and companies to show name and address, subject of the material offered, and symbols that indicate whether the agency has a catalog and whether the information is in the form of print, audiovisual, or both.

Health Care and the Consumer: A Guide to Informational Materials. Washington, DC: Pharmaceutical Manufacturers Assn., n.d. 29 pp.
The guide describes more than 200 publications, films, and teaching aids produced for the public by PMA and its member companies. Contains an extensive list of pamphlets under topics such as diabetes, hepatitis, spastic colon, epilepsy, and hypertension with the addresses for ordering items. A good source for ordering free pamphlet materials from large pharmaceutical companies such as Abbott, Lilly, and Robins.

Health Education Films: An Annotated Guide. Cambridge, MA: Community Health Information Network (CHIN), n.d. 89 pp. $20.
Reviews over 200 16mm films on topics such as accident prevention, death and dying, aging, nutrition, physical fitness, and so forth. Information on rental fees and recommended audiences is included.

Health Education Materials and the Organizations Which Offer Them. Washington, DC: Health Insurance Inst., n.d. 25 pp.
List is based upon a survey by the Health Insurance Institute, "which asked insurance companies, health organizations, medical associations, health-related businesses, private publishers, and government agencies to list their available publications." More than 200 sources of free or low-cost materials are identified and grouped under headings such as aging, alcoholism, cerebral palsy, child care and development, drug abuse, genetic disease, heart disease, mental health, nutrition, and venereal disease. Indicates availability of pamphlets, films, books, posters, and so forth. A good assortment of organizations, yet lacks inclusion of the numerous information sources in federal agencies concerned with health and health promotion.

Lang, Lucille. *Health Materials for the Non-Medical Library. A Selected Bibliography.* Cleveland, OH: Cleveland Area Metropolitan Lib. System (CAMLS), 1978. 19 pp.
A nonevaluative compilation of publications arranged in 44 subject areas, such as arthritis, dentistry, migraine, pain, stress, and vitamins. Presented at a workshop held in November 1978.

Martin, Rebecca, and Yee, Sen. *List of Books.* San Francisco: Veterans Admin. Hospital, Patient Educ. Resource Center, 1978. 17 pp.
Contains some 250 titles of books relating to alcoholism, drug abuse, cancer, diet and nutrition, physical handicaps, stress, and other popular health topics. Useful as a checklist.

"Media for Consumer Health Care." *Previews* 8 (October 1979): 2–17.
Presents short descriptions of some 100 16mm films, audiocassettes, videocassettes, slides, and filmstrips on a variety of health topics including medical consumerism, nutrition, physical fitness, personal hygiene, emergencies, health problems and their control, coping, and death and dying. The selection is based upon what was received from producers and distributors of audiovisuals. This is a very limited compilation since many of the major producers evidently chose not to cooperate. Moreover, the basis for selection of individual items is not identified. The descriptions are nonevaluative and do not comment upon audience level, technical accuracy, substance, balance, authority, or other criteria.

Philbrook, Marilyn M. *Medical Books for the Layperson: An Annotated Bibliography.* Boston, MA: Boston Public Lib., 1976. 113 pp. $2.
Brief annotations of some 236 books selected from the collection of the Boston Public Library representing titles published from 1969 through mid-1975. Topics covered include aging, alcoholism, bed-wetting, cancer, cataracts, deafness, epilepsy, mental illness, nursing homes, and vasectomy. Useful despite the lack of evaluation. A subject index is provided.

Philbrook, Marilyn M. *Medical Books for the Layperson: An Annotated Bibliography. Supplement.* Boston, MA: Boston Public Lib., 1978. 46 pp. $1.
An update of the earlier bibliography by the same author to include books from mid-1975 through 1977. Short descriptions are provided for more than 100 books listed under Library of Congress subject headings.

"Physical Fitness Books." Library Journal (June 15, 1979): 1318–1323.
Four reviewers—Jerry Holtz, William Hoffman, Paula Strain, and Howard Miller—present a highly selective list of books on running, exercise, walking, and body building. Short annotations justify their selections.

Polidora, Jim. "Holistic Health Reading Guide—Parts I and II." *Holistic Health Review* 2 (Spring 1979): 22–28; (Summer 1979): 17–25.

Short annotations are provided on a selection of books relating to holistic health, wellness, self-health care, healing for the whole person, health activation, spiritual exercise, enlightenment, and mind expansion. An attempt is made to blend conventional with unconventional sources of information. Also includes lists of journal articles, periodicals, and holistic health organizations.

Selected Bibliographies. Los Angeles: Consumer Health Information Program and Services (CHIPS)/Salud y Bienestar, 1978–.

A series of eleven bibliographies have been published by the CHIPS program on key health topics. Each bibliography lists books, pamphlets and booklets, and resource organizations. These bibliographies also contain the best available listings of Spanish-language materials on consumer health. Lists are divided into general subject areas. No annotations or evaluations are provided. Titles of bibliographies are as follows:

A Selected Bibliography on Diet, Nutrition, and Diet Therapy. CHIPS Bibliography No. 1, January 1978. 5 pp.

A Selected Bibliography on Cancer. CHIPS Bibliography No. 2, March 1978. 17 pp.

A Selected Bibliography on Prenatal, Postnatal, and Infant Care. CHIPS Bibliography No. 3, March 1978. 16 pp.

A Selected Bibliography of Government Publications on General Health. CHIPS Bibliography No. 4, March 1978. 16 pp.

A Selected Bibliography on Diabetes. CHIPS Bibliography No. 5, March 1978. 6 pp. *Update,* October 1978. 2 pp.

A Selected Bibliography on Allergy. CHIPS Bibliography No. 6, October 1978. 4 pp.

A Selected Bibliography on Women's Health Care. CHIPS Bibliography No. 7, December 1978. 16 pp.

A Selected Bibliography on Death and Dying. CHIPS Bibliography No. 8, June 1979. 14 pp.

A Selected Bibliography on Phencyclidine Hydrochloride—PCP. CHIPS Bibliography No. 9, June 1979. 6 pp.

A Selected Bibliography on Hypertension and Stroke. CHIPS Bibliography No. 10, January 1980. 6 pp.

A Selected Bibliography on Cancer. Update. CHIPS Bibliography No. 11, March 1980. 10 pp.

Simons, Anne. "Medical Textbooks I Have Known." *Medical Self-Care* 6 (Fall 1979): 23–29.

A selection by a young resident physician of basic reference books suitable for those who would like to go beyond the lay medical literature. Contains recommended books on anatomy, pharmacology, microbiology, pathology, physical diagnosis, internal medicine, surgery, pediatrics, psychiatry, and medical and surgical subspecialties. Full bibliographic citations are supplied for 63 books.

Social Issues Information List. Washington, DC: Natl. Audiovisual Center, General Services Admin., n.d. 15 pp.
A listing of federally produced audiovisual materials in a number of health-related areas: aging, child abuse, death and bereavement, family planning and sex education, mental health, and parenting. Purchase and rental information is supplied with cost for each item and booking and film shipment procedures.

Suggested Consumer Health Information Resources. Chicago: Amer. Hospital Assn., Center for Health Promotion, 1978. 3 pp.
Listing of books on nutrition, low cholesterol diets, physical fitness, stress, self-health care, and perspectives on health care. No annotations or evaluations are provided.

Ulene, Art, and Feldman, Sandy. *Help Yourself to Health: A Health Information and Services Directory.* New York: Putnam's, 1980. $10.95 (paper).
This is an ambitious, and successful, attempt to assemble the vast array of inexpensive pamphlet and booklet materials, information clearinghouses, referral hotlines, self-help workshops, disease detection programs, treatment clinics, and health resource organizations available to the public. The guide is divided into five sections: publications, services, organizations, addresses, and a subject index. The publications section, consisting of some 3,000 brochures and pamphlets, does not include books. It is arranged by topics such as teeth and gums, kidney and urinary tract, cancer, diabetes , alcoholism, infections, allergies, and so forth. Since addresses of organizations and services are listed separately, a fair amount of switching from one section to another is required. The directory is comprehensive in coverage and is the best compilation to date of the pamphlet and booklet literature, a product of more than two years' research effort. It is of more use, however, for the ultimate consumer to browse through and use than as a tool for systematic collection development. Highly recommended.

Walker, William D., and Hirschfeld, Lorraine. "Sources of Health Information for Public Libraries." *Illinois Libraries* 58 (June 1976): 459–502.
Contains a number of bibliographies prepared for the one-day workshop "Sources of Health Information for Public Libraries" sponsored by the Library of the Health Sciences at the University of Illinois Medical Center in Chicago. In addition to a listing of general materials, special bibliographies cover topics such as aging, death and dying, alcoholism and drug abuse, cancer, heart disease, health statistics, and cancer information. Selection tools for health education media and distributors are listed. The annotations are informative, and an attempt has been made to select the best materials available. Many listings are, however, obsolescent, and the publication is slanted toward organizations and sources in Illinois.

Wood, M. M. "300 Valuable Booklets to Give Patients and Their Families: A
   Source Guide." *Nursing 74,* April 1974, pp. 43–50, May 1974, pp 59–66.
A good selection of pamphlet and booklet materials available on many topics
of major health interest: alcoholism, allergies, arthritis, hypertension, mental
health, nutrition, pregnancy, sickle cell disease, varicose veins, and so forth.
Available materials are listed and annotated under the organizational source.
Although many of the items listed are obsolescent, superseded, or no longer
available, this is still a most useful guide to health-related organizations that
distribute educational materials. Covers printed and audiovisual items.

PATIENT EDUCATION MATERIALS

Ash, Joan, and Stevenson, Michael. *Health: A Multimedia Source Guide.* New
   York: Bowker, 1976. 185 pp. $16.50
An annotated guide to 700 organizations that deal with health-related
matters—publishers, audiovisual producers and distributors, libraries, government agencies, and professional and voluntary societies. For each organization listed, the availability of publications and other media is indicated.
Three indexes are provided: an alphabetical listing; an index to sources that
provide free or inexpensive pamphlet material to the layman; and an index to
sources by subject. This publication is useful to those desiring to develop
health information collections either within the hospital or in public library
settings.

Bibliography of Patient and Community Health Education. Chicago: Amer. Society
   for Health Manpower Educ. and Training, 1980.
A comprehensive bibliography of patient and community health education
resources.

*Commercially Produced Patient and Community Health Education Audiovisuals Used
   by 224 Hospitals.* Chicago: Amer. Hospital Assn., Center for Health Promotion, 1979. 209 pp.
Listing was compiled under the American Hospital Association-Bureau of
Health Education contract by the Mental Health Materials Center. Six
hundred audiovisuals are listed that are used by 244 hospitals in their patient
and community health education programs. No evaluation has been attempted. Audiovisuals are grouped by subject such as arthritis, mastectomy, prenatal care, and so forth. In each instance, brief information is supplied with
respect to source, cost, format, running time, primary audience, and context.
Particularly helpful is the indication of the number of hospitals that report
the use of each audiovisual. An appendix lists the names and addresses of
distributors.

Duke, Phyllis, comp. "Audiovisuals: Patient Education." In *Journal of Biocom-
   munication* 5 (March 1978): 18–23.

A list of some 80 producers of patient education materials. Most of the major suppliers are noted with a brief description of the principal health topics covered by each source. Types of media available, such as films, audiocassettes, charts, models, and videocassettes are indicated. Addresses are provided for the ordering of 21 university catalogs of rental films for general public education.

Gotsick, Priscilla, Branham, Janice, and Conley, Bruce. *Sources of Patient Education Materials.* Detroit: Kentucky-Ohio-Michigan Regional Medical Lib. Network, Health Information Lib. Program, 1979. 17 pp.
Contains 121 health-related organizations, professional associations, and companies that produce and/or distribute patient education materials. Each entry indicates available formats (slides, filmstrips, videocassettes, films, audiocassettes, and so forth) and the major subject areas covered, such as muscular dystrophy, nutrition, and family planning. A good selection of the many sources currently available.

Martin, Rebecca, and Yee, Sen. *Patient Education Audiovisuals: A Core List.* San Francisco: Veterans Admin. Hospital, n.d. 5 pp.
A core list of highly recommended programs from the collection of the Patient Education Resource Center, Veterans Administration Hospital, San Francisco. The composition of the list reflects the common medical problems of a veterans population, as encountered in a general hospital. The programs cover alcoholism, arthritis, colostomy, diabetes, diet and nutrition, eye, gastrointestinal tract, heart disease, hip replacement, lung disease, medication, surgery, and general health. The total cost of the programs listed is approximately $8,000. Purchase of the basic items, indicated by an asterisk, would amount to $2,200.

Martin, Rebecca, and Yee, Sen. *Sources for Patient Education Materials.* San Francisco: Veterans Admin. Hospital, August 1977. 14 pp.
A good summary of 140 voluntary health organizations, professional associations, media producers, publishers, government agencies, pharmaceutical companies, and universities that supply audiovisuals, books, and pamphlet materials relating to patient education.

Martyn, Dorian, Spencer, Dorothy, and Duke, Phyllis. *Source List for Patient Education Materials.* Milledgeville, GA: Health Services Communications Assn. (HESCA), Education Committee, 1978. 47 pp. $3.
The most comprehensive listing to date of organizations that supply books, pamphlets, or audiovisual materials. The 530 entries were derived from an extensive survey of health organizations designed to identify available materials. Each entry contains the name and address of the organization, types of materials available, availability of catalogs, and the source from which the entry was obtained for inclusion. The list is not selective and includes all organizations that reported the availability of educational materials. A subject

index is provided utilizing subject headings modified from MeSH (Medical subject headings used by the National Library of Medicine). Apart from the subject indexing of each source there is no listing of specific materials available. The objective of the publication is, however, to serve as a list of sources rather than as a compilation of materials. Highly recommended.

Some Sources for Patient Education Videotape Programs: Some Commercial Suppliers
   of Patient Education Materials. Chicago: Amer. Hospital Assn., February
   1977. 4 pp. (Distributed by the Center for Disease Control, Bureau of
   Health Education, Atlanta, GA).
Lists the names, addresses, and phone numbers of the principal suppliers of audiovisual materials.

The Videolog: Programs for the Health Sciences, 1979. New York: Esselte Video,
   1979. 399 pp. $35.
Contains descriptions of over 7,000 videotape and videocassette programs and series for both professional and patient health education. An annotated description is provided for each entry. A subject index lists titles of programs. Reference to the alphabetical listings then provides a short description of each item together with price and ordering information. Patient health education programs, over 800 in number, are listed by title under the heading "Patient Education." This section is further divided into topics such as alcoholism and drug abuse, cardiology and cardiovascular system, dental health, nutrition, obstetrics, and so forth.

SPANISH-LANGUAGE MATERIALS

Guide to Audiovisual Aids for Spanish-Speaking Americans: Health-Related Films,
   Filmstrips and Slides, Descriptions and Sources. Health Services Admin., 1974.
   DHEW Pubn. No. (HSA) 74-30. 37 pp.
Materials, mainly films, are grouped by topics such as aging, cancer, diabetes, heart disease, multiple sclerosis, venereal disease, mental health, and prenatal and infant care. Short nonevaluative descriptions are provided. Also contains names and addresses of 44 distributors of materials. The dates of the materials are from 1940 to 1973.

Korzdorfer, Kamala, and Yeh, Irene, comps. *Spanish Language Health*
   Materials: A Selected Bibliography. Hayward, CA: California Ethnic Services
   Task Force, 1978. 41 pp.
This bibliography is designed for use by medium-sized public libraries in either initiating or expanding a Spanish-language materials collection in health. The materials listed (books, pamphlets, and texts) are either in Spanish or bilingual Spanish-English form and represent a wide range of reading levels and interests. Most of the annotations include a critical description of contents and an evaluation in terms of language and reading level. The major

topics covered are alcohol and drugs, consumer health information, diseases, human physiology, medical care, medicinal plants and herbs, mental health, nutrition, pediatrics and child care, physical fitness, pregnancy and child-birth, sex education, and women's health. Also included is a list of titles only of materials that were unavailable for examination and names and addresses of sources. An excellent guide—evaluative and informative.

Spanish-Language Health Communication Teaching Aids: A List of Printed Materials and their Sources. Health Services and Mental Health Admin., 1973. 55 pp. DHEW Pubn. No. (HSM) 73-19.
A compilation of pamphlet, book, poster, and other information materials available from state health agencies, pharmaceutical companies, publishers, and community health organizations. Although many of the teaching aids may now be unavailable because of the age of the listing, this is still a useful guide to some 90 sources of such materials. Annotations are nonevaluative.

GOVERNMENT PUBLICATIONS

Consumer Information Catalog: A Catalog of Selected Federal Publications of Consumer Interest. Pueblo, CO: Consumer Information Center. Qtrly. Free.
Each issue lists, with short descriptions, more than 200 selected federal publications on a variety of popular topics, including an extensive assortment of free or low-cost publications in general health, diseases and common ailments, drugs and medicines, and food, diet and nutrition. Many of the publications are reprints of articles that orginally appeared in the *FDA Consumer.* A limit of 20 publications is imposed on each order. Orders are filled by the Consumer Information Center.

MEDOC: A Computerized Index to U.S. Government Documents in the Medical and Health Sciences. Salt Lake City, UT: Eccles Health Sciences Lib., Univ. of Utah. Qtrly. $35/yr.
MEDOC lists health-related government documents received at Eccles Health Sciences Library. The coverage is broad and includes a large number of health-related topics. Four indexes are provided: Superintendent of Documents Number Index; Title Index; Subject Index; and Series Number Index. Consumer health and patient education publications are indicated as such by the use of "G" for general. MEDOC contains many omissions; some lay health publications fail to receive the "G" designation; and the materials listed are in many instances not current. Nevertheless, MEDOC is a useful guide to health-related government publications and is worth the price.

Monthly Catalog of United States Government Publications. Washington, DC: Superintendent of Documents, Government Printing Office. Monthly. $55/yr.
Each issue contains between 1,500 and 3,000 entries of new items for sale.

Entries are arranged by the Superintendent of Documents classification number and contain four indexes: author, title, subject, and series report. Complete bibliographic data are provided for each document. A rich source for health-related documents.

Newsome, Walter L. *New Guide to Popular Government Publications.* Littleton, CO: Libraries Unlimited, 1978. 370 pp. $18.50.
Includes a fairly representative listing of consumer-oriented publications on alcoholism, allergies, cancer, cardiovascular diseases, dental health, drug abuse, eye disorders, genetic disorders, infectious diseases, mental health, organ transplants, smoking and health, and miscellaneous health problems. The criteria for inclusion or exclusion are not clear.

NIH Publications List. Natl. Insts. of Health, Div. of Public Information, October 1979. DHEW Pubn. No. (NIH) 80-6. 64 pp.
Many of the publications listed are oriented toward the general public. Nineteen component divisions of the National Institutes of Health are included, such as the National Cancer Institute, the National Heart, Lung, and Blood Institute, and the National Institute of Arthritis, Metabolism, and Digestive Diseases. In most cases, one copy of each publication listed is available free from the Public Inquiries Office of the NIH component listed at Bethesda, Maryland 20205. Some are for sale from the Superintendent of Documents although GPO numbers are not given. Several hundred publications are listed. Contains a title index.

Schorr, Alan Edward. *Government Reference Books 76/77: A Biennial Guide to U.S. Government Publications.* Littleton, CO: Libraries Unlimited, 1978. 355 pp. $18.50.
Contains a selection of bibliographies, directories, pamphlets, and other publications on a variety of health topics. Does not differentiate between professional and consumer-oriented materials.

Subject Bibliography Index. Washington, DC: Superintendent of Documents, Government Printing Office, SB-999, April 1, 1977. 8 pp.
A listing of over 270 subject bibliographies intended to provide subject access to the more than 24,000 publications, periodicals, and subscription services for sale by the Superintendent of Documents. To include the 3,000 or more new titles made available each year, the subject bibliographies are updated periodically. Currently, there are 19 subject bibliographies of interest to consumer health and patient education:

Alcoholism. SB-175, January 27, 1979. 10 pp.
Care and Disorders of the Eyes. SB-028, July 10, 1978. 3 pp.
Consumer Information. SB-002, June 27, 1978. 34 pp.
Dentistry. SB-022, September 12, 1978. 6 pp.
Diseases in Humans. SB-008, July 28, 1978. 18 pp.

Drug Education. SB-103, January 11, 1979. 15 pp.
Food, Diet, and Nutrition. SB-291, January 30, 1979. 22 pp.
The Handicapped. SB-037, May 1977. 5 pp.
Hearing and Hearing Disability. SB-023. 4 pp.
Heart and Circulatory System. SB-104, May 31, 1979. 4 pp.
Hospitals. SB-119, January 18, 1979. 8 pp.
Medicine and Medical Science. SB-154, May 17, 1978. 26 pp.
Mental Health, SB-107, August 11, 1978. 12 pp.
Nurses and Nursing Care. SB-019, July 14, 1978. 9 pp.
Occupational Safety and Health. SB-213, March 28, 1979. 4 pp.
Physical Fitness. SB-239, February 1, 1979. 3 pp.
Public Health. SB-1222, March 9, 1979. 6 pp.
Smoking. SB-015, August 1, 1978. 2 pp.
Vital and Health Statistics. SB-121, November 1, 1978. 8 pp.

Washington Information Directory 1979–80. Washington, DC: Congressional
  Qtrly, 1979. 931 pp. $22.50.
A comprehensive point of entree into the information resources and services
of agencies of the executive branch, the Congress, and private or nongovern-
mental organizations. Contains a chapter on health and consumer affairs
which provides a good selection of information sources under headings such
as alcoholism, drug abuse, family planning, mental health, and so forth.
However, it has many ommissions, such as many of the federal health information clearinghouses. Contains also a short reference bibliography.

Chapter 4

Bibliographies of Major Health Topics

In addition to the general bibliographies of consumer health information materials described in Chapter 3, a number of bibliographies are available on special health topics. This chapter brings together bibliographies, catalogs, compilations, publications lists, and guides that note books, pamphlets, booklets, and audiovisual materials on 12 major health topics: Alcoholism, Arthritis, Birth Control and Family Planning, Cancer, Children's Health, Death and Dying, Diabetes, Diet and Nutrition, Drug Abuse, Heart Disease and Hypertension, Mental Health, and Women's Health.

The selection of these topics for coverage in this chapter reflects the popularity of these areas and the fact that considerable effort has been made by bibliographers to assemble and organize available publications. The subject scope of each bibliographic compilation is indicated together with the presence or absence of evaluative comments.

ALCOHOLISM

AA Conference-Approved Literature and Other Service Materials, 1979. New York: Alcoholics Anonymous World Services. Pamphlet. Updated periodically.
A listing of books, booklets, pamphlets, directories, wallet cards, posters, and other materials related to alcoholism and recovery. A short description of each item is provided.

Al-Anon and Alateen Publications List. New York: Al-Anon Family Group Headquarters. Pamphlet. Updated periodically.
Contains some 100 pamphlets and other materials designed to treat and rehabilitate alcoholics.

Alcoholism. (Subject Bibliography SB-175). See *Subject Bibliography Index* in the Government Publications section of Chapter 3.

Grouped Interest Guides. Rockville, MD: Natl. Clearinghouse for Alcohol Information. Updated biannually.
This series of bibliographies in 15 subject areas contains references and annotations for recent documents that have been judged significant because of their technical content. Current titles include:

Alcohol, Accidents, and Highway Safety
Alcohol and Mental Health
Alcohol Treatment Modalities
Animal Research on Alcohol Effects
Drugs and Alcohol
Education and Training about Alcohol
Heredity, Genetics, and Alcohol Abuse
Legal Aspects of Alcohol Use and Abuse
Occupational Alcoholism Programs
Physiologic Concomitants of Alcohol Use and Abuse
Psychological Studies of Alcohol and Alcoholism
Rehabilitation Strategies for Alcohol Abusers
Sociocultural Aspects of Alcohol Use and Alcoholism
Statistical and Demographic Research of Alcohol Use and Abuse
Teenagers and Alcohol

Hazelden 1980 Educational Services Catalog. Center City, MN: Hazelden Foundation, 1980. 74 pp.
A publication of the Hazelden Literature Department, a division of Hazelden Foundation, which is a leading resource center for the publication and distribution of educational and therapy materials in the field of alcoholism, other drug dependencies, and personal growth. The materials are addressed to the needs of recovering persons, their families, professionals in the field, treatment centers and hospitals, clergy, libraries, and schools. Covers books, pamphlets, and audiovisuals. Short descriptions are provided. Hazelden also distributes some Alcoholics Anonymous and Al-Anon Materials.

Selected Guide to Audiovisual Materials on Alcohol and Alcoholism. Rockville, MD: Natl. Clearinghouse for Alcohol Information, 1974. DHEW Pubn. No. (ADM) 74-32. 36 pp.
A comprehensive list, somewhat outdated.

ARTHRITIS

Audiovisual Materials on Arthritis for Patient Education. Bethesda, MD: Arthritis Information Clearinghouse, June 1979. 15 pp.
Catalogs from producers of audiovisual materials were examined to prepare a

list of patient education audiovisuals. The major producers included are the Arthritis Foundation, Core Communications, Graphics Plus Associates, Milner Fenwick, Modern Talking Picture Service, National Safety Council, Professional Research, PBS, Soundbooks, Therapy Graphics, University of Michigan, and Wright/Dow Corning. A very brief description of each item is given with an indication of format and rental or purchase price.

"A Guide to Books on Arthritis." *Consumer Reports* 44 (July 1979): 393.
A description of some dozen recommended books selected according to Arthritis Foundation criteria.

Patient Education Resources on Arthritic Conditions: Booklets and Brochures.
Bethesda, MD: Arthritis Information Clearinghouse, October 1979. 37 pp.
An excellent comprehensive bibliography with short descriptions of booklets, brochures, and pamphlets on arthritis in general, rheumatoid arthritis, osteoarthritis, back and spine disorders, gout, lupus erythematosus, psoriasis, and psychosocial aspects, including daily living, nutrition, and quackery. Source, price, and ordering information are supplied together with a title index, source and producer index, and a directory of Arthritis Foundation chapters. The following bibliographies are also available from the clearinghouse:

> *Activities of Daily Living: A Selected Bibliography,* 1979. 2 pp.
> *Arthritis and Employment: A Selected Bibliography,* 1979. 14 pp.
> *Costs, Risks and Benefits of Joint Replacement,* 1979. 13 pp.
> *Directory of Organization and Information Resources,* 1979. 28 pp.
> *Juvenile Rheumatoid Arthritis: A Selected Bibliography: Patient Management and Information for Patients and Teachers,* 1979. 2 pp.
> *Osteoarthritis: Patient-Oriented Materials,* 1979. 2 pp.
> *Patient Education-Program Design: A Selected Bibliography,* 1979. 2 pp.
> *Patient Education Programs in Arthritis: A Selected Bibliography,* 1979. 2 pp.
> *Psychological Factors in Arthritis: A Selected Bibliography,* 1979. 20 pp.
> *Selected Patient Information References on Nutrition and Arthritis,* 1979. 2 pp.
> *Selected References on Sexuality and Rheumatic Disease,* 1979. 2 pp.

BIRTH CONTROL AND FAMILY PLANNING

See also Women's Health, this chapter.

Bibliography Series. Rockville, MD: Natl. Clearinghouse for Family Planning Information.
Bibliographies on the following topics are available from the clearinghouse: barrier methods and spermicidal agents; birth defects, genetics, and genetic counseling; common reproductive tract infections; contraceptive methods; contraceptive research and technology; family planning for adolescents; family planning for the handicapped; family planning motivation and practice;

family planning programs and services; human sexuality and sex education; infertility; intrauterine devices; legal aspects; men and family planning; natural methods; oral contraceptives; reproduction and reproductive health; sterilization.

Catalog of Family Planning Materials. Rockville, MD: Natl. Clearinghouse for Family Planning Information, 1979. DHEW Pubn. No. (HSA) 79-5606. GPO No. HE 20.5102:F21/8. 144 pp.

Lists approximately 1,000 print and audiovisual patient education and staff training materials. The catalog is divided into four sections—print materials and audiovisual materials for the general public and for professional audiences. Topics covered include contraceptive methods, human sexuality, infertility, sex education, sterilization procedures, adoption, breast and pelvic examinations, menstruation and menopause, pregnancy and childbirth, and venereal disease. Short descriptive annotations are provided for each book, pamphlet, poster, model, bumper sticker, and audiovisual listed. Title, author, and distributor indexes are also supplied. A most useful compendium of information resources.

Catalog of Family Planning Materials: Supplement—September 1979. Rockville, MD: Natl. Clearinghouse for Family Planning Information, 1979. DHEW Pubn. No. (HSA) 79-5606-1. 41 pp.

This is a supplement to the catalog listed in the preceding entry. The supplement is also divided into four sections—print and audiovisual materials for the general public and for professional audiences. Short descriptive annotations are accompanied by title, author, and distributor indexes.

CANCER

Asbestos and Health: An Annotated Bibliography of Public and Professional Education Materials. Natl. Cancer Inst. Bethesda, MD: Cancer Information Clearinghouse, 1978. DHEW Pubn. No. (NIH) 78-1842. 60 pp.

Compilation of 162 references with annotations on regulation and control, safety monitoring, smoking cessation, public action materials, and control technology. Lists industry and government agency publications covering books, brochures, newspapers, journal articles, and audiovisuals. Complete ordering information is contained in each entry. Author, title, and subject indexes are provided.

Breast Cancer: Annotated Bibliography of Public, Patient, and Professional Information and Educational Materials. Natl. Cancer Inst. Bethesda, MD: Cancer Information Clearinghouse, 1979. DHEW Pubn. No. (NIH) 79-2002. 71 pp.

Comprehensive listing of book, pamphlet, and audiovisual materials to assist health educators and health care providers to identify and select appropriate materials. Topics covered include general information, benign breast disease, breast self-examination, treatment methods, and rehabilitation.

Cancer Information in the Workplace: Annotated Bibliography of Educational Materials for the Public and Health Professionals. Natl. Cancer Inst. Bethesda, MD: Cancer Information Clearinghouse, 1979. DHEW Pubn. No. (NIH) 79-2001. 58 pp.
Bibliography is intended to assist health educators, industrial hygienists, and health care providers in identifying and selecting appropriate educational materials. Covers carcinogens, cancer hazards in the workplace, prevention, screening, and surveillance.

Coping with Cancer: Annotated Bibliography of Public, Patient, and Professional Information and Education Materials. Natl. Cancer Inst. Bethesda, MD: Cancer Information Clearinghouse, 1980. Pubn. No. (NIH) 80-2129. 113 pp.
A bibliography designed to assist health educators and health care providers identify and select appropriate materials. Includes books, pamphlets, and audiovisuals produced subsequent to 1971. Provides short descriptions and ordering information. Principal topics covered are cancer in adults, cancer in children, coping with breast cancer, lung cancer, head and neck cancer, colorectal cancer, and leukemia. Good coverage and informative descriptions of available materials. Public and patient information materials are contained in separate sections.

Information Bibliography: Cancer Education Materials. Natl. Cancer Inst. Bethesda, MD: Cancer Information Clearinghouse. Monthly. Free.
A listing with short annotations of new publications designed for public education, patient education, and professional education. Typical topics include breast cancer, smoking, prevention, nutrition, radiation therapy, and Laetrile. The source of each item listed is indicated to facilitate ordering.

Nutrition for the Cancer Patient: Selected Annotations of Educational Materials. Natl. Cancer Inst. Bethesda, MD: Cancer Information Clearinghouse, 1977. DHEW Pubn. No. (NIH) 78-1511. 13 pp.
Annotations are provided for both patient education and professional education purposes. Brochures and booklets on food selection, diets, recipes, home care, and nutritional tolerance are described. In each instance the source is indicated to facilitate acquisition. A subject index is provided. Useful for health care providers and communicators.

Oral Cancer Education: Selected Annotations. Natl. Cancer Inst. Bethesda, MD: Cancer Information Clearinghouse, 1977. DHEW Pubn. No. (NIH) 78-1514. 17 pp.
Short descriptions of materials for public education, patient education, and professional education. Print and nonprint materials are listed on prevention and early detection, self-examination, smoking and oral cancer, and self-care suitable for lay use. Annotations are nonevaluative. Contains index and ordering information.

Patient Education Materials for Ostomates: Selected Annotations. Natl. Cancer Inst. Bethesda, MD: Cancer Information Clearinghouse, 1977. DHEW Pubn. No. (NIH) 78-1512. 10 pp.

Short, nonevaluative annotations of print and nonprint materials on colostomy, ileostomy, urostomy, and ostomy. The relevant source, such as the United Ostomy Association, is indicated for each item.

Public and Patient Cancer Education Materials in Spanish: Selected Annotations. Natl. Cancer Inst. Bethesda, MD: Cancer Information Clearinghouse, 1977. DHEW Pubn. No. (NIH) 78-1513. 18 pp.

Annotations and sources are supplied for 77 booklets, brochures, leaflets, newsletters, motion pictures, and other materials on cancer of the breast, gastrointestinal tract, skin, and head and neck; leukemia prevention and detection; and smoking.

Public Education Materials Catalog 1979–1980. New York: Amer. Cancer Society, 1980. 157 pp.

A complete listing of cancer materials currently available from the American Cancer Society for use by the general public. Includes pictures and short descriptions of books, booklets, pamphlets, folders, leaflets, posters, kits, displays, exhibit materials, and audiovisuals. Supplementary lists of materials specifically designed for youth are also indicated. An excellent resource for those persons desirous of building a pamphlet collection or designing an education program.

A Selected Bibliography on Cancer. (CHIPS Bibliography Nos. 2 and 11). See *Selected Bibliographies* in the General Materials section of Chapter 3.

Skin Cancer Education Materials: Selected Annotations. Natl. Cancer Inst. Bethesda, MD: Cancer Information Clearinghouse, 1978. DHEW Pubn. No. (NIH) 78-1551. 35 pp.

Contains 85 annotations of materials that present a variety of approaches to cancer education. No attempt has been made to evaluate the entries. Most of the items listed are for professional education purposes, although a few public education materials are included.

Smoking and Health: An Annotated Bibliography of Public and Professional Education Materials. Natl. Cancer Inst. Bethesda, MD: Cancer Information Clearinghouse, 1977. DHEW Pubn. No. (NIH) 78-1841. 82 pp.

Contains approximately 300 citations to U.S. and Canadian print and nonprint materials and programs on smoking. Among the topics covered are education, risk and prevention, cessation ("How to Kick the Habit"), nonsmokers' rights, and legislation. Spanish- and French-language materials are included together with serial publications, reports, and teaching aids. Complete source, cost, and order information are provided for each entry.

Smoking and Health: An Annotated Bibliography. School Edition. Natl. Cancer Inst. Bethesda, MD: Cancer Information Clearinghouse, 1979. DHEW Pubn. No. (NIH) 79-1908. 36 pp.
A resource for the identification and selection of materials that will help students think about, and understand, the smoking problem. Includes annotations for some 125 print and nonprint items relating to risk and prevention, cessation, nonsmokers' rights, Spanish-language materials, and teaching resources such as curriculum guides. Contains source, cost, and ordering information for each entry.

CHILDREN'S HEALTH

Altshuler, Anne. *Books That Help Children Deal with a Hospital Experience.* Health Services Admin., Bureau of Community Health Services, 1978. DHEW Pubn. (HSA) 78-5224. 30 pp.
Prepared in response to requests from parents, nurses, teachers, pediatricians, and physicians in family practice for an up-to-date, comprehensive bibliography of children's books on the subject of illness and hospitals. The purpose is to enable adults to select books most suitable to the needs of the child to be hospitalized. The publication contains a guide to selecting books for preschool and elementary school children. The annotated list of available books evaluates both the overall quality and the accuracy of medical information included. Contains titles such as *Man I Broke My Arm,* and *Wendy Well and Bill Better ask a 'Mill-Yun' Hospital Questions.* A list of publishers is included.

Aradine, C. R. "Books for Children about Death." *Pediatrics* 57 (March 1976): 372–378.
Books about death for preschool and school-aged children are reviewed in terms of child development, children's understanding of death, and literary quality. The subject content includes death as a concept; death as a permanent loss of, and separation from, someone or something loved; the feelings that result when death, loss, separation occur; and how feelings are managed by the child and adults important to him. Book descriptions are provided for those aimed at the preschool child, the young school-aged child, the older school-aged child, and adolescents. Highly useful for pediatricians, pediatric nurses, and childlife workers.

Baskin, Barbara H. and Harris, Karen H. *Notes from a Different Drummer: A Guide to Juvenile Fiction Portraying the Handicapped.* New York: Bowker, 1977. 375 pp. $17.50.
Summarizes and evaluates over 400 children's and young adult fiction titles dealing with a wide range of physical, emotional, and intellectual handicaps.

Entries note suggested reading levels and indicate the type of disability represented in each book. Includes a discussion of selection criteria. With entries arranged by author, the book contains a title index and a subject index.

Bernstein, Joanne E. *Books to Help Children Cope with Separation and Loss.* New York: Bowker, 1977. 255 pp. $16.25.
A bibliographic guide to 1,438 children's books that deal with emotional deprivation and how to help children adjust to the stress of loss. Titles are arranged under categories such as accepting a new sibling, going to a new school, death, divorce and marital separation, desertion, serious illness, facing foster care, accepting stepparents, and understanding adoption. Introductory chapters define the nature of loss and discuss the technique of bibliotherapy. Author/title and subject indexes included.

Campbell, Patricia J. *Sex Education Books for Young Adults, 1892–1979.* New York: Bowker, 1979. 169 pp. $15.95.
This monograph is a history and analysis of sex education books written for American teenagers from the late Victorian era to the present. Each of the first eight chapters covers the literature of roughly a decade; the final chapter is an annotated guide to current recommended titles and includes a discussion of selection criteria. Index.

Chabon, Shezly, and Chabon, Robert. "Annotated Bibliography of Health Care Books for Children." *American Journal of Diseases of Children* 133 (February 1979): 184–186.
Ratings are given for books written on children in preschool through sixth grade (aged 3 to 11 years). Short annotations are presented on topics such as visits to the doctor, hospital visits, eyeglasses and eye surgery, chicken pox, and lumps, bumps, and rashes. Useful to help physicians, other health care providers, and parents prepare children for medical contacts.

Galligan, Ann Costello. "Books for the Hospitalized Child." *American Journal of Nursing* 75 (December 1975): 2164–2166.
Recommended books are calculated to provide comfort and elicit feelings of security, promote quiet relaxation, give information and correct misconceptions, help the child develop self-awareness, moderate withdrawal, and stimulate his imagination. The author claims that books can have a positive effect on a child's mental health, development, and perception of life, especially in an anxiety-provoking situation such as hospitalization.

Moore, Coralie, and Morton, Kathryn. *A Reader's Guide for Parents of Children with Mental, Physical, or Emotional Disabilities.* Health Services Admin., Bureau of Community Health Services, 1979. DHEW Pubn. No. (HSA) 79-5290. GPO No. HE 20.5108: R22/979. 144 pp.
Publication prepared by Family and Community Services, Montgomery County, Maryland Association for Retarded Citizens, under contract with the

Bureau of Community Health Services. Major topics included are learning disabilities, mental retardation, autism, emotional disturbances, physical handicaps, epilepsy, visual handicaps, hearing impediments and speech handicaps, cleft palate, and multiple handicaps. Books described are those that tell how to teach, train, and play at home; those written by parents who have "lived it"; those for children about children with handicaps; and those on particular disabilities. Particularly useful is a listing of national organizations and agencies concerned with disability, together with the titles of directories, journals, and publishers of printed materials. Each major topic covered includes details as to where to write for further information. Indispensable.

Murphy, Diane. "The Therapeutic Value of Children's Literature." *Nursing Forum* 11 (February 1972): 141–164.
The purpose of the bibliography is to demonstrate when, where, and why children's literature can help to improve the nursing care of children. Books may serve as a means of establishing rapport between nurse and child and may assist in the recovery of the child. Also, reading, and being read to, can help a child cope with fears and adjust to his or her environment. The bibliography is geared to kindergarten through sixth grade reading levels. Books are listed by problem topics, such as personal appearance, new child in the family, character and personality adjustments, and temporarily or permanently broken homes. Price and publisher information are not given.

Van Vechten, Doris, Satterwhite, Betty, and Pless, Barry. "Health Education Literature for Parents of Physically Handicapped Children." *American Journal of Diseases of Children* 131 (March 1977): 311–315.
A comprehensive compilation of books and pamphlets on a number of topics, such as allergies, asthma, birth defects, cerebral palsy, cleft palate, congenital heart disease, diabetes, muscular dystrophy, and sickle cell anemia. The audience level, source, and cost are indicated for each item listed.

DEATH AND DYING

Duke, Phyllis, comp. *Media Guide on Death and Dying.* New York: Biomedical Communications, 1978. 32 pp. $6.
Descriptive bibliography lists more than 200 audiovisual materials dealing with death and dying. Each citation provides information on format, running time, audience, source, and content.

Hospices and Related Facilities for the Terminally Ill: Selected Bibliographic References. Health Resources Admin. Bureau of Health Planning, 1979 DHEW Pubn. No. (HRA) 79-14022. GPO No. HE 20.6112/2:15. 52 pp.
A hospice program is defined as providing palliative, supportive care to the terminally ill person, offering an alternative to the sometimes impersonal, detached atmosphere of traditional institutional care for the dying. This publication provides highly informative detailed abstracts, prepared by the

National Health Planning Information Center staff, for both journal articles and books on hospice facilities, hospice services, and home health care for the terminally ill. Bibliographies, pamphlets, and newspaper articles are also listed. An excellent guide for those interested in acquiring publications on this topic.

Kutscher, Martin L., and others. *Comprehensive Bibliography of the Thanatology Literature.* Edison, NJ: Mss. Information, 1976. 285 pp. $16.50.
Contains approximately 4,800 entries. The references are arranged alphabetically by author. Entries in the compilation are most numerous under the broad headings of abortion, the family, hospitals, and the law and under the more specific headings of euthanasia, fear of death, the dying child, cancer patients, and bereavement.

A Selected Bibliography on Death and Dying. (CHIPS Bibliography No. 8). See *Selected Bibliographies* in the General Materials section of Chapter 3.

Simpson, M. A., ed. *Dying, Death, and Grief.* New York: Plenum, 1979. 288 pp. $21.95.
Critical review and annotated bibliography cites 800 books available dealing with death, dying, bereavement, suicide, and terminal and cancer care. Journal articles, films, videotapes, audiotapes, and teaching materials are covered.

The Thanatology Librarian: News of Books on Death, Bereavement, Loss, and Grief. Brooklyn, NY: Highly Specialized Promotions. $3.50/yr.
Provides annotations of recent books on topics such as widowhood, death by violence, suicide, gerontology, loss and grief, and hospices. Includes news of free pamphlets.

The Thanatology Library: Annotated Catalog of Books and Audiovisual Materials of Thanatology. Brooklyn, NY: Highly Specialized Promotions, 1979. 32 pp. $1.
The catalog contains annotated citations of books on death and dying, classifying them under subject headings such as bibliographies, death, terminal care, the funeral, grief and mourning, gerontology, and widowhood. Contains sections on thanatology periodicals, audiovisual materials, educational materials, hospices, and a recommended basic collection. Title, author, and publisher indexes are included.

DIABETES

Audiovisual Resources for Diabetes Education. Ann Arbor, MI: Univ. of Michigan Medical School, Michigan Diabetes Research and Training Center, 1979. $15.

Compilation designed to assist health professionals in the identification and selection of audiovisual materials for diabetic patients and public education. Includes program titles, bibliographical information, and descriptions of 350 programs located by a search of indexes and producer/distributor catalogs. Also provides a directory of distributors and addresses of American Diabetes Association affiliates.

Care of the Diabetic Foot: Selected Annotations. Washington, DC: Natl. Diabetes Information Clearinghouse, March 1979. Pubn. No. (NIH) 79-1870. 23 pp.
Lists leaflets and brochures and 11 audiovisual programs. Source and price information is supplied for each item, with a short description of the content.

Cookbooks for Diabetics: Selected Annotations. Washington, DC: Natl. Diabetes Information Clearinghouse, July 1979. 32 pp.
Lists 33 cookbooks available from commercial publishers and American Diabetes Association affiliates. Provides price and source data together with short descriptions of each item.

The DAC Index of Diabetes Education Materials. Cleveland Heights, OH: Diabetes Assn. of Greater Cleveland, 1973. 186 pp. $10. Updated 1977 with looseleaf inserts.
Comprehensive list of books, pamphlets, journal references, and audiovisual materials. Covers blindness, detection, employment, exercise, juvenile diabetes, nursing, nutrition, and pregnancy. Items have short descriptive annotations.

Diabetes Educational Materials for Adults with Limited Reading Skills: Selected Annotations. Washington, DC: Natl. Diabetes Information Clearinghouse, August 1979. 9 pp.
Contains short descriptions of 19 print and 2 nonprint items. Source and price information is given together with a readability rating utilizing the SMOG index.

Diet and Nutrition for People with Diabetes: Selected Annotations. Washington, DC: Natl. Diabetes Information Clearinghouse, November 1979. NIH Pubn. No. 80-1872. 57 pp.
Listing of 160 pamphlets, books, booklets, audiovisuals, journal articles, and games. Items are divided into two sections: materials suitable for public and patient education and those for professionals.

Educational Materials for and about Young People with Diabetes: Selected Annotations. Washington, DC: Natl. Diabetes Information Clearinghouse, July 1979. NIH Pubn. No. 79-1871. 43 pp.
Materials are divided into two sections: those suitable for professionals and those for public patient education. No attempt is made to judge the educa-

tional value of each item listed. Annotations are provided for both print and nonprint materials. Sources and prices are indicated.

Teaching Guides for Diabetes Education Programs: Selected Annotations. Washington, DC: Natl. Diabetes Information Clearinghouse, June 1979. 10 pp.
Descriptions of manuals, reference books, guides, and booklets available for patient education. Source and price information is supplied for each item listed.

A Selected Bibliography on Diabetes. (CHIPS Bibliography No. 5). See *Selected Bibliographies* in the General Materials section of Chapter 3.

DIET AND NUTRITION

Audiovisual Guide to the Catalog of the Food and Nutrition Information and Educational Materials Center, 2nd ed. Beltsville, MD: Food and Nutrition Information and Educ. Materials Ctr., Natl. Agricultural Lib., 1977. 132 pp.
Listing and description of available audiovisuals relating to human nutrition research and education. Subject, title, and corporate indexes are supplied together with an index by media format—audiocassettes, slides, videocassettes, and so forth.

Audiovisual Resources in Food and Nutrition: 1970–1978. Rockville, MD: Oryx, 1979. 210 pp. $18.95.
Successor to the *Audiovisual Guide to the Catalog of the Food and Nutrition Information and Educational Materials Center* (see above). Includes the current 1978 cumulation of audiovisual materials plus a full retrospective listing of all currently available audiovisual materials listed for the nine-year period 1970–1978. Lists and describes approximately 1,200 motion pictures, filmstrips, videocassettes, and other materials relating to human nutrition research and education and cognate topics.

Audiovisuals for Nutrition Education. Berkeley, CA: Society for Nutrition Educ., April 1979.
Evaluative reviews of more than 250 audiovisuals produced from 1974 to 1978. Lists media type, audience level, availability, and prices as of December 1978. Includes all audiovisual reviews published in the *Journal of Nutrition Education.*

Casale, Joan T. *The Diet Food Finder.* New York: Bowker, 1975. 304 pp. $21.50
An annotated bibliography of more than 200 cookbooks, brochures, and other materials, such as periodicals, selected by means of a consensus of registered dietitians. Recipe indexes list 15,000 recipes from 86 cookbooks with author,

title, and subject indexes together with a bibliography. Recommended by
Journal of Nutrition Education.

Catalog of the Food and Nutrition Information and Educational Materials Center.
   Supplements 1–8, 1974–1978. Beltsville, MD: Food and Nutrition Information and Educ. Materials Ctr., Natl. Agricultural Lib.
Abstracts with detailed subject descriptions for books and journal articles,
acquired by the Food and Nutrition Information and Educational Materials
Center of the Department of Agriculture, relating to human nutrition research and education and food science and food service management. The
center lends books, provides photocopies, answers specific questions, and
offers comprehensive reference and referral services. Since 1979, catalogs are
being published by Oryx Press.

Coble, Yank. "Nutrition References for You and Your Patient." *Journal of the
   Florida Medical Association* 66 (April 1979): 489–491.
Much of the information on nutrition is disseminated by self-acclaimed experts, faddists, and hucksters anxious to sell megavitamins and liquid protein.
The author, a physician, presents selected references on nutrition, food faddism, quackery, physical fitness and nutrition, and obesity. Useful as a guide
to authoritative sources of nutrition information.

Food, Diet and Nutrition. (Subject Bibliography SB-291). See *Subject Bibliography
   Index* in the Government Publications section of Chapter 3.

Index of Nutrition Education Materials. Washington, DC: Nutrition Foundation,
   Office of Education and Public Affairs, 1977. 237 pp. $8.75.
Lists more than 2,000 books, pamphlets, and audiovisual aids available from
over 400 government agencies, trade associations, professional societies, and
health and educational organizations and foundations. There are four major
sections: two of these contain entries for publications and teaching aids according to subject and include readership level, publication information, and
price. There is extensive coverage of most aspects of health in children,
adolescents, the handicapped, and the elderly. Braille and foreign language
materials are included. The third section is by source and contains names and
addresses of major organizational sources of nutrition education materials
and lists items available grouped by topic. The fourth section gives
state offices of nutrition-related agencies together with brief descriptions
of services offered by nutrition information centers in the United States.
Invaluable.

"Nutrition Education and the Spanish-Speaking American: An Annotated
   Bibliography (1961–72)." *Journal of Nutrition Education* 5 (April–June
   1973): 159–179.
Bibliography includes background information for and about Spanish-
speaking groups that may aid in preparing nutrition education messages.

There are three major groupings: nontechnical materials in Spanish or Spanish and English; nontechnical materials in English for Spanish cultural groups; and materials for professional and paraprofessional workers in Spanish or English. Audiovisual materials and games are included.

Nutrition Education Materials. Rosemont, IL: Natl. Dairy Council, 1979. 15 pp.
A catalog of booklets, leaflets, films, filmstrips, slides, transparencies, and other educational materials that provide authentic information about dairy foods and their contributions to nutritional well-being. Topics include coronary heart disease, nutrient composition of food, nutritional deficiencies, obesity and weight reduction, physical fitness, and pregnancy and lactation. Contains lists of regional Dairy Councils from which materials can be ordered.

Nutrition Information Resources for the Whole Family. Berkeley, CA: Natl. Nutrition Educ. Clearinghouse, April 1979. 11 pp.
Purpose of the brochure is to provide a guide to reliable nutrition information. Resources listed include individuals, societies, journals, basic references, and selected current books. Guidelines for judging information are also given. Book reviews are drawn from the *Journal of Nutrition Education.* Provides a listing of recommended periodicals and sources of pamphlet materials with addresses. Bibliographies available from the clearinghouse include *Infant Nutrition and Feeding* (December 1976), *Pregnancy and Nutrition* (December 1978), and *Aging and Nutrition* (May 1978).

Nutrition References and Book Reviews. Chicago: Chicago Nutrition Assn., 1975. 53 pp. $2.
An explosive growth can be observed in the number of nutrition books published. Librarians called upon to advise on the choice of reading matter for the public are offered a list of publications with critical reviews prepared by qualified nutritionists. Most of the reviews have appeared in professional journals. Four lists are supplied: recommended; recommended for special purposes; recommended only with reservations; not recommended. Titles not recommended include *Dr. Atkins' Diet Revolution* and Stillman's *The Doctor's Quick Weight Loss Diet.*

A Selected Bibliography on Diet, Nutrition, and Diet Therapy. (CHIPS Bibliography No. 1). See *Selected Bibliographies* in the General Materials section of Chapter 3.

Wanzek, Carol S., and Lindren, Martha J. *Publications List 1977.* Chicago: Chicago Nutrition Assn. 136 pp.
This annotated bibliography of educational materials on food, nutrition, and related topics is intended for educators, nutritionists, and consumers. More than 400 items from 156 companies are listed by title, subject classification,

and source. The source section contains an annotated bibliography of all publications listed, arranged in alphabetical order by the organization making the publication available. Information on author, publication date, type of publication, cost, suggested age group, subject classification, and other pertinent information is provided. This is an update of *Nutrition References and Book Reviews,* annotated above.

Woods, Ralph. *Government Guides to Health and Nutrition: Compiled with Commentaries.* New York: Pyramid Books, 1977. 127 pp.
This practical bibliography shows how to utilize federal agencies to get the latest information (either free or low-cost) on the entire spectrum of health, nutrition, and safety. Topics covered include pregnancy, childbirth, diets, food additives, diseases, Medicaid, clinics, and contraception.

DRUG ABUSE

Drug Abuse Prevention Films: A Multicultural Film Catalog. Natl. Inst. on Drug Abuse. Rockville, MD: Natl. Clearinghouse for Drug Abuse Information, 1979. DHEW Pubn. No. (ADM) 79-791. 52 pp.
This film catalog (filmography) supplies an annotated list of films that can be used by drug programs, community centers, schools, libraries, and other groups concerned about the primary prevention of drug abuse within five minority groups—Asian/Pacific Islanders, blacks, Mexican-Americans, Puerto Ricans, and Native Americans. Primary prevention films are those that can be used to promote personal and social growth and thereby reduce the physical, social, and emotional problems resulting in or from the use of drugs. Brief descriptions are provided for each film together with an indication of the audience. Also included are a short list of recommended films and other sources of film reviews and evaluations, together with names and addresses of film distributors.

Drug Education. (Subject Bibliography SB-103). See *Subject Bibliography Index* in the Government Publications section of Chapter 3.

Publications Listing of the National Clearinghouse for Drug Abuse Information. Rockville, MD: Natl. Clearinghouse for Drug Abuse Information, June 1979. 7 pp. Updated periodically.
Contains a complete inventory of prevention and education materials, posters, report series, reference series, research issue series, research monograph series, technical papers, and special reports currently available from NCDAI.

A Selected Bibliography on Phencyclidine Hydrocholoride—PCP. (CHIPS Bibliography No. 9). See *Selected Bibliographies* in the General Materials section of Chapter 3.

Where the Drug Films Are: A Guide to Evaluation Services and Distributors. Natl. Inst. on Drug Abuse. Rockville, MD: Natl. Clearinghouse for Drug Abuse Information, 1977. DHEW Pubn. No. (ADM) 77-429. 19 pp.

Attempts to provide a guide to sources of evaluation of the numerous audiovisuals dealing with drug abuse. Lists the major evaluators: Addiction Research Foundation, Iowa Drug Abuse Information Center, Mental Health Materials Center, National Institute on Drug Abuse Pretest Service, National Coordinating Council on Drug Education, the Pyramid Project and its publication *Prevention Resources,* and the Wisconsin Substance Abuse Clearinghouse. Provides also a list of film libraries and state lending agencies from which federally produced materials can be borrowed. Also included is a list of the principal commercial and nonprofit distributors.

HEART DISEASE AND HYPERTENSION

Audiovisual Aids for High Blood Pressure Education. Natl. High Blood Pressure Educ. Program. Bethesda, MD: High Blood Pressure Information Ctr., October 1979. DHEW Pubn. No. (NIH) 80-1663. 195 pp.

This listing is divided into three main sections, which focus on target audiences: public education, patient education, and professional education. Each entry provides the title of the production, any consultants who helped produce it, the producer, the production date, a brief (nonevaluative) content summary, the program's format, the recommended audience, and ordering information (source, order number, cost, and availability). Since many of the listings can be used with more than one kind of audience, they may appear in more than one section. With very few exceptions, audiovisuals have a production date of 1974 or later.

Cardiac Disease: A Selected Bibliography of Print and Audiovisual Materials for the Patient. New York: New York Univ. Medical Ctr., Patient Educ. Ctr., October 1978, 16 pp.

Comprehensive compilation of books with very short annotations of audiovisual materials and pamphlets. Valuable as a selection tool.

Catalog of Audiovisual Aids in Hypertension. Natl. High Blood Pressure Educ. Program. Bethesda, MD: High Blood Pressure Information Ctr., 1975. DHEW Pubn. No. (NIH) 75-719.

A catalog of films, videotapes, cassettes, and slides covering information on hypertension for the general public, patients, and health care professionals. A description of each item in the catalog is included, as well as information on the availability of materials.

Catalog of Audiovisual Aids (Supplement). Natl. High Blood Pressure Educ. Program. Bethesda, MD: High Blood Pressure Information Ctr., 1975. DHEW Pubn. No. (NIH), 76-1055.

Updates the *Catalog of Audiovisual Aids in Hypertension,* described above, with changes, corrections, and additional items. Lists slides, audiotapes, videocassettes for the general public and patient education. Title, author, description of content, recommended use, source, and availability are given for each item listed.

Catalog of Information and Education Materials. Bethesda, MD: Natl. Heart, Lung, and Blood Inst., April 1978. DHEW Pubn. No. (NIH) 78-926. 35 pp.
Lists professional and consumer education materials produced by the National Heart, Lung, and Blood Institute, the National High Blood Pressure Education Program, and the National Sickle Cell Disease Program. A short description is given of each item. Instructions on how to order documents are also supplied. Typical titles include: "High Blood Pressure Facts and Fiction," "If You're Black, Here Are Some Facts You Should Know about High Blood Pressure."

Educational Materials for Hypertensive Patients: A Catalog of Evaluated Publications. Natl. High Blood Pressure Educ. Program. Bethesda, MD: High Blood Pressure Information Ctr., 1977. DHEW Pubn. No. (NIH) 77-1244. 56 pp.
Evaluates 57 pamphlets and booklets on hypertension produced by pharmaceutical manufacturers, universities, and other organizations. Each publication is reviewed in terms of content, technical accuracy, timeliness, concept load, overall effectiveness of presentation, appropriateness for particular target audiences, usage in treatment (initiation of treatment, long-term maintenance, and so forth), and special strengths and weaknesses. Publications reviewed are arranged in four groups: Very Good; Excellent; Good; and Adequate. Subgroupings include Very Easy Reading Level; Easy Reading; Average Reading; Fairly Difficult Reading; and Difficult Reading. Materials are also listed by title and producer/distributor. A most useful publication for the selection of materials for various audiences and purposes.

Publications List Order Form. Natl. High Blood Pressure Educ. Program. Bethesda, MD: High Blood Pressure Information Ctr., June 1979. 4 pp. Updated periodically.
Checklist and order form for pamphlets and booklets issued free by the National High Blood Pressure Education Program.

A Selected Bibliography on Hypertension and Stroke. (CHIPS Bibliography No. 10). See *Selected Bibliographies* in the General Materials section of Chapter 3.

MENTAL HEALTH

Guide to Mental Health Education Materials: A Directory for Mental Health Educators. Natl. Inst. of Mental Health. Rockville, MD: Alcohol, Drug

Abuse, and Mental Health Admin., 1975. DHEW Pubn. No. (ADM) 75-35. 56 pp.

A comprehensive compilation of pamphlets, leaflets, reports, periodicals, bibliographies, films, radio programs, and posters. Topics covered are aging, alcohol, child mental health, community mental health, crime and delinquency, crises, death, depression, drugs, family planning, family relations, halfway houses, health and safety, homosexuality, infants, mental illness, retardation, physical handicaps, racism, recreation, sex, suicide, and therapy. An appendix lists and describes the organizations active in producing mental health education materials.

Mental Health. (Subject Bibliography SB-107). See *Subject Bibliography Index* in the Government Publications section of Chapter 3.

Mental Health Materials Center. *Current Audiovisuals for Mental Health Education.* Chicago: Marquis, 1979. $8.50 (paper).

A comparative guide to more than 700 films, filmstrips, videotapes, and other audiovisuals released between 1974 and 1978. Summaries, evaluations, and comparative ratings designed to aid professionals in the selection of released educational materials. Primary audience, distributor, and purchase or rental costs are specified.

Mental Health Materials Center. *The Selective Guide to Audiovisuals for Mental Health and Family Life Education,* 4th ed. Chicago: Marquis, 1979. 511 pp. $24.50.

Detailed evaluations are supplied to facilitate the selection and effectiveness of more than 400 films, filmstrips, videotapes, and audiocassettes, arranged by subject and cross reference. Each entry includes a summary of content, primary audience, evaluation, and suggestions for use with target audiences, together with full title, running time, color or black and white, producer, date, and ordering information. This publication is updated by *Sneak Previews,* a quarterly publication, from which the next edition of the *Selective Guide* is compiled.

Mental Health Materials Center. *The Selective Guide to Publications for Mental Health and Family Life Education,* 4th ed. Chicago: Marquis, 1979. 912 pp. $34.50 (paper).

Topics covered include marriage and family life, early and middle childhood, adolescence, school mental health, drug abuse, alcoholism, aging, child abuse, suicide and crisis intervention, and death and dying. Provides detailed evaluations, summary of content, and designation of audience level for more than 470 books, pamphlets, and other publications.

Mental Health Media Center. *Film Catalog.* Bethesda, MD: Re-runs Unlimited. Lists films available through mental health audiovisual service contracted to the Mental Health Association. Includes short descriptions and ordering information for sale or rental.

Publications List. Rosslyn, VA: Natl. Assn. for Mental Health, 1978. 23 pp. Updated periodically.
Free and low-cost publications available on a large number of topics, such as civil rights, citizen participation, homosexuality, community mental health centers, depression, and mental illness.

Publications of the National Institute of Mental Health. Rockville, MD: Natl. Clearinghouse for Mental Health Information, June 1979. 4 pp. Updated periodically.
A listing of several hundred publications produced by the National Institute for Mental Health, many of which are designed for the layperson. Typical listings include: "Plain Talk about Feelings of Guilt," "Caring About Kids: Helping the Hyperactive Child." Bulk copies (more than ten) can be ordered from the Superintendent of Documents, U.S. Government Printing Office.

Selected Mental Health Audiovisuals. Natl. Inst. of Mental Health, Rockville, MD: Alcohol, Drug Abuse, and Mental Health Admin., 1975. DHEW Pubn. No. (ADM) 76-259. 223 pp.
Contains abstracts of approximately 2,300 nonprint materials arranged by topics such as aging, child mental health, depression, mental retardation, schizophrenia, and treatment. Includes price, format, and ordering information for each item.

WOMEN'S HEALTH

See also Birth Control and Family Planning, this chapter.

Childbirth Education: Sources of Audiovisual Aids. Chicago: Amer. College of Obstetricians and Gynecologists, Resource Center, 1978. 10 pp.
Lists audiovisuals in a variety of formats available from some 78 producers and distributors.

Cowan, Belita. *Women's Health Care: Resources, Writings, Bibliographies.* Washington, DC: Natl. Women's Health Network, 1978. 57 pp. $4.
This is a compilation of book annotations, journal articles, booklets, pamphlets, audiovisuals, and other information materials selected to reflect the point of view of the women's health movement. The listings are arranged according to major topics: women and the health care system; women's rights as patients; gynecological self-help; sterilization abuse; women and drugs; childbirth; pregnancy; birth control; synthetic estrogens; DES and cancer; sexuality; aging; and rape. Each section has a short introductory explanation.

Recommended magazines and films are also provided together with a directory of organizations. Comprehensive and thought provoking.

Educational Materials for Obstetrics and Gynecology. Chicago: Amer. College of
   Obstetricians and Gynecologists, Resource Center. 184 pp. $5.
Includes extensive listings for teaching aids, many with reviews.

Health Resource Guides. Washington, DC: Natl. Women's Health Network,
   1980. $3 each; $20 for set of nine.
A series of nine books on the following subjects:

   No. 1. *Breast Cancer.* 69 pp.
   No. 2. *Hysterectomy.* 67 pp.
   No. 3. *Menopause.* 57 pp.
   No. 4. *Maternal Health and Childbirth.* 85 pp.
   No. 5. *Birth Control.* 108 pp.
   No. 6. *DES* (Diethylstilbestrol). 49 pp.
   No. 7. *Self-Help.* 62 pp.
   No. 8. *Abortion.* 85 pp.
   No. 9. *Sterilization.* 74 pp.

Each guide contains a discussion of the major issues; extracts from relevant
medical literature; governmental regulations; legal decisions; bibliography
and references; audiovisual materials; resource groups; resource people; and
other sources of information. Extensive lists of books, periodicals, newsletters,
and newspapers are provided on each topic. These include both professional
and lay publications. The guides are highly informative and bring together a
vast compendium of useful information. The objective of this series is to
supply information to women to enable them to be more active participants in
the protection and promotion of their own health.

Ruzek, Sheryl K. *Women and Health Care: A Bibliography with Selected Annotations.* Evanston, IL: Northwestern Univ., Program on Women, 1976. 75 pp.
   $3.50.
A collection of a wide variety of information material relevant to women and
health care. Part I provides annotations of material covering the broad range
of basic issues in women's health care while Part II describes material available
on health care issues of particular interest to women—gynecological exams,
contraception, abortion, pregnancy and childbirth, menstruation, menopause, surgery, drugs, and experimentation. Other sections cover sexuality
and mental health, health collectives, free clinics, self-help groups and
women's health directories, lay referral systems, and communication networks. Both lay and professional literature are covered. This is essentially an
academically oriented bibliography and is less informative to peruse than the
Cowan work *(Women's Health Care)* listed above.

A Selected Bibliography on Prenatal, Postnatal, and Infant Care. (CHIPS Bibliography No. 3). *A Selected Bibliography of Women's Health Care.* (CHIPS Bibliography No. 7). See *Selected Bibliographies* in the General Materials section of Chapter 3.

Chapter 5

Magazines, Journals, and Newsletters

The publications listed in this chapter are popular magazines, journals, and newsletters that endeavor to bring health-related information to the lay public. They share the common purpose of presenting interesting and comprehensible information calculated to improve health, engender more healthy life-styles, and produce more knowledgeable consumers of health care services. Several of the publications listed are oriented toward professionals who provide consumer health information to the layperson. Entries provide subscription address, frequency, and price.

America's Health. (World Wide Medical Pr., 641 Lexington Ave., New York, NY 10022) Qtrly. Free.
This is a scientifically oriented publication on medicine and health for the general public. The Spring 1979 issue, volume 1, no. 4, contains articles on emergency services, tooth implants, acne, the pituitary gland, how babies learn to love, the limits of national health insurance (guest editorial by Dr. Ted Cooper) and "Is America in the Grip of a Cancer Epidemic?" by Dr. Elizabeth Whelan. The articles are authoritative and well written but require concentrated reading. Very suitable for high school assignments.

Consumer Reports. (Consumers Union, Box 1000, Orangeburg, NY 10462) Monthly. $12/yr.
A variety of health-related subjects has come under the scrutiny of *Consumer Reports.* Recent issues have analyzed blood pressure kits, cutting the risk of childbirth after 35, mistreatment of arthritis, safety of hair dyes, cancer insurance, prescription drugs, self-administered pregnancy tests, nutrition, breast feeding, hay fever, and medical malpractice. An excellent source of authoritative information with helpful suggestions for further study.

Current Health. (Curriculum Innovations, Box 310, Highwood, IL 60040)
    Monthly, September–May. $3.95/yr.
An excellent magazine designed for a high school audience. Information is
presented in a tutorial manner, with good illustrations and cartoons. As a
supplement to school health education, it presents highly useful information
on basic topics such as nutrition, drugs, and the environment. Includes
quizzes, answers to questions, and a section on health careers. Recommended
for teenagers.

Employee Health and Fitness. (American Health Consultants, 67 Peachtree Pk.
    Dr. N.E., Atlanta, GA 30309) Monthly. $87/yr.
A new publication concerned with health promotion in an industrial context.
The content covers the cost-effectiveness of employee programs, stress on the
job, running and exercise, incentives to stop smoking, hypertension, screening and control in the work place, employee counseling services for alcohol,
drug, and emotional problems, and health hazard appraisal. Expensive, but of
interest to health promotion personnel, corporate benefits managers, and
those in management concerned with escalating health insurance costs.

Executive Fitness Newsletter. (Rodale Press, 33 E. Minor St., Emmaus, PA 18049)
    Biweekly. $24/yr.
This newsletter contains short articles and stories on running, exercise, and
diet. A more academic presentation than is found in *Prevention* magazine,
from the same publisher.

Executive Health Report. Formerly *Executive Health.* (Executive Health Publica-
    tions, Box 589, Rancho Santa Fe, CA 92067) Monthly. $24/yr.
A publication with a highly prestigious editorial board, consisting of Sir Hans
Krebs, Linus Pauling, Hans Selye, Albert Szent-Gyorgi. Despite the Nobel-
laden board, the content seems focused upon expounding the benefits of
vitamin C, vitamin B_6 (pyridoxine), and related causes.

Family Health. (Portland Pl., Boulder, CO 80302) 10 issues/yr. $12/yr.
The most popular of all the consumer health magazines, with the largest
circulation. The writing is slick, if not simplistic, containing elementary information on a variety of topics such as Caesarean births, diet and nutrition,
health insurance, needless surgery, biofeedback, aging, dental care, dandruff,
and so forth. Although many of the columnists are well qualified, the treatment of most topics is superficial and little guidance is given on information
sources for further exploration.

FDA Consumer. (Superintendent of Documents, Government Printing Office,
    Washington, DC 20402) 10 issues/yr. $12/yr.
This magazine is an official publication of the Food and Drug Administration.
The articles are prepared in most cases by members of the FDA's Public

Affairs staff and have a high standard of accuracy and understandability. The *FDA Consumer* is a primary source of information on food additives, prescription drugs and generic equivalents, food labeling, carcinogenic agents and cancer risks, drug recalls, radiation hazards, medical devices, and related topics that fall under the general jurisdiction of the FDA. Recommended.

The Harvard Medical School Health Letter. (Harvard University Press Building, 79 Garden St., Cambridge, MA 02138) Monthly. $12/yr.
Well written and informative summaries of information prepared by the members of the Harvard Medical School faculty. Topics covered include: diabetes, back sprain, x-ray hazards, sudden infant death syndrome, child restraints in automobiles, first aid for choking, excessive sun exposure, and so on. Authoritative and calculated to appeal to the more sophisticated reader; highly useful for students. Recommended.

Health Activation News. (Health Activation Network, Box 923, Vienna, VA 22180) Qtrly. $7.50/yr.
The newsletter of the Health Activation Network, this publication presents news of the health activation and wellness movement. Information is presented on educational materials and equipment, the Family "Black Bag" Program, and the contents of the ideal medicine chest. Also contains short articles by Keith Sehnert, M.D., and interviews with principals in the wellness movement such as John W. Travers. However, the publication is rather thin in terms of substantive content.

Health Facts. (Center for Medical Consumers and Health Care Information, 237 Thompson St., New York, NY 10012) Bimonthly. $8.50/yr.
A consumer newsletter published bimonthly. Each issue focuses upon a single topic, using the most current medical journals, texts, opinions, and sources. The publication endeavors to produce an informative summary of the best available information on a variety of topics for the purpose of enabling its readers to participate more intelligently in medical decisions. Individual issues are devoted to a detailed analysis of current knowledge in a specific area, such as hypertension, exercise, psychotropic drugs, depression, and the annual physical. Of special value and merit are the issues covering health care choices (acupuncture, homeopathy, naturopathy, osteopathy, and so forth); nonmedical therapies (biofeedback, herbal medicine, meditation, megavitamin therapy, and Shiatsu); three surgeries (risks of unnecessary tonsillectomy and adenoidectomy, hysterectomy, and coronary artery bypass surgery); and nutrition and health. An excellent publication, well written and informative, which can be placed in loose-leaf binders for reference purposes.

The Health Letter. (Communications, Box 326, San Antonio, TX 78292) 24 issues/yr. $19.50/yr.
Clear explanations of common health problems given by Lawrence Lamb, M.D., a syndicated medical columnist. Back issues are available that allow the

accumulation of a loose-leaf file covering a wide variety of popular subjects, such as asthma, female hormones, diverticulosis, obesity, varicose veins, and gall bladder disease. Similar to *Health Facts,* but contains more technical detail.

Health/PAC Bulletin. (Human Sciences Pr., 72 Fifth Ave., New York, NY 10011) Bimonthly, $14/yr. individuals; $28/yr. insts.
An antiestablishment publication designed to demystify medicine and to topple the image of the omnipotent physician. Contains information on a variety of subjects, such as diseases, treatment, free clinics, and so forth.

Holistic Health Review. (Human Sciences Pr., 72 Fifth Ave., New York, NY 10011) Qtrly. $15/yr. individuals; $35/yr. insts.
This publication is sponsored by the Holistic Organizing Committee and the Berkeley Holistic Health Center. The publication contains articles reflecting the holistic point of view, reviews of recent holistic health conferences, interviews with persons prominent in holistic health, and book reviews. The Spring 1979 issue contains a Holistic Health Reading Guide. Contributing editors include Tom Ferguson, M.D., Dr. Kenneth Pelletier, C. Norman Shealy, M.D., and David Sobel, M.D.

Life and Health. (Review & Herald Publishing Assn., 6856 Eastern Ave. N.W., Washington, DC 20012) Monthly. $11.95/yr.
This magazine presents significant, interesting, health-related information calculated to motivate readers to adopt and practice sound principles of healthy living. The emphasis is on prevention rather than treatment. Contains good, interesting articles on alcoholism, nutrition, adolescence, bed-wetting, cancer, and other topics. Clear and readable presentations. Publication is affiliated with the Health Department of the General Conference of the Seventh Day Adventists. Recommended.

The Medical Letter on Drugs and Therapeutics. (Medical Letter, 56 Harrison St., New Rochelle, NY 10801) 24 issues/yr. $22.50/yr.
This is an authoritative advisory newsletter for physicians. Summary information is presented on one key topic per issue. Among the topics covered are: hypoglycemics, treatment of lice, rabies vaccine, tennis elbow, coffee and cardiovascular disease, treatment of urinary tract infections, traveler's diarrhea, drugs for parkinsonism, toxic reactions to plant products sold in health food stores, and adverse interactions of drugs. An excellent source of information on a wide variety of medical problems, drugs, and treatments understandable by most laypersons. Highly recommended.

Medical Self-Care: Access to Medical Tools. (Box 717, Inverness, CA 94937) Qtrly. $15/yr.
The editor of this publication is a graduate of Yale Medical School, Tom Ferguson, M.D. Typical topics covered in this unconventional magazine are

how to be your own doctor (sometimes); your health and how to manage it; Rx running; teaching medicine to kids; menopause; self-care and alternative medicine; doing your own vaginal exam; dealing with stress; a field guide to men's reproductive health. Of particular value are excellent book reviews—several dozen in each issue. Also featured are nontraditional views on medical education. A warm, sensitive, and provocative publication, rich in ideas and sources of further information. Highly recommended.

The Nation's Health. (Amer. Public Health Assn., 1015 15th St. N.W., Washington, DC 20005) Monthly. $5/yr.
This is the official newspaper of the American Public Health Association, which is an excellent and valuable source of information relating to federal health legislation, health planning, mental health services, funding priorities, new health care programs, and so forth. Summarizes current appropriations and legislative highlights. Also contains news of meetings, book announcements, and a Washington report. Summarizes information not readily available elsewhere.

Physician's Patient Education Newsletter. (Univ. of Alabama, 930 S. 20th St., Birmingham, AL 35294) Bimonthly. $10/yr. individuals; $18/yr. insts.
This publication is supported in part by a grant from the Andrew J. Mellon Foundation Health Alliance Program. Although primarily designed for health professionals, it has a number of articles on how to establish patient education programs in a variety of settings, the use of mass media for health promotion, and needs assessments in patient education programs. Contains short, informative, and readable comments on patient education objectives and methodology.

Prevention: The Magazine for Better Health. (Rodale Press, 33 E. Minor St., Emmaus, PA 18049) Monthly. $10/yr.
This magazine relates the causes and symptoms of most health problems to nutrition, diet, and life-style. Consequently, yogurt, vitamin C, vitamin E, bran, brewer's yeast, exercise, sunshine, trace minerals, and so forth are recommended to prevent and treat a variety of ailments ranging from cancer and hypertension to the common cold. By way of example, l-tryptophan is preferred over Dalmane for the treatment of insomnia, and the high fiber diet is considered the best protection against colorectal cancer. The publication is highly readable and interesting. However, its scientific merit is cast into doubt by the mass of advertisements for vitamins, minerals, and food supplements that crowd the content.

PROmoting HEALTH. (Center for Health Promotion, Amer. Hospital Assn., 840 N. Lake Shore Dr., Chicago, IL 60611) Bimonthly. $24/yr.
A new publication from the Center for Health Promotion of the American Hospital Association, this newsletter is primarily designed for health professionals concerned with patient education, community health, and employee

health programs. It also contains material of interest to the public: reviews of latest books and periodicals, descriptions of health promotion resources, and news of innovative physical fitness programs.

Taking Care. (Center for Consumer Health Education, 380 West Maple Ave., Vienna, VA 22180). Monthly. $15/yr.

A clearly written and useful newsletter covering a wide variety of topics. The principal emphasis in on wellness, physical fitness, exercise and preventive medicine. The publication spells out how to stay healthy and what to do about common problems such as ear pain, fever, bee stings, colds and flu, hypertension and heart stroke. Contains contributions by Donald M. Vickery, M.D., author of *Take Care of Yourself: A Consumer's Guide to Medical Care* and president of the Center for Consumer Health Education. Excellent, inexpensive guide to effective decision making. Highly recommended.

Chapter 6

Professional Literature

Most of the health information needs of the American public can be satisfied by popular publications especially designed for lay usage. Sometimes, however, more detailed and specific information is required that transcends simple, generalized explanation. In these cases, it is necessary to locate authoritative and accurate information. Recourse must be made to the professional literature of medicine. If, for example, information is needed on the moving research frontier of new treatment modalities, specific drugs, or surgical procedures, a search of the technical literature will be required. It is also required where a topic may not have been described to date in popular books or pamphlets.

To satisfy these more complex information requirements, consumer health collections can be supplemented by a small number of authoritative, technical publications, which can be highly useful in responding to specialized information needs. But what are the "best" reference publications in the health sciences? A number of information specialists have produced core lists of recommended textbooks and reference sources covering the broad spectrum of basic and clinical sciences. However, these lists were created not for lay use, but rather for collection development for professional library use. The techniques used for identifying the "best" publications include citation analysis, journal usage counts, surveys, and so forth.

For the purpose of selecting a small number of recommended professional publications appropriate to serve as a back-up to popular consumer health collections, seven core lists are available. These are:

1. Allyn, R. A. "A Library for Internists III: Recommended by the American College of Physicians." *Annals of Internal Medicine* 90 (March 1979): 446–477.
2. Bell, J. A. "The Academic Health Sciences Library and Serials Selection." *Bulletin of the Medical Library Association* 62 (July 1974): 281–290.

3. Brandon, A. N. "Selected List of Books and Journals for the Small Medical Library." *Bulletin of the Medical Library Association* 65 (April 1977): 191–215.
4. Cormier, J. "Medical Texts for Public Libraries." *Library Journal* 103 (October 15, 1978): 2051.
5. Moll, W. "Basic Journal List for Small Hospital Libraries." *Bulletin of the Medical Library Association* 57 (July 1969): 267–271.
6. Natl. Lib. of Medicine. "List of 100 Titles for *Abridged Index Medicus.*" January 1980.
7. Stearns, Norman, and Ratcliff, Wendy. "An Integrated Health Science Core Library for Physicians, Nurses, and Allied Health Practitioners in Community Hospitals." *New England Journal of Medicine* 283 (December 31, 1970): 1489–1498.

The principal conclusion that emerges from an examination of these lists is the large amount of agreement on titles. Moreover, it is evident that the criteria for selecting technical publications for lay usage must necessarily be the same as those utilized for professional usage. In both cases, one must take into account factors such as technical accuracy, balance, validity, currency, clarity, and comprehensiveness. Therefore, it is possible to lean heavily upon the judgments reflected in the core lists noted above for the identification of authoritative texts useful as references in relation to complex lay health information requests.

Based upon an examination both of these lists and of the actual publications, a number of monographs, journals, and indexes have been identified for use in consumer health collections. An attempt has been made to cover the total field of medicine and surgery, including specialties. Emphasis has been placed upon clinical books rather than those in the basic sciences. In each instance, the most comprehensive and authoritative works have been selected. The books, journals, and indexes considered as basic to any collection are marked by an asterisk. These include twelve basic books with a total list cost of $396.70; four journals with a total annual cost of $124; and one index with a total annual cost of $24. This may be considered a modest investment.

BOOKS

General Reference

Dorland's Medical Dictionary, 25th ed. Philadelphia: Saunders, 1974. $24.50.
*Dreisbach, Robert M. *Handbook of Poisoning: Prevention, Diagnosis and Treatment*, 10th ed. Los Altos, CA: Lange, 1978. $9.
*Kruzas, Anthony. *Medical and Health Information Directory*. Detroit: Gale, 1980. $78.
Merck Manual of Diagnosis and Therapy. 13th ed. Rahway, NJ: Merck, 1977. $9.95.
Physicians' Desk Reference, 33rd ed. Oradell, NJ: Medical Economics, 1979. $14.25.

Medical Specialties

Cardiology

*Hurst, John Willis. *The Heart: Arteries and Veins,* 4th ed. New York: McGraw-Hill, 1978. 2 vols. $65.

Dermatology

Fitzpatrick, Thomas B., ed. *Dermatology in General Medicine,* 2nd ed. New York: McGraw-Hill, 1979. $85.

Endocrinology

American Diabetes Association, Committee on Professional Education *Diabetes Mellitus,* 4th ed. Karl E. Sussman and Robert J. Metz, eds. New York: Amer. Diabetes Assn., 1975. $6.50.
Williams, Robert H. *Textbook of Endocrinology,* 5th ed. Philadelphia: Saunders, 1974. $32.50.

Gastroenterology

Sleinsenger, Marvin H., and Fordtran, John S. *Gastrointestinal Disease: Pathophysiology, Diagnosis, Management,* 2nd ed. Philadelphia: Saunders, 1978. 2 vols. $65.

Geriatrics

Reichel, William, ed. *Clinical Aspects of Aging: A Comprehensive Text.* Prepared under the direction of the Amer. Geriatric Society. Baltimore, MD: Williams & Wilkins, 1978. $38.50.

Hematology

Williams, William J. and others. *Hematology,* 2nd ed. New York: McGraw-Hill, 1977. $48.

Human Sexuality

Kaplan, Helen Singer. *The New Sex Therapy: Active Treatment of Sexual Dysfunction.* New York: Brunner-Mazel, 1974. 544 pp. $17.50.

Infectious Diseases

Top, F. H., and Wehrle, P. F., eds. *Communicable and Infectious Diseases.* St. Louis, MO: Mosby, 1976. $48.50.

Internal Medicine

Isselbacher, K. J., ed. *Harrison's Principles of Internal Medicine,* 9th ed. New York: McGraw-Hill, 1980. 2 vols. $55.
*Krupp, Marcus A., and Chatton, Milton J. *Current Medical Diagnosis and Treatment.* Los Altos, CA: Lange, 1979. $19. Rev. annually.

Rakel, Robert, and Conn, Howard F. *Family Practice,* 2nd ed. Philadelphia: Saunders, 1979. $38.50.

Nephrology

Brenner, B. M., and Rector, F. C. *The Kidney.* Philadelphia: Saunders, 1976. 2 vols. $95.

Nutrition

Goodhart, Robert S., and Shils, Maurice E., eds. *Modern Nutrition in Health and Disease: Dietotherapy,* 6th ed. Philadelphia: Lea & Febiger, 1980. $47.50.

Obstetrics and Gynecology

*Danforth, David N., ed. *Obstetrics and Gynecology,* 3rd ed. New York: Harper, 1977. $45.

Oncology

*Del Ragato, Juan, and Spjut, Harlan. *Ackerman and Del Ragato's Cancer: Diagnosis, Treatment, and Prognosis,* 5th ed. St. Louis, MO: Mosby, 1977. $67.50.

Ophthalmology

Newell, Frank W. *Ophthalmology: Principles and Concepts,* 4th ed. St. Louis, MO: Mosby, 1978. $29.50.

Orthopedics

Brashear, Robert H., and Raney, Richard Beverly. *Shand's Handbook of Orthopedic Surgery,* 9th ed. St. Louis, MO: Mosby, 1978. $23.50.

Pediatrics

*Silver, Henry K., and others. *Handbook of Pediatrics,* 13th ed. Los Altos, CA: Lange, 1980. $9.50.

Pharmacology

*Goodman, L. S., and Gilman, A., eds. *The Pharmacological Basis of Therapeutics,* 5th ed. New York: Macmillan, 1975. $36.

Psychiatry

Freeman, Alfred M., and others. *Comprehensive Textbook of Psychiatry,* 2nd ed. Baltimore, MD: Williams & Wilkins, 1975. 2 vols. $100.

Rheumatology

McCarty, Daniel J., and others, eds. *Arthritis and Allied Conditions: A Textbook of Rheumatology,* 9th ed. Philadelphia: Lea & Febiger, 1979. $55.

Surgery

*Dunphy, J. E., and Way, L. W. *Current Surgical Diagnosis and Treatment,* 4th ed. Los Altos, CA: Lange, 1979. $19.

Sabiston, David G., ed. *Davis-Christopher Textbook of Surgery,* 11th ed. Philadelphia: Saunders, 1977. 2 vols. $53.

Urology

Smith, Donald R. *General Urology,* 9th ed. Los Altos, CA: Lange, 1978. $14.50.

JOURNALS

Hospitals. Variant title: *Journal of the American Hospital Association.* (American Hospital Association, 840 N. Lake Shore Dr., Chicago, IL 60611) Semimonthly, $30/yr.

JAMA: The Journal of the American Medical Association. (American Medical Association, 535 N. Dearborn St., Chicago, IL 60610) Weekly. $36/yr.

Lancet, North Amer. Ed. (Little, Brown, 34 Beacon St., Boston, MA 02106) Weekly. $45/yr.

Medical World News. (McGraw-Hill, 1221 Ave. of the Americas, New York, NY 10020) 26 issues/yr. $28/yr.

New England Journal of Medicine. (Massachusetts Medical Society, 10 Shattuck St., Boston, MA 02115) Weekly. $30/yr.

Nursing 80. (Box 3744, One Health Rd., Marion, OH 43302) Monthly. $18 yr.

INDEXES

Abridged Index Medicus. (Superintendent of Documents, Government Printing Office, Washington, DC 20402) Monthly. $24.

Hospital Literature Index. (American Hospital Association, 840 N. Lake Shore Dr., Chicago, IL 60611) Qtrly. $60.

Chapter 7

Federal Health Information Clearinghouses

A number of clearinghouses exist to provide health information services to the public. A clearinghouse may be defined as an organization whose primary purpose is to provide information products and materials about current knowledge, programs, services, and sources of further assistance in a prescribed subject area. Its key function is linkage or brokerage between individuals and organizations seeking assistance and the resources that fulfill their requests. Typical functions performed by clearinghouses are locating, acquiring, screening, abstracting, and indexing publications; conducting information searches; and distributing copies of documents in the form of articles, booklets, pamphlets, brochures, bibliographies, and research syntheses.

Despite problems with respect to relevance and quality of materials, duplication and gaps in service, the absence of effective announcement mechanisms, the impersonal style of disseminating documents, the lack of coordination and fragmented coverage, the federal health information clearinghouses can be a most useful resource for identifying and acquiring materials.

The principal health information clearinghouses are:

Arthritis Information Clearinghouse, Box 34427, Bethesda, MD 20034.
The Arthritis Information Clearinghouse is a service of the National Institute of Arthritis, Metabolism, and Digestive Diseases, designed to help professionals and educators in their interaction with patients, their families, and the public. The clearinghouse provides a single access point for identifying print and nonprint educational materials concerned with arthritis and related musculoskeletal diseases.

The clearinghouse collects, organizes, and disseminates information on arthritic conditions. It reviews, abstracts, indexes, and analyzes bibliographic and audiovisual materials and maintains a retrievable data base.

85

The clearinghouse distributes the Arthritis Information Clearinghouse *Bulletin* to announce new programs and to highlight holdings. It compiles and distributes bibliographies and fact sheets on topics of interest to its users and maintains contact with voluntary and professional organizations, other health-related clearinghouses, government agencies, and various information resources. It refers information requests from patients to the Arthritis Foundation or other appropriate agencies. The *Bulletin* is a good source of patient education on materials including books, pamphlets, audiovisuals, and other materials. Popular articles on arthritis are also noted.

A number of bibliographies and catalogs of patient education materials are available on specialized topics, such as juvenile rheumatoid arthritis, nutrition and arthritis, and public information resources on arthritic conditions. These bibliographies are enumerated in the Arthritis section of Chapter 4.

Also available is a series of reference sheets on *Patient Education Programs in Arthritis, Patient Education References on Nutrition and Arthritis,* and on *Osteoarthritis.* Literature searches are conducted, on request, of the clearinghouse data base and other bibliographic sources concerning patient, public, or professional education about arthritis. An Arthritis Information Clearinghouse *Thesaurus* was published in December 1979.

Cancer Information Clearinghouse, Office of Cancer Communications, National Cancer Institute, 7910 Woodmont Ave., Suite 1320, Bethesda, MD 20014.

The Cancer Information Clearinghouse is a service of the National Cancer Institute's Office of Cancer Communications. The clearinghouse collects and disseminates information on materials, programs, and resources related to public, patient, and professional education. Documents collected are abstracted, indexed, and stored. Bibliographic information is made available upon request and by active dissemination.

The clearinghouse offers a variety of services to organizations involved in cancer education. These services include:

1. Routine information searches—individually tailored searches of the clearinghouse files and other data bases
2. Referral services—referral to sources of educational materials and services
3. Topical bibliographies—lists of educational materials on specific subjects
4. Special information packages—packets of materials available on a specific topic
5. Current awareness services—bulletins alerting cancer-concerned organizations to new publications, programs, services, data bases, and audiovisual materials
6. Selective dissemination of information—distribution of pertinent information to organizations working on specific topics
7. Monthly accessions list—covering print and nonprint materials

Of particular value are the specialized bibliographies on topics such as *Asbestos and Health, Breast Cancer, Cancer Information in the Workplace,* and others. All these bibliographies are described in the Cancer section of Chapter 4.

The clearinghouse also distributes the *What You Need to Know about Cancer Series* (1979) of pamphlets on topics such as bladder, bone, breast, colon, and rectum cancers, childhood leukemia, and multiple myeloma. Booklets are also available on *Drugs vs. Cancer, Chemotherapy and You, What You Can Do to Protect Yourself Against Cancer, Breast Self-Examination,* and other subjects. A complete list is given in the Pamphlets section of Chapter 13.

The Cancer Information Service responds to information requests made by the public. An 800 (toll-free) number is covered by a staff person, who will answer questions such as: "What does a Pap smear tell?" or "My mother died of breast cancer. Does that increase my risk of getting breast cancer?" Relevant pamphlets will be mailed to those requesting information, or other appropriate pamphlet resources, such as those of the American Cancer Society and the Leukemia Society of America, will be recommended. Call Directory Assistance 800-555-1212 for the specific number for the state from which the request originates.

Clearinghouse on the Handicapped, Office for Handicapped Individuals, 200 Independence Ave. S.W., Washington, DC 20201.
The clearinghouse serves handicapped individuals by referring inquiries to appropriate information sources, including other government agencies and voluntary organizations. A number of publications are available, including a *Pocket Guide to Federal Help for the Disabled Person* and *Selected Federal Publications Concerning the Handicapped.* The clearinghouse also recently issued a 236-page *Directory of National Information Sources on Handicapping Conditions and Related Services.* In the directory, "handicapped" is interpreted broadly to include physical disorders and disabilities and emotional problems. Consequently, coverage includes cancer, heart disease, cystic fibrosis, Down's syndrome, epilepsy, leukemia, alcoholism, spinal cord injury, and a wide variety of health-related topics. Descriptions are provided of relevant advocacy, consumer, and voluntary health organizations; federal clearinghouses; database vendors; federal government organizations other than information units; professional and trade organizations; and service organizations. A valuable and informative listing. When ordering, request DHEW Pubn. No. (OHDS) 80-22007.

Consumer Information Center, Pueblo, CO 81009.
The center was established by presidential order in 1970 to encourage federal agencies to develop and release useful consumer information and to increase public awareness of this information. Consequently, the Consumer Information Center distributes federal consumer publications and advertises their availability in the mass media. The center publishes quarterly the *Consumer Information Catalog,* a listing of more than 200 selected federal consumer

publications on a variety of topics such as automobiles, gardening, housing, and home maintenance. Health-related topics are prominently represented. The catalog is further described in the Government Publications section of Chapter 3. The center is an agency of the General Services Administration.

High Blood Pressure Information Center, National Heart, Lung and Blood
    Institute, 120/80 National Institutes of Health, Bethesda, MD 20014.
The High Blood Pressure Information Center (HBPIC) acquires, indexes, maintains, and disseminates all types of data in the area of high blood pressure (hypertension). It provides reference and referral services; publishes a bimonthly newsletter; distributes publications and pamphlets produced by the center or other agencies (selected titles are annotated in the Pamphlets section of Chapter 12); supplies current awareness notices for a variety of subjects related to high blood pressure; and coordinates the activities of other organizations involved in high blood pressure control. It is part of the National High Blood Pressure Education Program (NHBPEP), which is dedicated to educating the public about the dangers of and treatment for high blood pressure.

In responding to public inquiries, the information center uses publications and prepared packets of reprints and resource materials on current topics; conducts special searches to provide access to the information center data base as well as resources of other libraries and information clearinghouses; consults with appropriate specialists; and provides referral to appropriate sources for additional information or assistance. Technical assistance from the community development service of the national program may also be requested through the information center for program planning or workshop development.

Informational materials produced and distributed by the information center include a series of timely literature searches (in cooperation with the National Library of Medicine) on topics of current interest in hypertension; a series of special information bulletins for key professional groups involved in hypertension control (pharmacists, dentists, and so forth); and a regular *Information Memorandum,* which features ongoing projects and activities, as well as new materials available, from national, state, and local groups involved in hypertension control activities. The center also distributes the *Catalog of Audiovisual Aids in Hypertension* and *Educational Materials for Hypertensive Patients: A Catalog of Evaluated Publications,* which are described in detail in the Heart Disease and Hypertension section of Chapter 4.

The information center also acts as the publishing arm of the national program for other educational materials developed by program staff and participants and maintains an extensive inventory of consumer and professional educational materials, which it distributes in quantity, free of charge, to local hypertension programs and health care providers upon request. The national program's objective in distributing free educational materials is to facilitate development of comprehensive high blood pressure control programs in communities throughout the nation.

National Clearinghouse for Alcohol Information, 1776 E. Jefferson St., Rockville, MD 20852. (Mailing Address: Box 2345, Rockville, MD 20852).
Established as a service of the National Institute on Alcohol Abuse and Alcoholism (NIAAA) for the purpose of making widely available current knowledge on alcohol-related subjects, the clearinghouse makes available pamphlets and directories on a variety of topics. It also offers a number of bibliographic and current awareness services:

1. *Grouped Interest Guides* provide bibliographic references and abstracts on recent publications in 15 topical areas, such as *Alcohol, Accidents and Highway Safety; Alcohol and Mental Health;* and *Drugs and Alcohol.* A full list of current titles appears in the Alcoholism section of Chapter 4.
2. *Individualized Interest Cards* is a monthly SDI (selective dissemination of information) service that offers continuing bibliographic updates in over 140 special interest areas covering both printed and audiovisual materials. Abstract slips provide complete bibliographic references and the source from which documents or audiovisuals can be ordered. The 140 special interest areas are arranged in 16 major groups, such as psychological studies, psychiatry; physiology and biochemistry; and mental health.
3. *The NIAAA Information and Features Service* is a news publication that presents articles on trends, opinions, and programs and spotlights topics of special interest to those interested in alcoholism.

National Clearinghouse for Drug Abuse Information, 5600 Fishers La., Rockville, MD 20857. (Mailing Address: Box 1635, Rockville, MD 20857).
The clearinghouse is a component of the National Institute on Drug Abuse. It has an extensive publication program producing both research studies and prevention and education materials for popular usage. Among the popular publications are a series on *Drug Abuse Facts* and booklets such as *Can Drug Abuse Be Prevented in the Black Community?* and *Growing Up in America: A Background to Contemporary Drug Abuse.* These and other titles are listed in the Pamphlets section of Chapter 16. The clearinghouse also makes available a number of bibliographies on the subject of drug abuse and catalogs of drug abuse prevention audiovisuals, which are described in the Drug Abuse section of Chapter 4.

National Clearinghouse for Family Planning Information, 6110 Executive Blvd. Suite 250, Rockville, MD 20852. (Mailing Address: Box 2225, Rockville, MD 20852).
The clearinghouse was established in July 1976 to collect and disseminate information on family planning and related topics. It provides the 5,000 federally funded family planning clinics with a centralized source for information about pamphlets, films, books, and other teaching aids that are available for patients, family planning workers, educators, and consumers. Patient and professional education materials are acquired and announced in areas such as contraception, teenage pregnancy and parenthood, human sexuality,

reproductive health, sex education, menstruation and menopause, steriliza-tion, infertility, abortion, venereal disease, and reproductive tract infections. The principal products and services are:

1. *Catalog of Family Planning Materials* and the September 1979 *Supple-ment* (annotated in the Birth Control and Family Planning section of Chapter 4).
2. Computer-produced bibliographies on a variety of topics, such as con-traceptive methods, infertility, oral contraceptives, and common repro-ductive tract infections.
3. Fact sheets on topics such as menopause, sterilization, and common reproductive tract infections.
4. *Health Education Bulletin* describing health education programs on a number of family planning topics such as programs for teenagers and school children. The monthly issues cover topics such as informed consent, pills, and sexually transmitted infections. Valuable.
5. *Information Services Bulletin,* an updating, alerting service that lists new printed and audiovisual materials for patient education. Short descrip-tive annotations are supplied, together with ordering information. High-lights new clearinghouse acquisitions. Highly valuable as an announce-ment mechanism and for locating materials.
6. Pamphlets and self-instructional booklets on family planning, steriliza-tion (male and female), contraception, and related topics. Further in-formation is provided in the Pamphlets section of Chapter 17.

National Clearinghouse for Mental Health Information, National Institute of Mental Health, 5600 Fishers La., Rockville, MD 20857.
The National Clearinghouse for Mental Health Information is the national center for the collection, storage, retrieval, and dissemination of scientific information in the area of mental health. It was established in 1963 in re-sponse to an overwhelming demand for a centralized resource to provide mental health information.

The clearinghouse has the following functions: acquiring and abstracting the world's mental health literature; collecting scientific, technical, and other information on mental illness and health from the staff and operating compo-nents of the National Institute of Mental Health (NIMH) and from sources outside the institute; classifying, storing, and retrieving information for dis-semination to the mental health community, private and lay organizations, and other components of NIMH; preparing special scientific publications; answering general inquiries from the public; and operating the mental health library.

The clearinghouse makes available to the general public a fairly large selection of publications designed for the lay public. Typical titles are *Citizen's Guide to the Community Mental Health Centers Amendments; Consumer's Guide to Mental Health Services; and Plain Talk about Stress.* Other titles are listed in the Pamphlets section of Chapter 15. *Publications of the National Institute of Mental Health,* annotated in the Mental Health section of Chapter 4, is also available from the clearinghouse.

National Clearinghouse for Smoking and Health, Office on Smoking and Health, 5600 Fishers La., Rockville, MD 20857.

The clearinghouse's Technical Information Center (TIC) collects, organizes, and disseminates the world's literature and special reports on smoking and its effects on health, including technical and general information.

Major resources of the center include an inquiry and reference service, which responds to written or phone inquiries on smoking and health. Persons may also visit the center from 8:30 A.M. to 5:00 P.M. weekdays. The center also conducts computer searches of over 26,000 hard copy files of research information from around the world. All items processed by TIC since 1970 are in a computerized data base. Users may request printouts on specific research topics by submitting Search Request Forms, available from the address above.

Among the center's publications are:

1. *Smoking and Health Bulletin,* which documents, abstracts, and indexes the latest additions to the TIC system. Issued eight times per year, it is available for free subscription. Some photocopies of articles listed in the *Bulletin* are available if the requester is unable to obtain them elsewhere.
2. *Bibliography on Smoking and Health,* an annual cumulative publication of the year's *Bulletins,* indexed by author and subject.
3. *The Health Consequences of Smoking,* HHS's annual report to Congress, which reviews the latest in research developments.
4. *Directory of Ongoing Research in Smoking and Health,* a biannual summary of worldwide current research, published in even-numbered years.
5. *State Legislation on Smoking and Health,* an annual summary and listing of states' bills and laws relevant to all aspects of smoking and tobacco commerce.

National Clearinghouse on Aging, Administration on Aging, 330 Independence Ave. S.W., Washington, DC 20201.

Provides information on programs for the aging and encourages establishment of area services to assist the elderly. The clearinghouse maintains a data base; collects, analyzes, and disseminates information; and publishes the periodical *Aging* (subscription available from the Superintendent of Documents). Other clearinghouse publications are described in the Pamphlets section of Chapter 11.

National Diabetes Information Clearinghouse, 805 15 Street N.W., Suite 500, Washington, DC 20005.

The National Diabetes Information Clearinghouse was established in 1978 by the National Institute of Arthritis, Metabolism, and Digestive Diseases to collect, organize, and disseminate information about diabetes programs and materials. In this endeavor, it serves diabetes research and training centers, local, state, and national diabetes organizations, hospitals, professional groups, state departments of health, and various federal agencies.

The clearinghouse is a joint venture with its users, functioning as the central point for the collection and dissemination of diabetes information. It strives to ensure the availability of patient education materials tailored to individual needs, to organize methods for providing the public with information concerning diabetes as a health problem, and to develop means to increase timely exchange of information among scientists and researchers.

The clearinghouse offers several direct services. Based on its own collection and other sources, it compiles and publishes annotated topical bibliographies providing an abstract, source, and pricing information for each item. To help improve the care of diabetic persons, to increase public awareness of diabetes as a health problem, and to enhance the timely exchange of current scientific and related information, it sponsors and coordinates conferences, workshops, and meetings about diabetes and its complications.

Diabetes Dateline is a printed current awareness service. Another valuable service is the publication of bibliographies on a number of subjects such as diet and nutrition and cookbooks for diabetics. These are annotated in the Diabetes section of Chapter 4.

National Health Information Clearinghouse, InterAmerica Research Associates, 1555 Wilson Blvd., Suite 600, Rosslyn, VA 22209. (Mailing Address: Box 1133, Washington, D. C. 20013).

This clearinghouse was established on November 1 1979, as mandated by Section 1706 of the National Consumer Health Information and Health Promotion Act (Title XVII of the Public Health Service Act) of 1976. The principal objective of the clearinghouse, which is funded by the Office of Health Information, Health Promotion, Physical Fitness and Sports Medicine, is to facilitate access to existing sources of health information for the general public and providers serving the public. The clearinghouse will identify existing health-related information sources, including libraries, community organizations, educational institutions, voluntary organizations, and government agencies at all levels.

It is intended that the National Health Information Clearinghouse should serve as a referral center, providing one focal point for access to all the consumer health information products and services available in the United States. Initially, efforts have been focused on identifying information sources, acquiring relevant materials, and designing and planning information services and products. A toll-free 800 number was recently established to service requests nationally. The number is 800-336-4797; Virginia residents should call 703-522-2590.

The first of a number òf planned directories was also recently published. *Health Information Resources in the Department of Health and Human Services* (DHHS Pubn. No. 80-50146; 100 pp.) lists 76 federal and federally sponsored health information resources on topics such as alcoholism, child abuse, health care financing, and patient education. Each entry provides a capsule description and a contact person, address and telephone number, information on serial publications, automated databases, and audiences served. A subject index facilitates the location of resources if the exact name is not known.

National Health Planning Information Center, Box 1600, Prince Georges Plaza Branch, Hyattsville, MD 20788.

The center acquires, screens, and stores information on published journal articles as well as books and other documents about health planning and resources development. Currently, the collection includes approximately 15,000 documents.

The center's collection includes information in the following areas: planning procedures and analytical methods; techniques of administration and financial management of health planning agencies; methods for determining community and population characteristics; standards and criteria for project review assessment and quality assurance; health system regulatory activities; health care technology and equipment impact; and health care delivery plans and projects.

Typical topics covered are health resources, health care utilization, health and consumer education, health care costs, and financing and environmental and occupational health. The center is located in the Health Resources Administration.

National Health Standards and Quality Information Clearinghouse, 6110 Executive Blvd., Suite 250, Rockville, MD 20852.

The National Health Standards and Quality Information Clearinghouse provides a bibliographic and current awareness service for the Health Standards and Quality Bureau of the Health Care Financing Administration. Documents relating to the bureau's mission are collected and organized for quick retrieval.

The clearinghouse issues a monthly *Information Bulletin* containing abstracts of recent technical documents, full reports of meetings and hearings, news summaries, and announcements of coming events. Topical bibliographies available include *Health Systems Agencies and PSROs* (Professional Standards and Review Organizations); *Health Maintenance Organizations: Assessment and Evaluation; Quality Assessment of Long Term Care; Necessity of Surgery; Continuing Education and Quality of Health Care;* and *Consumer Participation in Health Care.* These bibliographies cover many topics vital to the interests of consumers.

Part III

The Literature

Chapter 8

Wellness, Physical Fitness, and Self-Health Care

BOOKS

General Health Guides

See also the General Sections of Chapter 9, Children's Health; Chapter 10, Women's Health; and Chapter 11, Health of the Elderly.

The Ann Landers Encyclopedia A to Z. New York: Doubleday, 1979. 121 pp. $17.50.
Four hundred essays on a variety of topics by an assembly of distinguished physicians, psychiatrists, business people, attorneys, teachers, clergy, and psychologists. At least 65 percent of the total contents is medical. Ann Landers is a member of the Visiting Committee of the Harvard Medical School and a trustee of the Menninger Foundation. Consequently, she has had no difficulty in assembling many talented contributors. The article on heart transplants is by Norman Shumway of Stanford Medical School and the essay on hemorrhoids is by John Brooks, professor of surgery at Harvard Medical School. Topics covered include aging, baldness, bites, cancer, colitis, dandruff, dyslexia, gall bladder disease, hysterectomy, moles, obesity, stress, and venereal disease. Highly recommended.

Chesterman, John, and Marten, Michael. *Man to Man.* New York: Paddington, 1978. 252 pp. $8.95; London: Paddington. £3.95.
Using a question-and-answer format, the authors discuss such topics as weight control and appearance; fitness and exercise; care of the skin, hair, eyes, teeth, and feet; sexual activity and performance; contraception and conception; venereal disease; common health problems, such as hemorrhoids, ulcers, hernias, and prostate disorders; cardiovascular disease; risk factors such as diet, stress, alcohol, and smoking; various drugs; and aging. Annotated bib-

liography included. A useful but very elementary guide, heavily emphasizing sexual matters.

Diagram Group. *Man's Body: An Owner's Manual.* New York: Paddington, 1976. 250 pp. $6.95; $2.75 (paper); London: Paddington. £3.50; London: Corgi. £1.35 (paper).

Abundantly supplied with comparative diagrams and charts, this handbook discusses male physiology and development; life expectancy and major threats to health; various disorders, including those peculiar to men; care of the skin, hair, and teeth; eyesight and hearing; stress; sleep; physical fitness; nutrition and weight control; drugs, including alcohol and tobacco; reproductive organs and male sexuality; and aging. "Woman's body—a nonowner's guide" is also provided. Appended is an anatomical reference guide. Straightforward and comprehensive. Highly recommended.

Galton, Lawrence. *The Complete Medical, Fitness, and Health Guide for Men.* New York: Simon & Schuster, 1979. 333 pp. $12.50.

Although this book is addressed to men, many of the medical concerns it discusses are not exclusively male. A large amount of useful information is accumulated on work, stress, fatigue and sleep problems, exercise and sports, sexual problems, male climacteric, prostate disorders, heart disease, obesity and nutrition, gastrointestinal complaints, hair and skin, and so forth. The author has laboriously digested large amounts of the professional literature and interviewed many specialists. Most of Galton's material, however, has been more cogently and authoritatively discussed elsewhere for lay audiences by highly qualified specialists. Furthermore, the book does not indicate when medical assistance should be sought.

Good Housekeeping Family Health and Medical Guide. New York: Hearst, 1979. 928 pp. $17.95.

This book reflects an ambitious and lavish attempt to present a layperson's guide to the intelligent and effective use of medicine. Some 37 American and British medical specialists explain their specialized and general concerns as they would to a seriously interested patient if they had the time. The book is divided into four sections: 1) a "Survey of Medical Specialties," which describes the scope and area of concern of more than a dozen major areas of specialized practice; 2) the "A-Z of Medicine," an encyclopedic compilation of information on several hundred diseases, symptoms, procedures, conditions, and technical terms; 3) a "Complete Family Health Guide," which provides detailed articles on a variety of topics, such as diagnosis and therapy, psychotherapy, nursing, home care, health care of children, nutrition, drugs and medicines, fitness and health, and family planning, and answers to 250 questions often asked of physicians; and 4) an illustrated course in first aid. Also included are a color atlas of the human body, excellent illustrations, diagrams, charts and figure drawings, and a detailed index. A most attractively produced book, informative and authoritative. Highly recommended for reference purposes and for just browsing.

Heimlich, Henry J., with Galton, Lawrence. *Dr. Heimlich's Home Guide to Emergency Medical Situations.* New York: Simon & Schuster, 1980. 350 pp. $10.95.

The inventor of the Heimlich Maneuver (to prevent choking) presents information on more than 250 "emergency" situations, describing how to recognize what is wrong, how to cope, and when to seek medical help. Specific, detailed information is given on bleeding, shock, poisoning, chest pain, choking, cardiopulmonary resuscitation, burns, acute abdominal pain, and medical emergency kits. An alphabetical guide lists more than 250 emergency situations. The descriptions of fractures, acute gastroenteritis, appendicitis, fever, foreign bodies in the eyes, drowning, diarrhea, fishhook accidents, kidney infection, and so forth are of high quality. However, the inclusion of much material on minor medical ailments, such as tennis elbow, food allergies, hangover, heel pain, jock itch, and numbness and tingling defeats the purpose of the book, in that true emergency information is confused with relatively trivial problems. Nevertheless, highly informative.

Johnson, G. Timothy. *Doctor! What You Should Know about Health Care Before You Call a Physician.* New York: McGraw-Hill, 1975. 424 pp. $8.95.

Dr. Johnson has his own television "doctor show" and is the editor of the *Harvard Medical School Health Letter.* His book is a highly informative guide to the health care marketplace as well as a reference book on common medical problems, such as heart disease, lung disease, cancer, nutrition, women's health care problems, and so forth. Some of the explanation is technical and demands concentrated reading. The consumer's point of view is, however, predominant.

Marchetti, Albert. *Common Cures for Common Ailments.* Briarcliff Manor, NY: Stein & Day, 1979. 367 pp. $10.95.

More than 500 antacid preparations, over 800 cough products, and 100 sleep aids presently can be bought without prescription. Marchetti has produced a comprehensive consumer guide to these over-the-counter drugs. Each of Marchetti's 34 chapters is devoted to a single ailment, such as acne, allergies, colds and flu, constipation, diarrhea, fever blisters and cold sores, headaches, hemorrhoids, insomnia, and sunburn. The causes, symptoms, and courses of the ailment are described by a question-and-answer technique. The various generic drugs that can be used to cure or relieve the ailment are indicated, together with a listing of available over-the-counter products by brand names, including the ingredients of each. Recommended products are shown in boldface type. Of 96 cough suppressants listed, only 22 are recommended. Guidance is given on self-treatment, precautionary measures, and when to consult a doctor. Excellent reference guide on how to use drugs in an appropriate and judicious manner.

Neumann, Hans. *Foreign Travel Immunization Guide.* Oradell, NJ: Medical
　　Economics, 1979. 54 pp. $3.50; $2.95 (paper).
This annual guide is based on data from the World Health Organization, the
Center for Disease Control, sources within the countries themselves, and on
the author's investigations and personal experiences. Noted are two major
trends: a reduction in the official requirements for smallpox and cholera
immunizations and a resurgence of the threat of malaria. Listed are requirements and recommendations for some 175 countries. Also of great value is
information on specific immunizations, with details as to validity, effectiveness, reactions, and booster, and advice on food, drinking water, diarrhea,
pregnancy and travel, and how to find a doctor abroad. Authoritative and
useful in the jet age. Highly recommended.

Parker, Page, and Dietz, Lois N. *Nursing at Home: A Practical Guide to the Care of
　　the Sick and the Invalid in the Home, Plus Self-Help Instructions for the Patient.*
　　New York: Crown, 1980. 344 pp. $14.95.
In 60 concise chapters, the authors give detailed instructions and practical
advice on how to provide nursing care at home. Topics covered include
sickroom equipment and supplies, day-to-day patient care such as foot care,
bathing and hygiene, body rubs, feeding, prevention of bedsores, and special
diets. A list of sickroom equipment and supplies is provided together with a
reference index and 178 aid-giving photographs and drawings. The second
section of the book is for the patient and supplies advice on exercise and rest,
coping with pain, communicating needs, and measures that can be taken to
prompt a return to normal family life. Eminently practical and helpful. Highly
recommended.

Rosenfeld, Isadore. *The Complete Medical Exam: What Your Doctor Knows Is
　　Critical; What You Know Is Crucial.* New York: Simon & Schuster, 1978. 378
　　pp. $10.95.
A step-by-step account of an actual physical exam. Details the questions your
physician asks you and why. Enumerates details of the exam and routine
and nonroutine tests. These include electrocardiogram, blood, urine, chest
x-ray, GI series, CAT scan, and myelogram. As good an explanation of
heart arrythmias as in a medical text, but comprehensible to the layperson.
Recommended.

Sehnert, Keith W. *How to Be Your Own Doctor—Sometimes.* New York: Grosset,
　　1976. 353 pp. $9.95.
A splendid book designed to educate "activated patients"—hearty hybrids
who are three-quarters patient and one-quarter physician. Such persons have
learned to speak the doctor's own language and ask questions rather than
passively sit, honor, and obey. Activated patients play an important and
needed role in health partnership with their doctors. Sehnert presents a vast
compendium of information to assist consumers: how to recognize symptoms,
how to rate your doctor, how to speak your doctor's language, and what to

expect from an annual checkup. A "book within a book" outlines symptoms, treatment, and "call the doctor" signals for 14 illnesses, 13 injuries, and 9 common emergencies. Also provided is a list of more than 100 self-help freebies. A highly useful and sensitive book written with acute insight into the consumer point of view.

Shakman, Robert A. *Where You Live May Be Hazardous to Your Health: A Health Index to Over 200 American Communities.* Briarcliff Manor, NY: Stein & Day, 1979. 260 pp. $10.95.

What makes a community a healthy place to live? Air pollution usually receives the most attention, but there are other factors as well, such as allergies, altitude, climate, rainfall, wind, temperature, and natural disasters. The essence of choosing a healthy place to live is to relate one's list of personal health factors and climate preference to community profiles to arrive at a short list of possible choices. To aid in the process, Shakman offers a series of maps that deal with eight major influences on health: precipitation, wind, heat, air pollution, cold, allergies, natural disasters, and sunshine. The lighter shaded areas on the maps are the most desirable areas. Also, specific information on air pollution, climate, time, natural disasters, and major disasters is provided for 200 American cities. A valuable book that brings together information that can be difficult to find elsewhere.

Smith, Bradley, and Stevens, Gus. *The Emergency Book: You Can Save a Life!* New York: Simon & Schuster, 1978. 160 pp. $4.95.

An excellent, explicit guide to the most common emergencies: heart attack, choking, drowning, shock, poisoning, drug overdose, injury and accidents, burns, and childbirth. The text is clear and is accompanied by high-quality photographs. Each chapter contains information on what to look for and what to do. Calculated to help reduce the 600,000 deaths each year from heart attacks and the 100,000 deaths caused by accidents. Highly recommended.

Vickery, Donald M., and Fries, James F. *Take Care of Yourself: A Consumer's Guide to Medical Care.* Reading, MA: Addison-Wesley, 1976. 269 pp. $9.95; $5.95 (paper); London: Allen & Unwin. £6.50; £3.50 (paper).

The physician authors believe that "you can do more for your health than your doctor can. As an enlightened medical consumer, you can save money and time and provide for the best possible medical care for yourself and your family. You can learn to treat many medical problems at home. And you can learn to recognize when it's important to get to a doctor or hospital." To sharpen the skills of medical consumers, Vickery and Fries discuss the effect of personal habits on health, the annual checkup, finding the right physician, the office visit, choosing the right medical facility, reducing medication costs, the home pharmacy, and avoiding medical fraud. Specific guidance is provided for 68 of the most common medical problems, such as sore throats, impetigo, cold sores, measles, and vaginal discharge. Each problem includes a general discussion of the complaint, suggestions on how to treat it at home, and information on what to expect at the doctor's office. Particularly valuable is the innovative use of flow diagrams, which provide instructions for deciding when to use home remedies and when to seek professional care. A landmark book. Highly recommended.

Medical Consumerism

Auerbach, Melissa, and Bogue, Ted. *Getting Yours: A Consumer's Guide to Obtaining Your Medical Record.* Washington, DC: Public Citizens Health Research Group, 1978. 36 pp. $4.95.
Advocates the patient's right to access to his own medical record and emphasizes the positive benefits in improved patient education, a more open physician-patient relationship, and avoidance of repetitive costly tests and procedures. The booklet also provides a step-by-step guide to obtaining medical records. Legal rights to medical records vary among states, and a chart is provided summarizing the rights of access in each state. About a third of the states have statutes allowing for some sort of direct patient access, but half of them recognize only very limited rights. The Federal Privacy Act governs access to records held by governmental agencies such as the Veterans Administration, military and Public Health Service hospitals. Suggests what to do if the request for access is denied.

Barrett, Stephen, and Knight, Gilda. *The Health Robbers: How to Protect Your Money and Your Life.* Philadelphia: Stickley, 1976. 340 pp. $10.50.
A collection of outspoken and provocative essays on a number of "hot" topics: misery merchants, weight control and fad diets, make-believe doctors, health hustlers, spine salesmen, dubious dentistry, quackery, miracle merchants, and so forth. The book is a publication of the Lehigh Valley (Pennsylvania) Committee against Health Fraud, Inc. A vocal expression of medical consumerism with a terse message: *caveat emptor.* Interesting, if somewhat overstated.

Belsky, Marvin S., and Gross, Leonard. *How to Choose and Use Your Doctor.* New York: Arbor, 1979. 272 pp. $4.95 (paper).
A book that is "a prescription for a new kind of patient: assertive, questioning, capable of making the decisions that are vital for his survival. The physician informs, the patient decides. For such a patient to materialize, mystery and power must be removed from the medical sanctuary." Belsky devotes great attention to unraveling the psychological factors at work in the doctor-patient relationship and has an interesting classification of types of patients. He describes games not to play and how to be a smart patient. Relevant medical information is presented where appropriate.

Cornacchia, Harold J. *Consumer Health.* St. Louis, MO: Mosby, 1976. 310 pp. $11.50; London: Mosby. £7.50 (paper).
A professor of health education describes the intelligent consumer, reliable

sources of health information, and consumer protection. Other topics include quackery; psychological factors in consumerism; several alternative healing philosophies; medical care, including self-help measures; health frauds, as in the treatment of arthritis and cancer; food faddism and weight control; drug products, including both prescription and over the counter; health care economics; and insurance. A balanced and critical text.

Cousins, Norman. *Anatomy of an Illness as Perceived by the Patient.* New York: Norton, 1979. 173 pp. $9.95.
The author, an editor long associated with the *Saturday Review,* describes his self-devised therapy to cope with ankylosing spondylitis, arthritis of the spine. This successful treatment consisted of laughter and intravenous vitamin C. Cousins moved out of the hospital, finding it "no place for a person seriously ill." An inspirational book that illustrates the power of the mind over the body.

Directory of Medical Specialists, 1979–1980, 19th ed. 2 vols. Chicago: Marquis, 1979. 4,301 pp. $99.50.
First published in 1940, the *Directory of Medical Specialists* is an authorized referral guide to physicians certified by the 22 boards constituting the American Board of Medical Specialties. The two-volume, nineteenth biennial edition presents professional and biographical information on more than 221,000 specialists practicing in the United States and abroad. Sketches include educational background, specialty and date of certification, career history, teaching positions, military record, professional memberships, and office address. Within each specialty, individuals are listed by city and state (or country), and alphabetically within each city. An excellent reference tool for the purpose of doctor shopping.

Freese, Arthur S. *Managing Your Doctor: How to Get the Best Possible Health Care.* Briarcliff Manor, NY: Stein & Day, 1977. 191 pp. $2.95 (paper).
General advice on how to find and check a family doctor; finding and using the right hospital; how to get life-saving help in medical emergencies; how to select a psychiatrist, dentist, surgeon, and so forth; information on x-rays, medication, and a variety of topics. Good, sensible advice extracted from authoritative sources, but written from the viewpoint of a health professional rather than that of the typical consumer.

Gaver, Jessyca. *How to Help Your Doctor Help You.* New York: Pinnacle, 1975. 344 pp. $1.75 (paper).
A book written by a medical writer to make the point that it is not the physician who is at fault in health care delivery problems, but the patient who is guilty of ignorance or noncompliance. Gaver presents some useful information about symptoms, diseases, and medical practice, but her presentation is pedestrian, unauthoritative, and hardly likely to improve the decision-making capabilities of consumers.

Gotts, Ronald, and Kaufman, Arthur. *The People's Hospital Book.* New York: Crown, 1978. 211 pp. $8.95.

The authors are director of the National Medical Advisory Service and member of the Joint Commission on Accreditation of Hospitals, respectively. Their objective is to make readers better informed patients and more successful hospital consumers and thereby ensure a less anxious and more comfortable hospital stay. Their book describes how to deal with doctors, nurses, emergency rooms, hospitals away from home, tests, anesthesia, and costs and how to remedy dissatisfaction. The choice of a hospital should be made with consideration of its ability to take care of a patient's needs, which is dependent upon the gravity of the problem. An informative, readable volume on how to understand and deal with hospitals.

Hardy, Robert C. *SICK: How People Feel about Being Sick and What They Think of Those Who Care for Them.* Chicago: Teach'em, 1978. 361 pp. $14.95 (paper).

In this anthology of personal testimonies, a health planner and consultant interviews patients with both common and rare medical conditions. Among the 60 cases presented are four types of cancer, cystic fibrosis, skin problems, respiratory illnesses, hearing and vision disorders, sterilization and infertility, reproduction, prostate and kidney problems, hernias, penicillin reactions, arthritis, fractures, circulatory and heart problems, diabetes and hypoglycemia, gall bladder attack, appendicitis, muscular dystrophy, gangrene, influenza, psychiatric disorder, drug addiction, gum disease, ulcerative colitis, and perforated duodenal ulcer. Striking expressions of the emotions involved in illness.

Illich, Ivan. *Medical Nemesis: The Expropriation of Health.* New York: Pantheon, 1976, 294 pp. $8.95; New York: Bantam, 1977. $2.75 (paper).

The focal point of the author's discussion is the growth of iatrogenesis (illness caused by doctors). Illich maintains that medical practice sponsors sickness by reinforcing a morbid society that encourages people to become consumers of curative, preventive, industrial, and environmental medicine. He argues that the major improvements in modern health have come about not from improved medicine, but rather from other factors, and that the number of diseases that can be cured by medicine is nowhere near as great as the growing medical budgets would make us believe. Illich concludes that medical nemesis is bound to set in unless the autonomy of the individual is reestablished.

LeMaitre, George D. *How to Choose a Good Doctor.* Andover, MA: Andover Pub. Group, 1979. 169 pp. $8.95.

LeMaitre insists on a personal, human doctor-patient relationship. He recommends the selection of a primary physician to serve as the coordinator of a patient's health services and to act as confidant and teacher of a healthy way of life. On selecting a doctor, he argues that no amount of documentation with medical credentials proves professional excellence. "Most doctors are competent . . . . Concern, hard work, thoroughness, follow-through, caring, availability, affordability, teaching, sympathizing, and understanding . . . these are what you look for in a doctor." The author recommends the rejection of physicians over 60 years of age and those lacking board certification. Suggested criteria include the reputation of the physician, accessibility, cost, delay in obtaining an appointment, and length of time in the waiting room. Advice is given on how to avoid surgery and how to get the most out of a visit to the doctor. Sensible and realistic guide to doctor-shopping likely to promote healthy, patient-doctor dialogue. Recommended.

Levin, Arthur. *Talk Back to Your Doctor: How to Demand (and Recognize) High Quality Health Care.* New York: Doubleday, 1975. 238 pp. o.p.
The physician author believes that consumers must play a more active role in their own health care. His emphasis is on how to judge *quality.* Therefore, he focuses attention on criteria to be used in selecting doctors; how well doctors diagnose and with what degree of error; what to expect from an office visit; when to expect diagnostic tests; dangers in prescription drugs; how to identify "good" and "bad" hospitals and how to avoid unnecessary hospitalization; operations that involve the most risk; and problems involved in health care for women and children. Levin writes in a crisp, informative manner and highlights in each section basic one-sentence principles. His lucid tutorial style is calculated to assist the layperson in the exercise of his or her rights as a health care consumer.

May, Lawrence A. *Getting the Most Out of Your Doctor.* New York: Basic, 1977. $11.95.
The author believes that the consumer willingly overbuys medical services in a society where the benefits of medical care have been oversold. "Patients must stop demanding X-rays, lab tests, and prescriptions . . . Patients must develop skills to care for themselves and to purchase health services intelligently." The various medical specialties are described, together with guidelines on how to select a physician. Advice is given on how to assist the physician in diagnosis by providing an accurate description of symptoms. Other topics treated are the intelligent use of drugs; maintaining a healthy life-style with special reference to diet, exercise, alcohol, and smoking; how to recognize and treat common problems, such as flu and diarrhea, without recourse to doctors; the risks and benefits of surgery—"the scalpel makes the cash register ring louder, and this temptation leads to unnecessary surgery"; and the newer trends in medicine. The book is highly readable and informative and will probably succeed in improving doctor-patient relationships. Highly recommended.

Consumer Reports, Editors of. *The Medicine Show.* rev.ed. New York: Pantheon, 1980. 383 pp. $10; $5.95 (paper).
In addition to evaluating various commercial remedies and health products, this objective guide advises on medical issues such as estrogen therapy in

menopause, "miracles" and "cure-alls," quackery, stocking the medicine cabinet and handling prescriptions, and selecting a family doctor and hospital. Glossary included. Most reliable and candid. Highly recommended.

Pekkanen, John. *The Best Doctors in the U.S.: A Guide to the Finest Specialists, Hospitals, and Health Centers.* New York: Seaview, 1979. 290 pp. $10.95; New York: Wideview, 1980. $5.95 (paper).
The listings are based upon the results of a survey of 500 physicians, each of whom was asked: "If you or a member of your family were ill with a problem in your specialty, who would you go to for treatment?" For each specialty, identified specialists were interviewed in depth to confirm the recommendations. Specialists are listed according to broad categories: adult medical, surgical, and diagnostic specialists; childbirth; pediatric; cancer and blood diseases (pediatric and adult); and special centers (such as pain clinics). Under each broad category names are listed under subcategories, such as diseases of the cardiovascular system, diseases of the nervous system, endocrinology, digestive diseases, plastic surgery, and so forth. Of particular interest is the explanation of the criteria Pekkanen used. This is a landmark book that will prove to be most valuable. The only caveat might be that the most skilled and renowned doctors are not necessarily available and willing to deliver patient care on a day-to-day basis.

Schaller, Warren E., and Carroll, Charles R. *Health, Quackery, and the Consumer.* Philadelphia: Saunders, 1976. 426 pp. $14.95; Eastbourne, England: Holt-Saunders. £10.
Beginning with a positive definition of health, this text discusses common misconceptions about health; advertising and psychology; consumer action to reduce health costs; individual responsibility and prevention; alternate health systems and practitioners; consumer health protection; recognizing quackery; use and abuse of health products; health care delivery; and methods, materials, and resources of consumer health education. Under preventive health care, information is provided on immunizations and checkups, symptoms, breast examination, quitting smoking, control of cholesterol, prevention of problem drinking, and medications for minor ailments. Thorough and practical. Recommended.

Drugs and the Consumer

American Pharmaceutical Association. *Handbook on Nonprescription Drugs,* 6th ed. Washington, DC: The Association, 1979. 488 pp. $7.95.
An educational and reference tool for the pharmacist. Designed to provide pharmacists with background information, suggested approaches to better patient service, and rapid, accurate retrieval of specific information. Contains medical and product information on 32 topic areas, such as antacid products, cold and allergy products, weight control products, burn and sunburn prod-

ucts, acne products, and hemorrhoidal products. An excellent source of authoritative product information to facilitate comparison and selection. Highly recommended for both professional and lay use.

American Society of Hospital Pharmacists. *Medication Teaching Manual: A Guide for Patient Counselling.* Washington, DC: The Society, 1978. 168 pp. $10.

A compilation of 140 monographs providing information a patient should know about his drug therapy. The monographs, presented in an easy-to-understand question-answer format, are designed to assist the health care practitioner in answering commonly asked questions about drugs and drug therapy. Because the monographs are written in nontechnical language, the manual should be useful to practitioners in providing drug therapy information directly to their patients. Each monograph explains when and why the drug is prescribed, how the drug should be taken and stored, what should be done if a dosage is missed, the potential side effects of the drug, and how to counterbalance these side effects. Highly useful for reference purposes.

George, David. *Common Medicines: An Introduction for Consumers.* San Francisco: Freeman, 1979. 179 pp. $7.

This preliminary edition is produced by the author, a professor of pharmacology and toxicology at the University of Utah, for his students. George offers a textbook-style compilation of information relating to composition, generic equivalents, actions, therapeutic use, contraindications, adverse reactions, precautions, and recommendations with respect to analgesics, histamines and antihistamines, cough remedies, anticholinergics, cold remedies, antacids, laxatives, antidiarrheals, antiemetics, antibiotics, sleep aids, psychotherapeutic drugs, acne medication, sunscreen and suntan products, drugs and dietary aids used in weight reduction programs, and products for the care of teeth and gums. An excellent source of authoritative information that can serve as an introductory textbook of pharmacology for individuals with little or no background in the biological sciences.

Gossel, Thomas A., and Stansloski, Donald W. *Home Pharmacy.* Skokie, IL: Consumer Guide, 1979. 287 pp. $1.95.

An inexpensive compilation of information about how drugs work, when potential dangers may arise, and what actions to expect from drug use. Presents elementary explanations on reading prescriptions, buying and storing drugs, poisoning, how to take medication, and common side effects of drugs. Particularly useful are the profiles of the most commonly prescribed drugs. These include name, trade name equivalents, generic equivalents, dosage forms, use, minor and major side effects, contraindications, interaction with other drugs, warnings and precautions, and general comments. Useful as a most inexpensive source of basic, elementary information.

Graedon, Joe. *The People's Pharmacy: A Guide to Prescription Drugs, Home Remedies and Over-the-Counter Medication.* New York: Avon, 1977. 401 pp. $5.95 (paper).
A readable and informative guide to the use of drugs for a wide variety of ailments, including allergies, asthma, high blood pressure, headaches, sunburn, and nausea. Good advice is given on how to save money on prescriptions. The book is best in its treatment of over-the-counter medication, on which more than $3 billion is spent annually, with sobering truths about Preparation H, Alka-Seltzer, Rolaids, and Tums. Practical advice is given on self-treatment, "What to Do When the Doctor Won't Come." The chapter on drug interactions is particularly valuable. An authoritative and lucid compendium of drug information, which is, however, somewhat simplistic and opinionated.

Hafen, B. Q., and Peterson, B. *Medicines and Drugs.* Philadelphia: Lea & Febiger, 1978. 265 pp. $12.75 (paper); London: Lea & Febiger. £9.
A comprehensive overview of the therapeutic, legal, social, and economic implications of the consumer's use and abuse of drugs. The message that no drug is completely safe and that all drugs should be used only with complete understanding of the proper administration and potential adverse effects is clearly conveyed. The book indicates how the use and abuse of medications and drugs exact a staggering toll in needless suffering, punitive consequences, economic loss, and destruction of human life. The data have been accumulated from the literature and from government and industry. The authors endeavor successfully to provide information for the rational use of drugs. They point to the relationship between the potential for excessive use of drugs in the home and the frequency of drug abuse in young people. The book addresses an important subject in a meaningful manner.

Hughes, Richard, and Brewin, Robert. *The Tranquilizing of America: Pill Popping and the American Way of Life.* New York: Harcourt, 1979. 326 pp. $11.95.
The authors outline the great price being paid in the quest for chemical calm. In 1977 there were 57 million prescriptions written for Valium, 15 million for Librium and more than 12 million for Dalmane. The dangers inherent in the abuse of psychotropics, sedatives, hypnotics, and antidepressant drugs are vividly portrayed. The widespread use of Ritalin for the treatment of hyperactivity is condemned, as is the pacification of the elderly by Thorazine and Mellaril. The advertising and promotional activities of companies such as Roche and Smith, Kline, and French are especially condemned. The same misinformation, lack of information, deception, and fraud accompanies the promotion of over-the-counter preparations that promise quick relief from colds, coughs, indigestion, diarrhea, headache, insomnia, and other ailments. A stimulating, thought-provoking, and controversial book. Pill poppers take note. Recommended.

Paulina, Albert M. *The Family Prescription and Medication Guide.* Englewood Cliffs, NJ: Prentice-Hall, 1979. 367 pp. $13.95.
Provides relevant information in a condensed, understandable form. The

book's objective is to help the patient achieve the maximum benefit from prescribed medication with the fewest possible side effects. A product summary section lists generic names and equivalent brand names together with medication information and instruction for usage. Also contains a cross index of generic and trade names and a chapter on pharmaceutical definitions. Strives to improve communication between patient, physician, and pharmacist.

Physicians' Desk Reference. Oradell; NJ: Medical Economics, 1979. $14.25.
The best-known source of drug information, distributed free to the 350,000 practicing physicians in the United States. The *PDR* includes information on about 2,500 drug products. The information is supplied voluntarily by the pharmaceutical manufacturers, who decide which drugs to list. However, FDA regulations require full disclosure of how a drug works, what it is to be used for, possible adverse reactions or side effects, contraindications, and other precautions and warnings about hazards posed by the drug. Indexes are provided by manufacturers, alphabetically by brand name, by generic name, and by classification of product, such as antihistamine and anticholinergic. A product identification section contains actual size, full-color photographs of pills, capsules, and other dosage forms. Also included are names, addresses, and phone numbers of drug manufacturers, a list of poison control centers, and a guide for physician management of drug overdose in adults. Despite the highly technical nature of the *PDR* and the meticulous documentation of all possible adverse reactions required by federal regulation, it is nevertheless a valuable information resource for reference purposes—if it is not stolen or mutilated.

Rubenstein, Morton. *A Doctor's Guide to Non-Prescription Drugs.* New York: Signet, 1977. 195 pp. $1.95 (paper).
Chapters on 16 common ailments contain a short, tutorial explanation followed by three listings for common drugs—recommended, acceptable, and unacceptable. Cost comparisons, based upon Los Angeles prices, are somewhat outdated. Concise presentation, combined with low cost, makes this book highly suited to libraries that desire multiple copies.

Surgery and the Consumer

See also Cosmetic Surgery in Chapter 17, Other Health Problems and Concerns

Crile, George, Jr. *Surgery: Your Choices, Your Alternatives.* New York: Delacorte, 1978. 197 pp. $7.95.
The book is written to make patients aware of the legitimate differences of opinion among the best-qualified surgeons. Most types of surgery, including operations for cancer, ulcers, heart disease, hernia, varicose veins, and prostate enlargement are described. Dr. Crile reviews the controversy over mastectomy and coronary by-pass surgery. He urges that patients ask questions,

weigh the alternatives, and be intelligent participants in the decision to have surgery. On a very controversial note, Dr. Crile advocates the abolition of fee-for-service surgery and the substitution of salaries paid by hospitals. This, he argues, would eliminate unnecessary surgery. He advocates better quality control, improved peer review and the publication of mortality rates by hospitals for each type of surgical procedure. The book is most informative and will doubtless make individuals more intelligent consumers of surgical procedures. Unfortunately, it may encourage excessive "doctor shopping" and perhaps deter patients from obtaining necessary treatment. Another disadvantage is that information is mixed with polemics. As an example: "unless the medical profession reforms itself there are forces at work that may well drive this country into completely socialized medicine." Provocative reading. Highly recommended.

Denney, Myron K. *Second Opinion.* New York: Grosset, 1979. 201 pp. $8.95.
A consumer's guide to surgical problems, such as when and where to get surgery, who needs it, what can go wrong, anesthesia, and what you should know before you consent to surgery. Information is presented on 31 surgical procedures, including appendectomy, back surgery, breast biopsy, cataract removal, cosmetic surgery, hernia, kidney stones, prostate gland surgery, and vasectomy. An excellent book that proves the necessity of seeking second opinions in defined circumstances. Recommended.

Galton, Lawrence. *The Patient's Guide to Successful Surgery: How to Make the Best of Your Operation.* New York: Avon, 1977. 468 pp. $2.50 (paper).
A prolific writer of consumer health books covers a broad range of procedures. In the sections on chest and blood-vessel surgery, various cardiovascular problems and corrective operations are described, with attention given to such matters as causes and symptoms, prevention, diagnosis and treatment, anesthesia, surgical access route, length of operation, postoperative care, and success rate. Although the general nature of this work precludes extensive detail on any one procedure, it is a valuable introductory and reference work for the lay reader.

Melluzzo, Paul M., and Nealon, Eleanor. *Living with Surgery: Before and After.* Dayton, OH: Lorenz, 1979. 279 pp. $9.95.
Major surgery is especially devastating because of the emotional stress involved. In this unique book, the authors are concerned with the psychological impact of surgery. The major surgical procedures covered are mastectomy, ostomies, amputations, hysterectomies, neurosurgery, kidney transplants, birth defects, and open heart surgery. Technical details are presented incidentally to the principal concerns of patients: what is involved, what the risks are, what changes there will be in my way of life, whether I will be disfigured or disabled, who will support the family. The major emphasis is placed on discussion of feelings, fears, and hopes illustrated by actual case histories. The authors believe that patients and their families can cope better if they have

adequate information and if they can openly communicate their feelings. A warm, sensitive, and supportive discussion of fears and anxieties frequently overlooked by those who consider surgery in exclusively physical terms. Highly recommended.

Health Activation and Self-Health Care

Ardell, Donald B. *Higher Level Wellness: An Alternative to Doctors, Drugs, and Disease.* Emmaus, PA: Rodale, 1977. 296 pp. $5.95; Bantam, 1979. $2.25 (paper); Berkhamsted: Rodale. £2.95 (paper).
A former health planner explains the concept of wellness as promoted by the Wellness Resource Center in Mill Valley, California, and as practiced at several health centers around the country. According to the author, the "fine dimensions of high level wellness" are self-responsibility, strengthened through such programs as est (Erhard Seminars Training), transactional analysis, and Arica "psychocalisthenics"; nutritional purification; stress management through medication, massage, and other techniques; physical fitness through a personalized exercise regimen and effective breathing; and environmental sensitivity. There is also a section on working for a healthier nation by demanding more preventive medicine. Included are several measures of healthy life-style, numerous principles and guidelines, and an extensive, annotated list of recommended books. An excellent book for people who feel controlled by sickness-inducing habits and who are dependent on others for their health and well-being. The author's goal is to show that a healthy life-style can provide more joy, satisfaction, and zest in living than can ever be obtained from the predominant behavior patterns in contemporary America—smoking, eating junk foods, not exercising, living with uncontrolled stress, and refusing accountability for one's own health. It is a soaring and elevated statement of the wellness concept.

Bloomfield, Harold H., and Kory, Robert B. *The Holistic Way to Health and Happiness: A New Approach to Complete Lifetime Wellness.* New York: Simon & Schuster, 1978. 311 pp. $9.95; $4.95 (paper).
A psychiatrist and a lecturer on holistic health provide strategies for weight reduction, physical fitness, cessation of smoking, control of hypertension and the risks of heart disease, curing insomnia, controlling stress and depression, increasing energy, improving sexual performance, and cutting alcohol consumption. The authors strongly emphasize the value of silence and meditation in triggering the individual's natural healing abilities and facilitating behavior modification. Included are a holistic health survey, recommendations for reducing cholesterol and fat consumption, and an extensive bibliography.

Diekelmann, Nancy. *Primary Health Care of the Well Adult.* New York: McGraw-Hill, 1977. 243 pp. $7.95 (paper); Maidenhead: McGraw-Hill. £5.95.
Directed at nursing personnel, this work is divided into sections on the young,

middle-aged, and older adult. In addition to providing a health overview for each age, the author discusses exercise and activity, nutrition and dieting, sexuality, environmental health hazards, sleep and medications, smoking and alcohol, menopause, rest, safety, and retirement. Includes end-of-chapter bibliographies. A most worthwhile book, remarkably comprehensive and insightful. Recommended for both professionals and laypeople.

Farquhar, John W. *The American Way of Life Need Not be Hazardous to Your Health*. New York: Norton, 1979. 196 pp. $9.95.
A cardiologist, director of the Stanford Heart Disease Prevention Program, explains risk factors and offers brilliantly practical techniques to help people modify their behavior regarding stress, exercise, diet, and smoking. The author begins with stress management since skills used here improve a person's ability to change other habits. With numerous self-contracts and behavioral drills, Farquhar provides the means to achieve small victories that gradually add up to healthful living. Includes a guide to further reading. Systematic yet tactful, this self-help book is cleverly superior to most. Essential.

Ferguson, Tom, ed. *Medical Self-Care: Access to Health Tools*. New York: Summit, 1980. 320 pp. $8.95 (paper).
An attractive and convenient compilation of the best of the first eight issues of *Medical Self-Care* magazine (annotated in Chapter 5). Articles are arranged around major topics, such as the self-care concept, being your own paramedic, birthing, body work, couples, drugs, dying and grieving, eating, elders, exercise, human sexuality, medical consumerism, men's health, stress, and women's health. Book reviews and listings of information resources reflect the dominant themes of self-health care, wellness and medical consumerism. Recommended for those who do not have a complete run of *Medical Self-Care* magazine.

Galton, Lawrence. *How Long Will I Live? And 434 Other Questions Your Doctor Doesn't Have Time to Answer and You Can't Afford to Ask*. New York: Macmillan, 1976. 308 pp. $9.95.
Using a question-and-answer format, a medical writer provides information on numerous health factors—family history; sexual differences; childhood and early experience; body build and body rhythms; environment; work, income, social and marital status; personality; sex life; weight, diet, and physical activity; smoking, drinking, and other matters of life-style; hidden problems such as hypertension and diabetes; checkups; major killers such as heart disease and cancer; the effects of aging. Included are recommended readings and a chart for determining personal health status. Despite its reference value, the work is hardly comprehensive and is seriously hampered by its format.

Haimes, Leonard, and Tyson, Richard. *How to Triple Your Energy.* New York: NAL, 1978. 228 pp. $1.75 (paper).

Two physicians specializing in preventive medicine, overweight, and nutritional disorders discuss the causes of energy deficiency and suggest strategies for improvement. After describing the various functions of nutrients, the authors identify common energy robbers including caffeine, nicotine, air pollutants, alcohol, overweight, prescription drugs, food additives, and certain natural food substances. When specific ailments are not involved, fatigue also can be due to such factors as inadequate exercise, insomnia, and poor stress control. Haimes and Tyson include an energy program that contains nutritional recommendations, breakfast pointers, exercises, foot care, sexual information, and such relaxation methods as meditation and biofeedback. Also provided are suggestions for medical tests and consultation, 12 concise energy guidelines, and a bibliography. Balanced and practical. Highly recommended.

Linde, Shirley M. *The Whole Health Catalogue: How to Stay Well Cheaper,* 1st ed. New York: Rawson, Wade, 1978. 226 pp. $12.95; $6.95 (paper).

Stating that the individual should accept "primary responsibility for his own health," a medical writer provides a handbook for the consumer. Among the topics discussed are choosing and interacting with a doctor, increasing life expectancy, the killer diseases and how to cope with them; the whole health diet; special diets for medical problems; general and specific exercises; control of smoking, alcohol, and stress; accident prevention; healthful sleep without pills; birth control, pregnancy, and childbirth; home sex therapy; caring for children; slowing the clock of age; eye health; dental care; getting psychiatric help, medicines; hospitalization; health insurance; treatment of common ailments; emergency techniques for life-threatening crises and everyday problems; outdoor and travel health; home medical tests. In addition, the book contains an excellent "Directory of Free Health Information and Services Which Most People Don't Know About" arranged by major topics. The text is also interspersed with notations of relevant information sources and treatment centers. Highly valuable.

Matheny, Kenneth B., and Riordan, Richard. *Therapay American Style: Person Power through Self-Help.* Chicago: Nelson-Hall, 1979. 285 pp. $16.95.

Two professors of counseling collaborate on a handbook for self-directed change. In four parts the book discusses overcoming the sense of helplessness, developing the motivation and resources needed to change, fine-tuning the mind and body, communicating effectively, and influencing others. Advice on weight loss, physical conditioning, and control of drinking and smoking emphasizes identifying trigger situations and setting realistic and rewarding goals. Also covered are several physical and psychological methods of handling stress. A sane and practical aid to do-it-yourself behavior modification. Recommended.

Mazzanti, Deborah Szekely. *Secrets of the Golden Door.* New York: Morrow, 1977. 288 pp. $12.50.
Reminding readers that good health is their birthright, the founder of a famous health spa presents her "secrets" of vitality and well-being. Mazzanti emphasizes the need for physical activity and provides detailed advice on exercise, posture, tension reduction, massage, and body awareness. Also discussed are "creative sleep," meditation, control of smoking and drug use, skin care, weight control and nutrition, vegetarianism. One chapter is devoted to developing an individual health routine. Included are 74 pages of menus. Helpful but unexceptional.

Norfolk, Donald. *The Habits of Health.* New York: St. Martin's, 1977. 239 pp. $9.95; Avon, $1.95 (paper).
Described as "the prudent person's guide to well-being," this "encyclopedia" of health and hygiene offers rather superficial coverage of 71 topics. According to Norfolk, well-being is promoted through exercise, breast-feeding, breakfast, fasting, laughter, mastication, meditation, relaxation, roughage, vegetables, willpower, and zest. Also discussed are such health hazards as apathy, change, flies, hangovers, obesity, smoking, and stress. More appropriate for trivia buffs than for consumers of health information.

Roberts, Toni M., and others. *Healthwise Handbook.* New York: Dolphin, 1979. 250 pp. $6.95.
The authors have produced a practical manual of self-health care. The book's objective is to "save time, worry, and needless expense by knowing when to treat minor illnesses at home and how to recognize when more skilled care is needed." Major topics include home physical exams, descriptions of many common health problems and their treatment, dental care, eating wisely, "mental wellness," the medicine chest, and recommended equipment. Especially valuable is the chapter on "becoming healthwise" through exercise, stress reduction, expression of feelings, less reliance on chemicals, and diet. The text is simple, clear, and well illustrated. Recommended for those seeking very elementary explanations.

Seebohm, Caroline, and Pool, Mary, eds. *The House and Garden Book of Total Health.* New York: Putnam's, 1978. 442 pp. $11.95.
Composed of interviews with 51 experts, this compendium covers the relationship of different body systems to health, nutrition and weight control, physical fitness, and emotional health. Features of interest include a doctor's "do's and don'ts" for healthy living, working with and rating the personal physician, nutrition labeling, planning sound vegetarian meals, types of exercise, sleep and relaxation, self-control, and personal energy. Included are numerous beauty tips and recipes. A chatty presentation.

Shealy, C. Norman. *90 Days to Self-Health.* New York: Dial, 1977. 178 pp. $7.95; Bantam, 1978. $2.25 (paper); London: Bantam. £0.85.

The doctor who developed "biogenics" (a form of bioenergetic therapy designed to relieve muscular tension through self-regulation) presents a 90-day program designed to relieve the health consequences of stress and to free the person from harmful habits. Borrowing from autogenics and biofeedback, the author's method aims at achieving conscious control over the autonomic nervous system through mental exercises and relaxation. The relevance of nutrition and physical exercise is also recognized in two chapters that provide specific guidelines for these health areas. Toward habit regulation, Shealy suggests exercises for weight balance, freedom from smoking and alcohol, and sleep harmony. Also discussed are pain, hospitalization, surgery, drugs, light, and meditation. A clear and sensible presentation that includes a section on the medical limitations of biogenics.

Taylor, Robert B. *Dr. Taylor's Self-Help Medical Guide*. New Rochelle, NY: Arlington, 1977. 380 pp. $9.95; New York: NAL, 1978. $2.25 (paper).
A family practitioner provides a health manual that covers more than 200 medical conditions, presented alphabetically. Identifying problems for which self-help is appropriate, the author offers advice on treatment and recommends specific natural remedies or nonprescription drugs. For disorders requiring professional help, Taylor discusses diagnosis and treatments. In many instances, preventive behavior is suggested and organizational addresses are provided for those seeking further information. Special features include therapeutic exercises and diets, a weight-watcher's calorie guide, an appendix on reading a prescription, and measurement conversion tables. Well organized and readable.

Ulene, Art. *Feeling Fine: A 20-Day Program of Pleasures for a Lifetime of Health*. Los Angeles: Tarcher, 1977. 287 pp. $7.95; New York: Ballantine, 1978. $2.50 (paper); London: Souvenir, £4.25.
Feeling fine involves knowing how to take care of oneself physically, learning to use stress energies constructively, finding ways to expand oneself emotionally, and discovering that one can cope with change and employ it positively. In order to feel fine the individual must practice "well-medicine." A program of self-caring is outlined based on the development and fostering of growing pleasures, unstressing pleasures, eating pleasures, and body pleasures. Rather simplistic presentation that reads like a television script but contains relevant and sensible advice.

Upledger, John E. *An Osteopathic Doctor's Treasury of Health Secrets*. New York: Parker, 1976. 205 pp. $8.95.
Asserting that self-help techniques are effective for many conditions, a professor of osteopathic medicine provides a compendium of remedies and aids to optimum health. Broad topics include improved breathing and increased mental energy; better circulation and blood pressure; blood sugar control; spinal exercises; less fatigue; cold prevention; headache and allergy relief; improved digestion; help for arthritis; skin care; sex, aging, and hormones. In

addition to neural massage and other osteopathic therapies, Upledger emphasizes the benefits of nutrition and vitamins, drinking water and reducing salt intake, relaxation and physical activity, and reduction of drugs and smoking. Although some advice here is hardly conventional, the work's emphasis is on healthful practices that support the body's natural defenses.

Vickery, Donald M. *LifePlan for Your Health.* Reading, MA: Addison-Wesley, 1978. 318 pp. $10.95; $5.95 (paper); London: Addison-Wesley. £6.95; £3.95 (paper).
Dr. Vickery is the coauthor of the best-sellers *Take Care of Yourself* and *Taking Care of Your Child.* In this book, his emphasis is on health promotion and preventive medicine. His major point is that life-style and the environment are more important to health than medical care. Simple descriptions are given of the principal diseases—cancer, heart disease, stroke, arthritis. Directions are given for calculating a "life score." A worksheet is provided taking into account factors such as exercise, weight, diet, smoking, alcohol, mental health, and family living. From this score, Vickery shows how to develop a life plan that sets priorities for improvement in life and health. Sensible advice that puts the burden of health back on the individual.

Wade, Carlson. *Healing and Revitalizing Your Vital Organs.* New York: Prentice-Hall, 1978. 249 pp. $9.95.
A prolific medical writer describes hundreds of natural remedies for health problems involving the organs. Discussed here are methods to heal and stimulate the glands, skin, heart, digestive and intestinal organs, eyes and ears, liver, kidneys, gall bladder, pancreas, respiratory organs, brain, prostate, and female sex organs. Wade suggests both conventional and exotic health boosters, including the elimination of refined sugar, salt, and harsh seasonings; moderate exercise; massage and contrast baths; cessation of smoking and drinking; raw vegetable juices and salads with natural dressings; fresh fruit; sunshine; no caffeine; little meat and no animal fats; deep breathing; whole grains; quiet periods and sleep; and various folk concoctions. Includes a 21-day rejuvenation program and an organ-healer locator index.

Holism and Alternate Medicine

Bach, Marcus. *The Power of Total Living: A Holistic Approach to the Coming of the New Person for the New Age.* New York: Dodd, Mead, 1977. 201 pp. $7.95; New York: Fawcett, 1978. $1.95 (paper).
A noted proponent of holism philosophizes about its history, purpose, and processes. According to Bach, holistic living calls for "exercise through discipline as it pertains to the body, nutritional eating through willpower as it involves the mind, and fasting through meditation as it relates to spirit." Practical aids include ten reasons and a ten-step procedure for fasting; "10 commandments of nutritional eating," pompously worded; and numerous exercises and breathing routines. Rather tedious.

Biermann, June, and Toohey, Barbara. *The Woman's Holistic Headache Relief Book.* Los Angeles: Tarcher, 1979. 212 pp. $7.95.
Emphasizing the need for self-healing and a mental orientation to wellness, two medical writers review the various causes of headaches and urge holistic methods of treatment. Among the possible factors involved are allergies, postural problems, glandular and nutritional imbalances, chemicals such as caffeine and nicotine, climatic and environmental influences, stress, and bad bite (i.e., temporomandibular joint syndrome). In addition to temporary relief measures such as massage and acupressure, the authors also suggest relaxation and exercise techniques, and stress reduction through autogenic training, meditation, biofeedback, and guided imagery. Holistic headache specialists, pain clinics, and positive thinking are also covered. Resource lists; suggested readings provided. Down-to-earth and amusing.

Hill, Ann, ed. *A Visual Encyclopedia of Unconventional Medicine.* New York: Crown, 1979. 240 pp. $12.95; $6.95 (paper).
Described as "a health manual for the whole person," this superbly illustrated work is the product of 54 contributors. Its contents include comprehensive systems such as oriental medicine and homeopathy; diagnostic methods; physical therapies such as acupuncture and Shiatsu massage, osteopathy, chiropractic, rolfing, sauna baths, breathing, various electrotherapies, and mineral contact; hydrotherapy including baths, steaming, mineral water therapy; plant-based therapies such as herbal medicine; nutrition, including systems like vegetarianism and natural hygiene, supplementary diets, restricted diets, and fasting; wave, radiation and vibration therapies; mind and spirit therapies, including autosuggestion, autogenic training, biofeedback, meditation, Arica, bioenergetics, Gestalt, etc.; and self-exercise therapies such as yoga, sports, and T'ai Chi Ch'uan. Introducing the section on nutrition is an article on "the roles of eating," providing practical advice that is free of fanaticism. Contains a reading list, resource directory, and numerous explanatory charts. Although some articles contain caveats, most of the writers are clearly biased toward their subjects; but despite the lack of objective criticism, this is a comprehensive reference aid.

Hulke, Malcolm, ed. *The Encyclopedia of Alternate Medicine and Self-Help.* New York: Schocken, 1979. 243 pp. $12.95; $6.95 (paper); London: Rider. £4.95.
Divided into two parts, this work provides expert descriptions of 79 therapeutic systems and practices together with a directory of pertinent services and aids. Contents include acupuncture, applied kinesiology, biofeedback, chiropractic, encounter and Gestalt therapy, health foods, herbalism, homeopathy, jogging, naturopathy, orthomolecular psychiatry, osteopathy, rolfing, Shiatsu massage, T'ai Chi Ch'uan, vegetarianism, and yoga. Material on unconventional treatments is also listed by disorder, under autism, baldness, cancer, constipation, migraine and tension headache, and multiple sclerosis. The directory covers products, associations, training and treatment centers, health resorts, and magazines. A bibliography is included. Compact

and readable, this reference tool fails, nevertheless, to provide full credentials or affiliations for its contributors.

Jackson, Richard. *Holistic Massage.* New York: Sterling, 1977. 128 pp. $5.95 (paper).
Written by a physical therapist, this work applies holistic principles to the self-help practice of massage. According to the author, "holistic massage involves two people working together on physical and nonphysical levels to effect positive changes in each. This differs from conventional massage, in which there is a passive receiver who has surrendered responsibility to an active giver who is supposed to have the power to relieve discomfort through direct manipulations." Among the topics covered are breathing, muscle tension and pain, body awareness, sickness as a positive life-force, and massage as medication. Included are specific strokes and techniques, explicit photographs, and anatomical drawings. A most unconventional presentation.

Kaslof, Leslie J. *Wholistic Dimensions in Healing: A Resource Guide.* New York: Dolphin, 1978. 295 pp. $7.95 (paper).
With contributions from 62 authorities, this work describes the development and principles of various holistic systems and practices. Divided into eight sections, the guide covers childbirth; integrated medical systems such as homeopathy, osteopathy, chiropractic, and naturopathy; nutrition and herbs, including a chapter on "preventive nutrition and health maintenance"; heuristic directions in diagnosis and treatment, including acupuncture, biorhythms, astrology; biofeedback and self-regulation; psychic and spiritual healing; psychophysical approaches such as massage, Shiatsu, sensory awareness, and rolfing; humanistic and transpersonal psychotherapies such as Gestalt, art therapy, and hypnosis. For each topic the introductory article is followed by an annotated directory of groups and associations, centers and clinics, publications, products and services, and researchers. A suggested reading list is supplied. Although few methods receive objective scrutiny, this selective, carefully compiled work has undeniable reference value.

LaPatra, Jack W. *Healing: The Coming Revolution in Holistic Medicine.* New York: McGraw-Hill, 1978. 235 pp. $9.95; London: McGraw-Hill. £7.50.
Offering an articulate exposition of the movement toward holism, a health systems analyst describes the rituals of a medical system concentrating on illness, and reviews the nature and tools of folk healing and the development and flaws of scientific medicine. In discussing the mind-body connection, LaPatra considers such topics as voluntary control of involuntary processes, psychosomatic illness, biofeedback, and placebo therapy. Chapters on healing the body, mind, and spirit holistically use case histories to explore such methods as homeopathic medicine, chiropractic, acupuncture, bioenergetics, Jungian analysis, meditation, and biochemical analysis. Practical strategies for self-healing are also suggested, using the common cold for illustration. In

closing, the author discusses the future of holism and the role of health professionals. Includes a descriptive inventory of 115 varieties of "fringe medicine"; notes and bibliography. A well-structured review, balanced and realistic. Highly recommended.

Ledermann, E. K. *Good Health through Natural Therapy.* New York: Sterling, 1977. 147 pp. $8.95; London: Kogan Page. £3.95.
A veteran British physician explains the rationale and workings of natural therapy, which strives for wholeness and harmony by stimulating the body's own healing processes. Among the topics discussed are the need for personal responsibility; obesity and saccharine disease; nutrients and contaminants in the soil; degraded and unnatural food; various unusual diets, including fasting; the benefits of vitamins, minerals, and certain foods; psychodietetics; fiber and elimination; air pollution; breathing rhythm; natural stimulation through the skin; posture, exercise, aerobics, and autogenic training; homeopathy, acupuncture, osteopathy, chiropractic, and massage. Includes case histories. There is an excellent passage on the limitations of natural therapy. Interesting, but complex and most unconventional.

Liu, Da. *The Tao of Health and Longevity.* New York: Schocken, 1978. 178 pp. $10.50; $4.95 (paper); London: Routledge. £2.95.
The author describes the historical development of Taoism and Confucianism in relation to health, the effect of T'ai Chi Ch'uan exercises on different body systems, and various self-help practices. Contents include instructions on breathing, the shortened form of T'ai Chi Ch'uan, sitting meditation, and eight exercises that stimulate the inner organs. Also discussed are massage, acupressure, and other self-treatment techniques; the health effects of food, clothing, shelter, and daily activity; Chinese diets and health foods; sexual concerns; and "peace of mind." End-of-chapter notes. A practical and convincing presentation, remarkably compatible with Western medicine in its growing concern for wellness.

Miller, Emmett E., and Lueth, Deborah. *Feeling Good: How to Stay Healthy.* Englewood Cliffs, NJ: Prentice-Hall, 1978. 269 pp. $12.95; $4.95 (paper).
A physician specializing in psychosomatic medicine focuses on personal responsibility and natural healing abilities in the management of stress and various medical problems. In the process of "selective awareness," the individual uses relaxation, imagination, and imagery to change self-image and establish more healthful behavior patterns. A blending of hypnosis and meditation, Miller's technique is similar to other holistic approaches to unifying mind and body. Especially insightful is the book's final section, where Miller discusses the disease-health continuum and the ideal of "metahealth" through personal commitment. Included are several illustrative "fables," a list of "selective awareness" tapes, and bibliography. Highly recommended.

Otto, Herbert A., and Knight, James, W., eds. *Dimensions in Wholistic Healing: New Frontiers in the Treatment of the Whole Person.* Chicago: Nelson-Hall, 1979. 543 pp. $22.95; $11.95 (paper).
A series of 31 essays brings together information on the theories and framework of holistic healing; Western approaches, including self-regulation, biofeedback, meditation, and hypnosis; and non-Western approaches, including Chinese medicine, Kundalini yoga, the Tibetan art of healing, and Ayurvedic medicine. This is an excellent source book that furnishes a conceptual framework for understanding the scope and content of holistic healing, linking the totality of a person's being—the mental, emotional, physical, social, and spiritual dimensions.

Rolf, Ida. *Ida Rolf Talks about Rolfing and Physical Reality,* ed. by Rosemary Feitis. New York: Harper, 1978. 215 pp. $8.95.
In this collection of personal reflections, the developer of rolfing talks about her life, her philosophy, and her holistic technique. Also known as structural processing or structural integration, rolfing is a method of deep, often painful, massage designed to return the body to its natural posture and balance. The programs have ten hourly sessions and require a trained "rolfer." Enhancing the value of this introspective and fragmentary book is the information provided in both the introduction and the glossary.

Rosa, Karl Robert. *You and AT.* Transl. by Helen Tuschling. New York: Saturday Review/Dutton, 1976. 136 pp. OP.
Described as a "method of autohypnotic exercises," autogenic training (AT) is "a distinctive treatment involving the organic processes of the body, malfunctions of which can be alleviated by bringing the regulative functions . . . into harmony." By means of AT, the individual eventually can acquire some voluntary control over his or her body's automatic functions and over such obstinate health problems as overeating, hypertension, asthma, migraine, and alcoholism. Although the work provides elementary instruction in the method, the author, a German psychotherapist, stresses the need for a preliminary checkup and thorough training under the direction of a qualified doctor. Progressive; clearly oriented toward whole health. Recommended.

Shames, Richard, and Sterin, Chuck. *Healing with Mind Power: Living and Feeling the Way You Want to through Guided Meditation and Self-Hypnosis.* Emmaus, PA: Rodale, 1978. 182 pp. $7.95; London: Rodale. £4.95.
Instrumental in the development of the Wholistic Health and Nutrition Institute at Mill Valley, California, Shames and Sterin discuss the value of self-hypnosis in personal health care. After describing the nature and development of the technique, the authors explain several reliable induction methods along with relevant tips and cautions for its practice. Self-hypnosis can be used for stress reduction and relaxation; control of harmful habits such as drug and alcohol abuse, unhealthy eating, and smoking; and for various disorders as a form of self-healing. Through self-hypnosis, the authors assert, individual

commitment to wellness becomes a dynamic process; and illness, when it occurs, becomes more manageable on a personal level. An exciting and clearly valid proposition, although exclusive reliance on this technique is probably ill-advised.

Sharma, C. H. *A Manual of Homeopathy and Natural Medicine,* ed. by David Leland. New York: Dutton, 1976. 153 pp. $2.95 (paper); London: Turnstone. £2.95; £1.95 (paper).
Homeopathy is a healing system based on the belief that minute doses of toxic substances can cure certain ailments. In this book, a physician who gave up orthodox medicine for homeopathy describes its principles and remedies. Also discussed are various key nutrients; Hindu conceptions of medicine and diet; preventing disease by removing pollutants; first aid and emergency treatment; and care of the skin, hair, eyes, ears, teeth, and feet. Sharma provides both standard and homeopathic advice on such common disorders as headache, insomnia, influenza, constipation, menstrual pain, and rheumatism. The work ends with a bibliography and a catalogue of homeopathic medicines.

Sobel, David, ed. *Ways of Health: Holistic Approaches to Ancient and Contemporary Medicine.* New York: Harcourt, 1979. 497 pp. $12.95; $7.50 (paper).
In this most impressive anthology, 20 scientists contribute essays on holistic approaches to health, ancient systems of medicine, unorthodox medicine, techniques of self-regulation, and an ecological view of health. Topics addressed include the limitations of modern medicine, its evolution along holistic lines, Navaho Indian medicine, Chinese medicine, religious and secular nonmedical healing, laying on of hands, homeopathic medicine, yogic therapy, the relaxation response, biofeedback, biological rhythms, physical activity in health maintenance, and nutritional science. Extensive references and supplemental bibliography are provided. A conscientious and scholarly work that envisions medicine as the science of human ecology. Essential.

Stiller, Richard. *Your Body Is Trying to Tell You Something: How to Understand Its Signals and Respond to Its Needs.* New York: Harcourt, 1979. 128 pp. $6.95.
Aimed at adolescents, this health book stresses the need for attunement to the body's messages. The author discusses such topics as anxiety and stress; psychosomatic symptoms; various kinds of headaches; digestive, dermatological, and allergic reactions; sexual concerns; hormonal problems; drugs and alcohol; exercise and weight control; "health" foods and vegetarianism; insomnia; and coping with adolescent changes. Includes glossary and reading lists. A clear and practical guide, with a holistic slant.

Tubesing, Donald A. *Wholistic Health: A Whole-Person Approach to Primary Health Care.* New York: Human Sciences Pr., 1979. 232 pp. $14.95.
A minister and psychotherapist details the purpose and function of holistic

health centers. In the first five chapters, he discusses the shortcomings of standard health care and traditional concepts of health and illness. Tubesing presents the philosophy behind holistic centers and examines how this form of health care creates an atmosphere of teamwork for patients and professionals. Also discussed are modalities of care, the place of holistic centers in the community, their feasibility and future. References included. Despite a rather colorless presentation, this work may become a milestone.

Dental Care

See also Dental Care in Chapter 9, Children's Health.

Himber, Jacob. *The Complete Family Guide to Dental Health.* New York: McGraw-Hill, 1978. 147 pp. $2.95 (paper); London: McGraw-Hill. £2.20 (paper).
The author, a dentist, provides excellent advice on preventive dental care, through both diet and proper hygiene. Also covered are topics and issues concerning children's teeth, including preventive orthodontics, healthy foods, bottle-mouth syndrome, and the breast versus the bottle. Various remedial procedures are discussed, as are such special considerations as mouth guards, denture care, canker sores, headaches, and mouth cancer. Himber includes suggestions for choosing a dentist and determining when a specialist is needed. Most positive and instructive.

Nguyen, Thanh Nguyen, and de Roulf, Patty. *Your Mouth.* Radnor, PA: Chilton, 1978. 210 pp. $8.95.
Elementary, tutorial explanation of the teeth and how to avoid costly and painful dental problems. Simple descriptions are given of fluoridation, tooth decay and its causes, gum diseases, and the specialties of endodontics, pedodontics, periodontics, orthodontics, and oral surgery.

Wood, Norman. *The Complete Book of Dental Care.* New York: Hart, 1979. 336 pp. $12.95; $6.95 (paper).
Wood, a professor of oral surgery, aims to educate the consumer from the dentist's point of view and to arbitrate between the two factions, the dentist and the consumer. Wood tells how to cope with emergencies such as a toothache and bleeding gums and describes what a dentist can do for your teeth. Of special value is the advice given on how to choose and evaluate a dentist, reasonable fees, and the use of dental specialists. According to Wood, "If there are several teeth that need to be moved . . . you must go to an orthodontist. Many mouths have been destroyed by general dentists attempting to do orthodontic procedures." A unique, informative guide to dentistry from the consumer's point of view. Highly recommended.

Nutrition and Diet

Echols, Barbara E., and Arena, Jay M. *The Commonsense Guide to Good Eating.*
   Woodbury, NY: Barron, 1978. 174 pp. $4.50 (paper).
Concerned not only with weight control but also with healthful eating, the
authors provide a compact handbook on nutritional problems and issues.
Discussed are ideal nutritional requirements; five food selection goals; eating
habits; vegetarianism; health foods; weight, obesity, and dieting; shopping
and cooking tips; food equivalents and diet plans for fewer calories and better
nutrition; preventing atherosclerosis at an early age; diabetes; special problems such as food sensitivities, pregnancy, and so forth; warnings about food
poisoning. Included are notes, bibliography, and appendixes with recipes and
a detailed breakdown of vitamins and minerals. A well-written introduction
and a springboard for more thorough study.

Frank, Benjamin S., with Miele, Philip. *Doctor Frank's No-Aging Diet.* New
   York: Dell, 1978. 162 pp. $1.95 (paper).
Supporting the theory that high-quality nucleic acids can retard and even
reverse the aging process, a medical doctor provides a youth diet, heavy in fish
and legumes and other foods rich in ribonucleic acid (RNA). Vegetarians and
persons on restricted diets are also accommodated. According to Frank, the
program's benefits include glowing skin, restored health after alcoholism or
drug abuse, resistance to temperature extremes, improved breathing, cardiovascular vigor, lower cholesterol levels, better control of diabetes and
osteoarthritis. The author also reviews other theories of aging. Included are
26 pages of recipes and three appendixes that supplement Frank's thesis. An
intriguing but extreme proposition, requiring further investigation.

Fredericks, Carlton. *Carlton Frederick's High-Fiber Way to Total Health.* New
   York: Pocket Bks., 1976. 208 pp. $2.25 (paper).
A public health educator specializing in nutrition sings the praises of dietary
fiber in preventing a myriad of disorders and ensuring proper digestive
function. Claiming that even pigs eat better than most Americans, Fredericks
is especially enthusiastic about bran, wheat germ, and yogurt; especially condemning of sugar and commercially processed foods. Included are
weight control tips, high-fiber recipes, and recommended literature. A
reasonable presentation, although the astonishing claims for the value of bran
are questionable.

Galton, Lawrence. *The Truth about Fiber in Your Food.* New York: Crown, 1976.
   246 pp. OP; London: Crown. £5.40.
Reviewing the research of several scientists, a prolific medical writer explains
the crucial role of dietary fiber in disease prevention. Despite the growing
popularity of bran supplements, Galton adds, these are not as effective as

foods that retain their natural fiber content. Also included are chapters on the sugar controversy and on fiber as protection against the toxic effects of food additives and drugs. There are also a thorough chart of calorie and fiber contents in foods, numerous high-fiber recipes, and a selected bibliography. An exhaustive and complex history, simplified only in the final chapter, when Galton suggests "practicalities for the reader."

Goldstein, Jack. *Triumph Over Disease: By Fasting and Natural Diet.* New York: Arco, 1977. 245 pp. $5.95; 1978, $1.95 (paper); London: Arco. £4.50.
Because of the growing interest in the health benefits of fasting, works of this sort are inevitable. An exponent of natural hygiene, the author begins with a personal narrative of his struggle against ulcerative colitis. Attributing his recovery to the natural hygiene program of fasting and vegetarianism, Goldstein launches into a scathing review of fad diets and food additives. He then discusses the benefits of fasting, contraindications, the reasons for vegetarianism, and nine rules of food combining. Case histories and recommended literature included. Poorly organized and written. Sensationalistic.

Higdon, Hal, ed. *The Complete Diet Guide: For Runners and Other Athletes.* Mountain View, CA: World Pubns., 1978. 237 pp. $4.95 (paper).
Composed of articles by 22 contributors, this nutrition manual covers "basic nutrition, weight reduction, liquid requirements during competition," food restrictions, vegetarianism, and other special diets. Topics include common nutritional myths, such as the athlete's need for extra protein; the placebo effect of fad diets; the function and sources of essential nutrients from the athlete's point of view; food choices for competitors; pre-event meals; carbohydrate loading; the athlete's problems with sugar. Menus and recipes appended. This guide is well conceived, with nutritional wisdom for anyone concerned with rigorous exercise for total health.

McQueen-Williams, Morvyth, and Appisson, Barbara. *A Diet for 100 Healthy, Happy Years: Health Secrets from the Caucasus,* ed. by Norman Ober. Englewood Cliffs, NJ: Prentice-Hall, 1977. 220 pp. $9.95.
Contending that the longevity of the Caucasus (USSR) peoples is due primarily to their eating habits, the authors review the dietary fundamentals of this region and suggest seven nutritional tips ranging from use of fresh vegetables to pollen supplements. The work provides advice about essential vitamins and minerals, warnings about fad diets, Caucasian-based weight-loss suggestions, and information about the benefits of various herbs and botanicals. Also discussed are physical activities such as sex, walking, and gardening, for which the Caucasian life-style is the model. Appisson includes a lengthy collection of recipes, many borrowed from the Caucasus. Although many recommended dishes seem rather exotic, the authors believe that Americans can easily accept both the foodstuffs and the principles of the Caucasus. In any case, the work itself is fascinating.

Nach, Joyce D., and Long, Linda Ormiston. *Taking Charge of Your Weight and Well-Being.* Palo Alto, CA: Bull Publg. Co., 1978. 496 pp. $9.95 (paper).
Two psychologists provide a behaviorally oriented program for weight control and overall self-management. After reviewing the hazards and benefits of several diet techniques, the authors discuss setting goals, changing eating and other behavioral patterns, choosing foods the body needs, relaxing and thinking positively, coping with emotions, eating for a healthy heart, rewarding yourself, dieting with the constructive help of others, using imagery, improving self-image, managing special situations and weight maintenance, taking charge of other problem areas in your life. Included are numerous charts and forms for recording progress and mental exercises designed to reinforce resolve. A practical but somewhat complex manual.

Reuben, David. *Everything You Always Wanted to Know about Nutrition.* New York: Simon & Schuster, 1978. 287 pp. $9.95.
Dr. Reuben in this book denounces "the chemicalized, denutrified, contaminated, deeply embalmed garbage we incorrectly refer to as a 'modern diet.' " "People of America," he declares, "the greatest threat to your survival and that of your children is not some terrible nuclear weapon. It is what you are going to eat from your dinner plate tonight." In a most entertaining style, he discusses vitamins, minerals, trace elements, fats, carbohydrates, protein, sugar, and the ideal diet. For 99.9 percent of Americans, most of the dollars spent on vitamins are wasted; orange juice is a poor source of Vitamin C; taking iron supplements is expensive and hazardous and an adequate supply of minerals can be obtained from fresh, wholesome, unprocessed food; the amount of cholesterol ingested has nothing to do with heart attacks; eggs are good for you; "balloon" bread is devoid of all nutritional value and breakfast "cereal" is 88.18 percent refined sugar and starch; refined sugar has no benefit in the human diet and is poisoning the masses. Reuben outlines his ideal diet—the Carbohydrate Survival Plan—and provides a yes and no list of what to eat. Reserved for special condemnation are the big food processors, "who spend over two billion dollars each year to make you eat inferior, chemical-laden, artificial and imitation food" and the Food and Drug Administration, which, Reuben alleges, has ties with the food industry. Crisp, controversial, stimulating, opinionated—and food for thought.

Ross, Shirley. *Fasting.* New York: St. Martin's, 1975. 122 pp. $7.95; New York: Ballantine, 1976. $1.75 (paper); London: Sheldon. £3.50; Pan Bks. £0.70 (paper).
Fasting, according to the author, is a mystical experience. In discussing the various motives involved and reporting case histories, her enthusiasm is obvious. The merit of this book, however, rests on its health information. Not only does Ross detail the physical effects of fasting but she also spells out its contraindications, the need for medical supervision, and the safest ways to break the fast. The value of this information is undeniable, whether or not fasting is accepted as a healthy means of cleansing the body.

Sheinken, David, et al. *The Food Connection: How the Things You Eat Affect the Way You Feel.* Indianapolis: Bobbs-Merrill, 1979. 207 pp. $10.
Two psychiatrists and a medical writer collaborate on this work about brain sensitivity to certain foods and chemicals. Asserting that numerous physical and psychological symptoms can be so explained, the authors suggest various tests for identifying causal substances. Fasting, eliminating suspicious foods, a pulse test, kinesiologic testing, or four laboratory procedures can be used for diagnosis. Also discussed are combined sensitivities, stress, and other complications, as well as various treatments. Appendixes include information on common symptoms, food families, tests, diets, and resource organizations. Notes and bibliography included. A reasonable and dispassionate work, attuned to the ideal of total wellness.

Shute, Wilfrid E. *Health Preserver: Defining the Versatility of Vitamin E.* Emmaus, PA: Rodale, 1977. 167 pp. $7.95; London: Rodale. £4.75.
A Canadian cardiologist asserts that large doses of Vitamin E, alpha tocopherol, are instrumental in preventing or treating numerous disorders. Among these are circulatory problems such as varicose veins, intermittent claudication (limping), thrombophlebitis; various heart conditions; diabetes mellitus; multiple sclerosis; nephritis; rheumatoid arthritis; stomach ulcers; bone infections; vision problems; leukoplakia; shingles; and burns. Several case histories and letters support the author's arguments, but Shute admits that the medical establishment has been slow to endorse this "miracle" nutrient.

Stare, Frederick J., and Whelan, Elizabeth M. *Eat OK Feel OK! Food Facts and Your Health.* North Quincy, MA: Christopher, 1978. 320 pp. $9.75.
This book is well written and easy to read. Two nutrition experts with academic credentials describe the basic facts of good nutrition, explaining in detail the body's need for protein, carbohydrates, fats, minerals, and water. Also discussed are sodium, cholesterol, fiber, and alcohol; reading labels; food storage; beneficial and harmful additives; weight-loss advice and warnings; "the folly of fads"; and such special considerations as nutrition during pregnancy, breast-feeding, diet and the Pill, nutrition for children and the elderly, vegetarianism, and restricted diets. Appendixes include low-caloric and low-cholesterol menus, suggested readings and informational sources, glossary, and a nutrition quiz. Sane and comprehensive. Highly recommended.

Sussman, Vic S. *The Vegetarian Alternative: A Guide to a Healthful and Humane Diet.* Emmaus, PA: Rodale, 1978. 286 pp. $6.95 (paper); London: Rodale. £3.50.
In an effort to explain the rationale behind meatless eating, the author discusses the protein controversy, the form and function of human teeth, the hazards of eating meat, slaughter and other sins of the meat industry, ethical considerations, plant sensitivity, the world food crisis. Regarding the health

effects of vegetarianism, Sussman disputes the arguments that meatless eating is a risky and often complicated endeavor and contends that the vegetarian diet is naturally low in cholesterol and saturated fats. He promotes, further- more, a health regimen involving vegetarianism; regular exercise and rest, "plus the avoidance of highly processed and fabricated foods, excessive sugar and salt, tobacco, and excessive alcohol and drug use." Also included are descriptions of vegetarian types, foods of special interest, recipes, and an annotated bibliography. Although Sussman tends to overemphasize the ethi- cal issues, he documents his assertions well and eschews hysterical health claims.

Wordsworth, Jill. *Diet Revolution: Nutrition, Diets, and Food Fads: What the Experts Haven't Told You.* New York: St. Martin's, 1977. 188 pp. $7.95.
Warning against the "unscientific and over-simplified" arguments of many "self-styled experts," the author explores nutritional theories and controver- sies in order to separate fact from fallacy. Among the topics covered are nature cure, macrobiotics, vegetarianism, the case against excess protein, the whole-food theory, organic farming, the diseases of civilization and their various risk factors, nutritional deficiencies and "wonder" nutrients, additives and food pollution, and health foods. According to Wordsworth, the evidence points to the simple need to eat a balanced diet, emphasize whole foods, avoid those that are overly processed, and modify intake as the body ages. Bibliog- raphy included. With highly informative end-of-chapter "dialogues," this work offers a rational approach to selecting nutrition books and evaluating the claims of hobbyhorse riders.

Physical Fitness and Exercise

Agress, Clarence M. *Energetics.* New York: Grosset & Dunlap, 1979. 166 pp. $4.95 (paper).
The chief cardiologist at Cedars of Lebanon Hospital explains an exercise program that utilizes the principle of "dash training." Also called interval training, this is "a form of interrupted, rather than continuous, exercise; that is, periods of vigorous activity are alternated with periods of lesser activity." According to the author, this technique is ideal for heart patients and other high-risk individuals. Agress provides much valuable material on the benefits of exercise, safety in sports, tennis as dash training, coronary risk factors, and other cardiovascular concerns. Includes material on exercise testing, instruc- tions in cardiopulmonary resuscitation and pulse taking; extensive bibliog- raphy. A conscientious and articulate presentation, strongly emphasizing the relationship between exercise and heart health. Recommended.

Cooper, Kenneth H. *The Aerobics Way.* New York: Evans, 1977. 311 pp. $10; New York: Bantam, 1978. $2.50 (paper); London: Corgi, £0.85 (paper).
Called the "bible of the fitness movement," this work has extensive material on cardiovascular risk factors. The effect of aerobics on the heart and blood

vessels is explained, and advice on initiating a fitness program includes warnings against strenuous exercise when certain conditions exist. Exercise instructions are provided, along with several charts for marking progress. Also discussed is the importance of nutrition to cardiovascular health and the shortcomings of certain popular diets. Included in the appendix are coronary-risk factor charts, stress testing centers in the United States, and Cooper's point system tables. References provided. Conscientious and most persuasive; highly recommended.

Crabbe, Buster. *Energistics: The Simple Shape-Up Exercise Program.* Chicago: Playboy Pr., 1976. 158 pp. OP.
The author, an Olympic swimming champion and popular actor, presents his program for better general health and longer life through exercise, weight control, and relaxation. With a lenient, vitamin-conscious diet and a simple exercise routine, an individual can attain physical fitness regardless of initial condition. Crabbe reviews the necessary precautions that should be taken, especially when the novice is older, substantially overweight, or addicted to cigarettes. He also provides 16 workout tables from which personally tailored programs can be designed. Understandably, swimming and water exercises are prominently featured. A reasonable, but unexceptional work.

Getchell, Bud. *Physical Fitness: A Way of Life.* New York: Wiley, 1976. 300 pp. $7.45; Chichester, Sussex: Wiley, £4.30 (paper).
Divided into three sections, this text discusses the rationale behind physical fitness, methods, and related considerations. The author details the health benefits of exercise, provides a battery of tests for personal fitness appraisal, and supplies a thorough prescription for developing a personal program. Four exercise categories are considered: activities designed to loosen, stretch, shape, and strengthen the major muscle groups; those promoting cardiorespiratory endurance; weight training; and advanced procedures. Also discussed are the combined roles of nutrition and exercise in weight control, the role of activity in preventing heart disease, sports for a lifetime of fitness and fun. Included are supplementary readings and charts for further personal appraisal. A well-illustrated, extremely practical work.

Kuntzleman, Charles. *The Exerciser's Handbook.* New York: McKay, 1978. 276 pp. $10.95.
Using a question-and-answer format, the author discusses the physical benefits of exercise, plus several ways of getting the most return for the effort expended. Topics include tension and inactivity, aerobics and cardiovascular endurance, sexual improvement, the hazards of obesity, exercise and appetite, coronary-risk factors and prevention, relief of back pain, exercise and arthritis, respiratory problems, diabetes, longevity, psychological and intellectual benefits of exercise. Also discussed are frequency and length of exercise, pulse rates, blood pressure, quantifying aerobic exercises, sports for fitness,

shaping exercises, exercise for women and different age groups, weather considerations, nutrition, athletic ailments, the few who should not exercise. Warm-up and cool-down exercises are appended. An extremely detailed, reliable presentation, despite the format constrictions. Recommended.

Kuntzleman, Charles T., and the editors of *Consumer Guide. Rating the Exercises.* New York: Penguin, 1980. 348 pp. $2.95 (paper).
This informative book is designed to present the facts about exercise and discuss the advantages and disadvantages of specific sports and programs. Among the topics covered are the ways in which exercise helps the heart, aerobics and other cardiovascular exercise programs, and pulse-rated exercise plans. Citing various experts and studies, the authors rate popular activities for overall fitness benefits and issue warnings regarding their safety. Comparative rating chart; program outlines. An objective, encyclopedic reference aid.

Lyttle, Richard B. *The Complete Beginner's Guide to Physical Fitness.* New York: Doubleday, 1978. 152 pp. $6.95.
Directed at both children and adults, this work contains basic exercises and instructions; elementary information about physiology, metabolism, and nutrition; and two tests of physical fitness. The author suggests specific stretching and flexing exercises, aerobics, yoga movements, isometrics, and weight-lifting exercises. From the standpoint of health, this guide is uninformative and hardly worthy of the term "complete."

Mitchell, Curtis. *The Perfect Exercise: The Hop, Skip, and Jump Way to Health.* New York: Simon & Schuster, 1976. 189 pp. $6.95.
The author recommends jumping rope as an aerobic exercise that strengthens the heart, reduces weight, builds endurance, and improves agility and balance. In addition to singing the praises of this form of exercise, Mitchell provides practical advice about designing a personal program and issues appropriate warnings. Bibliography included. Suprisingly good.

Morehouse, Laurence, E., and Gross, Leonard. *Maximum Performance.* New York: Simon & Schuster, 1977. 353 pp. $8.95; St. Albans, Herts: Hart-Davis. £3.50.
A physiologist and professor of kinesiology, the study of human movement, Morehouse presents strategies designed to improve performance in every area of life, not merely in sports. Especially interesting are his 15 "kinesiological secrets," tips for moving like a champion. Emphasis is placed on balancing tension and relaxation. Also discussed are avoiding and managing illness and injury, coaching the child, and tips for specific sports. Although the work has some general applications, it is primarily devoted to body conditioning for "maximum performance" in sports. Extremely practical but written from

the perspective of an overly enthusiastic coach; not particularly oriented to wellness.

Pipes, Thomas V., and Vodak, Paul A. *The Pipes Fitness Test and Prescription.* Los Angeles: Tarcher, 1978. 186 pp. $8.95; $3.95 (paper).
The authors provide and interpret fitness tests for self-evalution of cardiovascular health, body composition and fat percentage, muscular strength and endurance, flexibility. For each of these crucial components of fitness, Pipes and Vodak then prescribe general goals and procedures. In a chapter on sports, warm-up and cool-down exercises are suggested and 16 popular activities are evaluated. Suggested readings are included. A highly instructive, health-conscious presentation.

Smith, David. *The East/West Exercise Book.* New York: McGraw-Hill, 1976. 224 pp. $7.95 (paper).
The author provides an illustrated exercise program based on such diverse systems as Hatha yoga, Kundalini, T'ai Chi Ch'uan, Arica, bioenergetic exercises, endurance training, mime, isometrics, and isotonics. Offering five "cycles" of increasingly difficult exercises, the program is ideal for beginners. Also included are suggested exercises for the office and a discussion of the physical fitness benefits of sports and games.

Solomon, Neil, and Harrison, Evalee. *Doctor Solomon's Proven Master Plan for Total Body Fitness and Maintenance.* New York: Berkley, 1978. 192 pp. $2.25 (paper).
Beginning with a review of the cosmetic and holistic benefits of exercise, the authors appraise various fitness "fads," including yoga, aerobics, and massage; and provide guidelines for assessing individual needs and preparing a suitable program. Recommended exercises are illustrated for eight anatomical areas of concentration. Also discussed are ways of coping with fatigue, exercises for back pain, exercises for sexual fitness, eating awareness, movement therapy, and relaxation techniques. Glossary is included. A conservative work that stresses caution and consultation with a personal physician; of little value to those concerned with cardiovascular exercises.

Spino, Dyveke. *New Age Training for Fitness and Health.* New York: Grove, 1979. 273 pp. $12.50.
The author, a clinical psychologist and cofounder of the Esalen Sports Center, describes health not only as the absence of disease but also as "the presence of adequate endurance, flexibility, strength, and mental powers." In this work, she provides a life-style review, exercises for training the will, nutritional advice emphasizing foods without chemicals or sugar, exercises for the spine, training guidelines for men and women, and a review of holistic healing modalities. References supplied. A positive, joyful presentation that stresses the need for natural balance through personal choices and a transcendental attitude.

Tulloh, Bruce. *Natural Fitness.* New York: Simon & Schuster, 1977. 192 pp.
$8.95; London: Arrow. £0.75 (paper).
Reviewing the natural life of the primitive hunter and farmer, the author
contends that urban dwellers are susceptible to degenerative diseases primarily because of their relative inactivity. Tulloh, a biologist and Olympic athlete,
discusses the physical and psychological benefits of exercise, muscular
strength, endurance, flexibility, body weight, the circulatory and respiratory
systems, smoking, stress tolerance, and sex. Included is advice on assessing
personal fitness, designing an exercise program, three 12-week programs for
different levels of performance, equipment and other practical considerations, specific indoor exercises. Caloric consumption and energy expenditure
charts and a bibliography are provided. A thorough and philosophical guide.

Van Aaken, Ernst. *Van Aaken Method,* trans. by George Beinhorn. Mountain
View, CA: World Pubns., 1976. 135 pp. $3.95 (paper).
A German physician, world-famous among runners, discusses health and
fitness, oxygen and endurance, training with his "pure endurance method,"
participation by women and children, and diet. According to the author, "the
central thought" of his method is "to continuously increase oxygen uptake
capacity by long, daily endurance exercise at a moderate, even slow pace."
More intense training is not recommended because it produces a harmful
"oxygen debt." Van Aaken also contends that the various "diseases of civilization" ultimately are caused by oxygen deficiency, overeating, and weakness of
will. With regular endurance running plus a diet of less than 1,600 calories,
the effects of stress can be alleviated and serious health problems avoided.
Even the risk of cancer is said to diminish when the body receives an optimal
oxygen supply through endurance training. A most intriguing proposition.

Zohman, Lenore R, Kattus, Alberta, and Softness, Donald G. *The Cardiologists'
Guide to Fitness and Health through Exercise.* New York: Simon & Schuster,
1979. 320 pp. $10.95.
The authors are exercise cardiologists who specialize in stress testing and
exercise therapy. They believe that exercise, together with a sound diet and no
smoking, is the simplest, most vital activity for maintaining good health. An
excellent, authoritative guide to walking, jogging, running, marathoning;
fitness activities; sports; health clubs, gymnasiums and fitness centers; exercise equipment; heart disease and sexual performance. Directions are given
for exercise as treatment for heart patients. Includes good diagrams, illustrations, and glossary. Highly recommended.

Running

Fixx, James F. *The Complete Book of Running.* New York: Random, 1977.
314 pp. $10.
This encyclopedic work has been lauded as one of the best available. In three
parts it discusses the "why," the "art," and the "world" of running. Though not

focusing on the health benefits of this exercise type, it presents relevant material in such chapters as "feeling better physically," "the longevity factor," and "the world's sickest running club." Appendixes covering the physiology of running and the Harvard Step Test, a stress test, are also valuable. Bibliography included.

Kostrubala, Thaddeus. *The Joy of Running.* Philadelphia: Lippincott, 1976. 159 pp. $8.95; New York: Pocket Bks., 1977. $1.95 (paper).
The author, a physician, endorses running as an exercise that lessens the risk of heart attack and promotes overall mental and physical health. A major topic is the relationship between exercise and heart function and disease. Describing his own "conversion" to running, Kostrubala provides tips to help others follow suit. Bibliography included.

Lance, Kathryn. *Running for Health and Beauty: A Complete Guide for Women.* Indianapolis: Bobbs Merrill, 1977. 193 pp. $8.95; New York: Bantam, 1978. $2.25 (paper); London: Proteus. £4.50.
Emphasizing the value of aerobics, this work explains why women need exercise and discusses both procedures and problems of running. Especially worthwhile are chapters on menstruation, pregnancy, rape, and other concerns unique to women; common injuries; warming up and other safety measures; nutrition and weight loss. Lance also covers such diverse topics as shoes, weather, scheduling, and competition. An enthusiastic, responsible presentation.

Mollen, Art. *Run for Your Life.* New York: Dolphin, 1978. 154 pp. $4.95 (paper).
Stressing the cardiovascular benefits of running, the author advocates a total exercise program, including cessation of smoking and adoption of a nutritious diet. Dr. Mollen, who prescribes exercise regimens for patients, details the positive physiological changes deriving from exercise. Included is an appendix with capsule advice for joggers. Most informative, but overemphasizing the marathon aspect of running.

Sheehan, George A. *Dr. George Sheehan's Medical Advice for Runners.* Mountain View, CA: World Pubns., 1978. 307 pp. $10.95.
A cardiologist and ardent exponent of running provides a medical encyclopedia that covers "diseases of excellence" and sports medicine; running for health; stress, overtraining, and exhaustion; illnesses such as mononucleosis and colds; the effects of weather, altitude, pollution, and running surface on health and performance; and psychological considerations. There are also chapters on the musculoskeletal, cardiovascular, respiratory, gastrointestinal, and other body systems. Among the topics discussed are foot care and shoes, bone and muscle injuries, breathing, nutrition and liquids, headaches, smoking, and concerns of women who run. A comprehensive, practical, and most enjoyable book.

Steincrohn, Peter. *How to Cure Your Joggermania! Enjoy Fitness and Good Health without Running.* Cranbury, NJ: Barnes, 1979. 206 pp. $9.95.

Steincrohn maintains that "if you're pushing forty, that's exercise enough." He doubts that jogging is the panacea sought for the control of obesity, anxiety, and hypertension and the myriad of other woes that beset us: "The normal-weighted, relaxed person who does not smoke, drink, or overwork and who lives without tension is more likely to be healthier and to live longer than his neighbor who tends to be overweight, jogs and goes through a variety of bodily contortions." Steincrohn recommends milder forms of exertion such as walking, gardening, swimming, and golfing—in moderation. The importance of controlling consumption of alcohol, cigarettes, and coffee is emphasized together with the need for relaxation. A provocative book.

Stress and Relaxation

Anderson, Robert A. *Stress Power: How to Turn Tension into Energy.* New York: Human Sciences Pr., 1978. 248 pp. $9.95.

A veteran physician involved in the holistic health movement discusses the possibility of avoiding the negative effects of stress by coping in positive and creative ways. Divided into three parts, the book covers the nature and manifestations of stress in mind and body, including specific disorders and self-destructive habits such as overeating and smoking; a functional model of humans, emphasizing the feedback process; and various kinds of coping behavior. Among these are such unsatisfying answers as medication, manipulation of the environment, and other surface changes; and such constructive responses as physical exercise, creative pursuits, conscious passive relaxation, meditation, goal setting, and positive visualizations. Notes and bibliography are provided. Recommended by Hans Selye (author of *Stress without Distress*), this challenging work is especially appropriate for the educated reader.

Benson, Herbert, and Klipper, Miriam Z. *The Relaxation Response.* New York: Avon, 1976. 222 pp.. $1.95 (paper); London: Fount Paperbacks. £0.75 (paper).

Benson provides insight into the nature of stress, the dangers of hypertension, and the elements essential for the success of the relaxation response—quiet environment, an object to dwell on, passive attitude, and a comfortable stance. He advocates the use of a meditation technique (relaxation response) to protect against the destructive effects of stress. Readable explanation of the importance of meditation techniques.

Brown, Barbara B. *Stress and the Art of Biofeedback.* New York: Harper, 1977. 298 pp. $12.50; New York: Bantam, 1978. $2.25 (paper); London: Bantam. £1.25 (paper).

An expert in psychiatry, pharmacology, and cardiovascular physiology presents a scholarly and comprehensive exposition of the value of biofeedback in controlling stress-related problems. According to the author, "biofeedback is a creation of the patient," rather than a tool of the health professional. "In its most elementary form, biofeedback is simply the providing of information about physiologic activities to the patient along with an instruction to change the physiologic activity in a specific direction. The patient does the rest." This form of therapy can be used to relieve muscle tension, headaches, insomnia, essential hypertension, bruxism (grinding teeth), hyperactivity, drug abuse, gastrointestinal complaints, and other problems. Appendixes include specific relaxation exercises; references and additional readings are listed. Although this work is intended for lay use, only the well-educated will comprehend many of its technical passages. An impressive book, nevertheless.

Dudley, Donald L., and Welke, Elton. *How to Survive Being Alive.* New York: Doubleday, 1977. 179 pp. $6.95; New York: NAL, 1979. $1.95 (paper).
A psychiatrist and a journalist collaborate on an excellent discussion of stress and its health effects. Subscribing to the holistic view that the mind and body are functionally inseparable, the authors explore psychobiological responses to frustration and life change. Reviewed here are several studies and stress scales, demonstrating that "the greater the amount of life change the worse the illness" that follows. Also discussed are several stress-related disorders and symptoms, both destructive and constructive coping behaviors, the need for moderate levels of both activity and relaxation, and beneficial responses to stressors. A nine-point "checklist for survival" and a lengthy bibliography are included. Pragmatic and readable; highly recommended.

Fast, Julius, with Fast, Barbara. *Creative Coping: A Guide to Positive Living.* New York: Morrow, 1976. 192 pp. $6.95.
These authors discuss stress and coping, using excellent anecdotes to illustrate their points. They review both destructive and healthful responses, including aggression, flexibility, empathy games, masking, and fantasy. Also explored are some of the predictable stress crises that people face during different stages of their lives. According to the authors, constructive coping involves certain basic steps: the gathering of information about a specific problem, internal organization, personal autonomy, and anticipation. References are provided. A perceptive and readable book that emphasizes the need for individuality and self-esteem.

Goldberg, Philip. *Executive Health: How to Recognize Health Danger Signals and Manage Stress Successfully.* A Business Week Book. New York: McGraw-Hill, 1978. 272 pp. $9.95.
An advocate of holistic living, Goldberg provides an encyclopedic handbook on recognizing and managing stress. Among the topics covered are the nature and causes of stress; physical and psychological symptoms of stress disorders; major illnesses such as atherosclerosis, hypertension, and other cardiovascular problems; ulcers; diabetes; headaches and migraines; medical checkups and care recommendations; tips for quitting cigarettes and for handling

alcohol; stress susceptible ("Type A") personalities; psychological strategies and services; exercise programs, precautions, and gear; nutrition, cholesterol, diet, sugar, vitamins, and minerals; mental relaxation techniques such as abdominal breathing, self-massage, progressive relaxation, biofeedback, transcendental meditation; sleep and insomnia; health management. Also provided are the Glazer stress-control questionnaire, Nathan Pritikin's maximum weight-loss diet, charts of life-change risks and of vitamins and minerals that affect stress control, and numerous other tools for evaluating and improving behavior. End-of-chapter references. An essential work.

Kinzer, Nora Scott. *Stress and the American Woman*. New York: Doubleday, 1979. 272 pp. $8.95.
Kinzer presents a most insightful and readable description of stress and its relationship to health and disease, marriage and children, drugs, alcohol, food, and mental illness. The book concludes with an excellent chapter on stress and coping. Well written, sensible, and devoid of jargon.

McLean, Alan A. *Work Stress*. Reading, MA: Addison-Wesley, 1979. 142 pp. $6.50.
The author is eastern area medical director of the IBM Corporation. McLean has produced a terse, well-written, informative summary on the vulnerability of individuals to stress, stressful events and conditions at work, and the broad social context of stress (health and safety practices of the employer, management attitudes, morale and employee participation in decision-making processes). Particularly helpful are chapters relating to personal coping strategies such as meditation, Benson's relaxation technique (*The Relaxation Response*), clinically standardized meditation, exercise, progressive relaxation, biofeedback, and professional intervention. A "coping checklist" is provided for readers to score their own strengths and weaknesses. Thought-provoking and relevant. Recommended.

Mitchell, Laura. *Simple Relaxation: The Physiological Method of Easing Tension*. New York: Atheneum, 1979. 163 pp. $8.95; London: Murray. £1.95 (paper).
Described as a series of "orders" that quickly relieve physical tension, the author's method of relaxation is designed for use during stressful periods. After discussing stress and the body's response to it, Mitchell explains in detail how to apply her technique, and when. Brief material is also provided concerning transcendental meditation and the relaxation response, biofeedback, and disassociation. References and suggestions for further reading are included. Satisfactory but uninspiring.

Norfolk, Donald. *The Stress Factor*. New York: Simon & Schuster, 1979. 224 pp. $8.95.
An analysis of the biology, origin, and control of stress by a management

consultant. Sensible advice is given on how to control and channel stress at work and at home. Norfolk believes that failure to adapt to stress leads to sickness, depression, loss of self-esteem, and low achievement. Readable, with a bibliography for further exploration.

Pelletier, Kenneth R. *Mind as Healer, Mind as Slayer: A Holistic Approach to Preventing Stress Disorders.* New York: Delacorte, 1977. $10; Dell, $4.95 (paper); London: Allen and Unwin. £5.95.
A clinical psychologist concerned with psychosomatic medicine discusses the health effects of stress and methods of controlling it. Among the topics covered are the individual's psychophysiological reactions to stress, including the fight-or-flight response and environmental stress triggers; personality types and afflictions such as hypertension and atherosclerosis, migraine, cancer, arthritis, and respiratory disease; and the value of meditation, biofeedback, autogenic training, and visualization in alleviating stress. In the final chapter, Pelletier reviews the progress toward a holistic medicine. Extensive bibliography is included. A scholarly and thought-provoking work, widely recognized as a holistic milestone.

Rosen, Gerald. *The Relaxation Book: An Illustrated Self-Help Program.* Englewood Cliffs, NJ: Prentice-Hall, 1978. 135 pp. $9.95; $3.95 (paper); London: Prentice-Hall. £6.95; £2.90 (paper).
Beginning with a review of the "relaxation response" and suggestions for self-assessment of tension, a psychologist provides a workbook for learning relaxation skills. Included are detailed instructions for relaxing different muscle groups, concentrating on a key word, and controlled breathing. Suggested program sessions, log sheets and assessment forms, quizzes, and recommended readings are also given. There is extremely little material on mental relaxation. Disappointing.

Selye, Hans. *Stress without Distress,* New York: NAL, 1975. 193 pp. $1.95 (paper); London: Hodder. £2.75; £1.25 (paper).
A guide to constructively managing stress. Good stress fosters creativity, well-being, and harmony while *distress* leads to ulcers, hypertension, and destructive effects on the body. Selye advocates self-responsibility and positive achievement. A philosophical rather than medical book that has become a well-deserved classic.

Speads, Carola H. *Breathing: The ABC's.* New York: Harper, 1978. 122 pp. $10.95; $4.95 (paper).
Contending that the quality of breathing has suffered as a result of the stresses of modern life, the author explains the respiratory process in detail and provides specific "experiments" by which breathing can be improved. In these experiments various movements, positions, or other "stimuli" are used to

trigger desired breathing reactions. Speads emphasizes, however, that there is no *one* way of breathing that is right for all situations, that breathing will vary depending on our needs of the moment. Sensitive yet down-to-earth; an ideal aid to stress control and body awareness. Highly recommended.

Weston, Lee. *Body Rhythm: The Circadian Rhythms within You*. New York: Harcourt, 1979. 170 pp. $8.95.
A free-lance writer discusses the daily rhythms that flow through every living creature. Although much of this book is devoted to the problem of jet lag, there are insightful chapters on such health concerns as sleep, stress, and the rhythms that affect us in sickness as well as in health. According to Weston, for instance, "stress, rhythms, fatigue, and some diseases appear to be as intertwined as a spider web." Physical or emotional problems can upset the body's rhythms, and disturbed rhythms likewise can adversely affect the state of health. Extensive notes and bibliography are supplied. An interesting work, though it offers little practical advice for self-help or personal adjustment.

Sleep

Coates, Thomas J., and Thoresen, Carl E. *How to Sleep Better: A Drug Free Program for Overcoming Insomnia*. The Self-Management Psychology Series. Englewood Cliffs, NJ: Prentice-Hall, 1977. 324 pp. $10.95; $4.95 (paper); London: Prentice-Hall. £8; £3.60 (paper).
In this scholarly self-help book, the authors discuss the rationale for behavioral approaches to insomnia, current scientific theories about sleep, and specific techniques for improving sleep. Contents include strategies for self-awareness, relaxation tips, and specialized skills such as cognitive focusing, improving sleep rhythms, and breaking out of the negative thinking cycle. Among the resource materials are a table of behavioral treatments for insomnia, a review of research issues, professionally oriented readings, and a directory of sleep-disorder centers. Although the work has technical sections, its many practical worksheets and diary forms clearly establish its value for the educated layperson.

Colligan, Douglas. *Creative Insomnia*. New York: Franklin Watts. 1979. 184 pp. $3.95.
A readable digest of current knowledge on sleep and sleep disorders. Colligan discusses the nature and causes of insomnia and describes the research conducted at sleep labs where insomnia is diagnosed and treated. Also covered are the various types of sleeping pills, methods of relaxation, and self-help checklists. As alternatives, Colligan suggests stargazing, reading boring books, genealogy, prayer power, and consumer activism. A list of sleep clinics is appended.

Gnap, John J., with Flaster, Nancy. *Easy Sleep*. New York: Stein & Day, 1978. 168 pp. $8.95; New York: Ballantine, 1979. $2.25 (paper).
A physician describes his method of overcoming insomnia without sleeping pills and other panaceas. Gnap's technique involves behavior modification by unwinding, directing energy toward conducive imaginary scenes, and drifting. In this way the brain's "can't sleep imprint" is eventually erased. Included are case histories, a question-and-answer section, notes and references. A simplistic approach to an often complex problem.

Goldberg, Philip, and Kaufman, Daniel. *Natural Sleep (How to Get Your Share)*. Emmaus, PA: Rodale, 1978. 328 pp. $10.95; $7.95 (paper); London: Rodale, £5.95; £3.25 (paper).
Focusing on the problem of insomnia, the authors discuss the function of sleep, causes of insomina, the case against sleeping pills, and possible treatments and strategies. These range from therapies for distinct medical problems; stress control through meditation, biofeedback, daytime names, and other relaxation techniques; helpful nutrients and foods to avoid; psychological approaches; living with a typical internal clock; courting sleep through regularity, bedtime rituals, ideal bedroom settings; massage, breathing techniques, sleep positions, and other in-bed considerations. For the chronic insomniac who finds no relief in this book, the authors provide a chapter on sleep centers, including a discussion by five specialists and a directory of sleep clinics and professionals. Also included are several charts and self-evaluation questionnaires, expert testimony on over-the-counter sleep aids, detailed materials on specific prescription drugs, concise descriptions of various sleep disorders, and a bibliography. Encyclopedic and thoroughly practical.

Trubo, Richard. *How to Get a Good Night's Sleep*. Boston: Little, 1978. 220 pp. $7.95.
It is estimated that 30 million Americans are currently taking prescribed or over-the-counter medications for sleep. Some 150 million dollars are spent on prescription sedatives annually. Trubo, in association with the editors of *Modern Medicine,* has compiled a highly readable compendium of current information on sleep and sleep disorders. Descriptions are also provided of sleep apnea, nocturnal myoclonus (restless legs syndrome), narcolepsy, and childhood disorders such as bed-wetting, tooth grinding, and sleep talking. Particularly valuable is the discussion of the common prescription drugs—barbiturates, benzodiazepines (Dalmane), chloral hydrate, methaqualone, glutethimide (Doriden), tranquilizers, and antidepressants. The author considers that the case against long-term use of most hypnotic drugs is overwhelming. Likewise, over-the-counter drugs such as Sominex offer little benefit to the average poor sleeper. L-Tryptophan, in dosages of 2 to 3 grams daily, offers great hope as being a substitute for hypnotics. A list of sleep-disorder clinics and a bibliography are provided. Informative and calculated to put you to sleep, on purpose. Highly recommended.

The Mind-Body Connection

Benson, Herbert. *The Mind/Body Effect.* New York: Simon & Schuster, 1979. 190 pp. $8.95.
A leading proponent of behavioral medicine documents the relationship between disease states and psychological factors. Among the topics covered are voodoo death and its modern equivalents, the dichotomy between mind and body in Western medicine, the placebo effect, the psychological aspects of pain sensation and relief, the relaxation response, and other approaches of behavioral medicine. The author also suggests that if emotional factors exacerbate hypertension, then some detection campaigns could start a course toward iatrogenic (physician-induced) hypertension. "Generally," Dr. Benson advises, "when you feel well, you are well. You should not seek excessive reassurance, such as repeated blood pressure recordings, when there are no medical complaints. You should not allow unwarranted worries about health to develop. The worries themselves may create a disease." A stimulating, readable book.

Bry, Adelaide. *EST: 60 Hours That Transform Your Life.* New York: Harper, 1976. 182 pp $7.95.
A favorable introduction to Erhard Seminars Training (est), this work by a counseling psychologist is an exposition of a technique designed to strengthen the sense of personal responsibility, to "transform the level at which you experience life so that living becomes a process of expanding satisfaction." According to Werner Erhard himself, this book is "readable, accurate, and gives a balanced view of est"; but the work, like the program, is clearly a subjective product of the author's own experiences and those of selected graduates. Relevant to Ardell's view (*Higher Level Wellness*), est is increasingly recognized as a legitimate holistic tool, but one that defies description.

Fredericks, Carlton. *Psycho-Nutrition.* New York: Grosset & Dunlap, 1976. 224 pp. $8.95; $3.95 (paper).
A prolific nutritionist proposes that nutritional deficiencies and sensitivities may affect mental and emotional health. Among the disorders covered are hypoglycemia, schizophrenia, psychoallergy depression, and hyperactivity. Fredericks also asserts that many of these disorders can be alleviated with special diets and supplements of vitamins and minerals. A resource directory is appended but no references are supplied. Although the author's arguments overemphasize nutritional factors, the work makes a good case for further study in this area.

Galton, Lawrence. *You May Not Need a Psychiatrist: How Your Body May Control Your Mind.* New York: Simon & Schuster, 1979. 292 pp. OP.
Galton, a medical writer, presents innumerable case histories to illustrate that many apparent psychological problems actually have physical causes. De-

scribed as "somatopsychic" by the author, these disorders are the reverse of those psychosomatic ailments where physical symptoms have emotional roots. Heart abnormalities, anemia, thyroid problems, scabies, tumors, epilepsy, water on the brain, allergies, hypoglycemia, nutritional deficiencies, and reactions to caffeine, tobacco, and other drugs are just some of the physical culprits identified in this work. Despite Galton's painstaking efforts and respectable references. the book offers too many case histories and too little practical information.

Lowen, Alexander, and Lowen, Leslie. *The Way to Vibrant Health: A Manual of Bioenergetic Exercises.* New York: Harper, 1977. 166 pp. $4.95 (paper).
According to the author, bioenergetics is "a way of understanding personality in terms of the body and its energetic processes." A method of psychotherapy developed by Dr. Lowen, bioenergetics employs specific physical exercises for relieving the muscle tension and energy drain caused by emotional stress. This work explains techniques for vibration and motility, breathing, sexuality, self-possession and self-expression, and sensing or "being in touch." Numerous exercises are detailed, but the author argues that these should be used in conjunction with therapy sessions. Resource addresses are appended. While several statements appear far-fetched, Lowen is reasonable in proposing that "the mind reflects what is happening in the body and vice versa."

Luby, Sue. *Hatha Yoga for Total Health: Handbook of Practical Programs.* Englewood Cliffs, NJ: Prentice-Hall, 1977. 254 pp. $16; $11.95 (paper); London: Prentice-Hall. £11.70; £8 (paper).
According to the author, hatha yoga "signifies the perfect knowledge of . . . the positive sun and negative moon energies, their joining in perfect harmony and complete equilibrium, and the ability to control their energies yoked within the control we have of our bodies." Unlike exercise programs for muscular development only, hatha yoga seeks the perfect functioning of all organs through controlled movement and breathing techniques. Luby, as an experienced instructor, provides various movements and poses for different body areas, basic and special breathing techniques, relaxation tips, five possible schedules, and recommended techniques for children and teens, expectant mothers, office workers, and older persons. Preparatory advice includes material on nutrition and fasting, sleep, smoking, and a section on special yoga covers the body's problem areas, fatigue and tension reduction, and yoga for special health problems such as arthritis, headaches, insomnia, and weight control. Selected references are included. A well-illustrated, valid aid to wellness. Recommended.

Marx, Ina. *Yoga and Common Sense,* rev. ed. Indianapolis: Bobbs-Merrill, 1977. 277 pp. $5.95 (paper).
After explaining why several other health therapies are not comparable to yoga, the author discusses the meaning and tradition of this system in its many variations. Chapters on meditation and mental health support the view that

yoga is a holistic tool. Among the physical benefits are weight control, a well-proportioned figure, firm muscle tone, good posture, flexibility, vitality, restful sleep, healthy skin, a harmonious sex life, freedom from smoking, and nutritional awareness. Marx illustrates numerous basic and advanced exercises in the book's final section. A thorough and enthusiastic treatment of the subject, including supportive statements by two medical specialists.

Longevity

Benet, Sula, *How to Live to Be 100: The Life-Style of the People of the Caucasus.* New York: Dial, 1976. 201 pp. $8.95.
An anthropologist provides a fascinating report on life-style and longevity in the Caucasus. In addition to sociological and demographic material, the author considers such health factors as heredity, diet, sexual activity, exercise and work, stress management, self-control, and social involvement. Although heredity and environment are significant factors, of equal importance are moderation and the rhythmic regularity of Caucasian life. Bibliography is included. Both intimate and scholarly.

Halsell, Grace. *Los Viejos: Secrets of Long Life from the Sacred Valley.* Emmaus, PA: Rodale, 1976. 186 pp. OP.; London: Bantam. £0.95 (paper).
The longest-living people in the western hemisphere dwell in the Andean mountains of Ecuador. In seeking the reasons for their longevity, the author explores their genetics, exercise, pristine environment, frugal diet, moderate smoking and drinking, sexual activity, self-esteem and social status, stress management, and their unselfish, remarkably content attitude toward life. A simple, moving account. Highly recommended.

Kugler, Hans J. *Dr. Kugler's Seven Keys to a Longer Life.* New York: Fawcett, 1979. 245 pp. $2.25 (paper).
Contending that the human life span is potentially much greater than "average" life expectancies indicate, a gerontologist focuses on improved nutrition, regular exercise, cessation of smoking, light drinking, stress management, environmental and economic factors. Kugler also describes research findings about the aging process and some proposed ways to retard it. Included are both commonly recognized and esoteric theories on preventing heart attack, cancer, senility and other mental disorders; advice on vitamin doses and the need for selenium; and such novel developments as cell therapy, nucleic acid therapy, and organ concentrates. Extensive chapter notes and longevity quizzes are provided. Despite several peculiar notions, the work offers sound anti-aging tactics.

Langone, John. *Long Life: What We Know and Are Learning about the Aging Process.* Boston: Little, 1978. 273 pp. $9.95.
A science journalist reviews ancient and modern quests for a longevity for-

mula. Examined are such diverse notions as organ regeneration, cooling the body to decrease metabolic rate, alleged "youth drugs" such as Gerovital H3, hormone therapy, brain chemistry research, autoimmunity, and possible genetic determination of cellular life spans. Discussing various health factors, Langone focuses on the benefits of proper diet, exercise, and stress management. A thoughtful, discriminating review.

McQuade, Walter, and Aikman, Ann. *The Longevity Factor: A Revolutionary New System for Prolonging Your Life.* New York: Simon & Schuster, 1979. 302 pp. $10.95.
Describes the new technique of health-hazard appraisal. The use of health profiling can answer two essential questions: how long is the individual likely to live and what can be done to lengthen the predictable life span. The health profile results in the calculation of the medical age, usually not the same as the calendar age, and pinpoints risks from diseases and accidents. The emphasis is placed on the fact that health profiles can be altered by modification of life-style and health practice. Tables and worksheets are provided for calculating one's own health profile. Specific advice is given on how to minimize threats to health. Provocative and challenging. A clear description of health risks analysis.

Rosenfeld, Albert. *Prolongevity.* New York: Knopf, 1976. 282 pp. $8.95; Avon. $2.50 (paper).
A science editor reviews current research on aging, its causes and possible postponement. After discussing the role of the gerontologist, Rosenfeld explores the likelihood that senescence is curable. Topics include the function of nucleic acid; theories concerning genetic switching, cross-linkage, free radicals, autoimmunity, etc.; diseases that accelerate aging; laboratory attempts to extend life spans; and experimental therapies involving hormones, enzymes, gene transplants, and special nutrients. Despite his emphasis on research, Rosenfeld also suggests such personal measures as eating lightly, limiting the intake of fats and sugar, regular exercise, moderate drinking and no smoking, controlling stress, working for a clean environment, and supporting research. The book's second part examines ethical considerations and the possible consequences of extended life spans. Heavily documented; rather dry.

PAMPHLETS

American Medical Association, 535 N. Dearborn St., Chicago, IL 60610.
ABC's of Perfect Posture, OP 320.
Basic Body Work for Fitness and Health, OP 428.
First Aid Guide, OP 015.
Fit for Fun, OP 249.
Healthy Way to Slimming, OP 003.

Helping Hands: The Challenge of Medicine, OP 418.
Home Accidents Aren't Accidental, OP 359.
Safety Belts Save Lives, OP 214.
Why Wait? Selecting a Family Doctor, OP 212.
Your Friend the Doctor, OP 068.

Blue Cross Association, 840 N. Lake Shore Dr., Chicago, IL 60611.

Food and Fitness, 1973, 96 pp.
Good Health: You Can Walk Away with It.
Help Yourself, 1978, 92 pp.
What Is Your Medical Age?

Consumer Information Center, Pueblo, CO 81009.

Adult Physical Fitness, 027G.
Exercise and Weight Control, 029G.
Facing Surgery? Why Not Get a Second Opinion? 587G.
How to Keep Your Family's Health Records, 581G.
An Introduction to Physical Fitness, 032G.
Successful Jogging, 586G.
Unless You Decide to Quit, Your Problem Isn't Going to Be Smoking; Your Problem's Going to Be Staying Alive, 034G.

National Institutes of Health, Publications, Bldg. 31, 9000 Rockville Pike, Bethesda, MD 20014.

Be Choosey: Pick a Lifestyle That Really Works for You, 1979, DHEW Pubn. No. (NIH) 79-50096.
A Guide to Medical Self-Care and Self-Help Groups for the Elderly, 1979, DHEW Pubn. No. (NIH) 80-1687, 23 pp.
You Can Reduce Your Risk of Heart Disease, Cancer, Stroke, 1979.

Physician's Art Service, Inc., Patient Information Library, 343-B Serramonte Plaza Office Center, Daly City, CA 94015.

An Apple a Year, 1976, 15 pp.
I Care, 1979, 15 pp.

Public Affairs Committee, Inc., 381 Park Ave. S., New York, NY 10016.

Better Health in Later Years, No. 446.
Health Hazard Appraisal: Clues for a Healthier Life Style, No. 558.
How to Keep Your Teeth after 30, No. 443.
How Weather and Climate Affect You, No. 533.
Vitamins, Food and Your Health, No. 465.
Watch Your Blood Pressure, No. 583.
Women and Smoking, No. 475.

AUDIOVISUAL PRODUCERS AND DISTRIBUTORS

**American Medical Association Film
 Library**
535 N. Dearborn St.
Chicago, IL 60610
First aid and safety; nutrition;
 physiology; preventive medicine.

Churchill Films
662 N. Robertson Blvd.
Los Angeles, CA 90069
Human development; nutrition.

Guidance Associates, Inc.
Communications Pk.
Box 300
White Plains, NY 10602
Physiology of exercise; nutrition and
 exercise; first aid.

Medcom
1633 Broadway
New York, NY 10019
The Human Body: I Am Joe's . . . (series).

Medfact, Inc.
1112 Andrew Ave. N.E.
Massillon, OH 44646
Physical fitness; weight control;
 nutrition.

Parents' Magazines Films
Distributed by PMF Films, Inc.
Box 1000
Elmsford, NY 10523
Food and nutrition, health and safety;
 family living.

Perennial Education, Inc.
477 Roger Williams
Box 855, Ravinia
Highland Park, IL 60035
Nutrition; good life habits, heredity.

Professional Research, Inc.
12960 Coral Tree Pl.
Los Angeles, CA 90066
Weight reduction and control; stress;
 physical fitness; dental health; oral
 hygiene.

Soundwords, Inc.
56-11 217 St.
Bayside, NY 11364
Healthy skin; weight reduction;
 nutrition; exercise; healthy feet;
 healthy hair and scalp; healthy teeth
 and gums.

RESOURCE ORGANIZATIONS

American Dental Association
Bureau of Health Education and
 Audiovisual Services
211 E. Chicago Ave.
Chicago, IL 60611

American Heart Association
7320 Greenville Ave.
Dallas, TX 75231

**American Holistic Medical
 Association**
Rte. 2 Welsh Coulee
La Crosse, WI 54601

American Hospital Association
Center for Health Promotion
840 N. Lake Shore Dr.
Chicago, IL 60611

American Lung Association
1720 Broadway
New York, NY 10019

American Medical Association
Department of Health Education
535 N. Dearborn St.
Chicago, IL 60610

American School Health Association
Kent State Univ.
Kent, OH 44240

Association for the Advancement of Health Education
1900 Associative Dr.
Reston, VA 22091

Blue Cross Association
840 N. Lakeshore Dr.
Chicago, IL 60611

Bureau of Health Education
Center for Disease Control
1000 Clifton Rd. N.E.
Atlanta, GA 30333

Center for Medical Consumers and Health Care Information
237 Thompson St.
New York, NY 10012

Gray Panthers
3700 Chestnut St.
Philadelphia, PA 19104

Health Activation Network
Box 923
Vienna, VA 22180

Health Research Group
2000 P St. N.W.
Washington, DC 20036

HealthRight
175 Fifth Ave.
New York, NY 10010

National Association for Mental Health
1800 Kent St.
Arlington, VA 22209

National Center for Health Education
211 Sutter St.
San Francisco, CA 94108

National Health Screening Council
4905 Del Ray Ave.
Suite 307
Bethesda, MD 20014

National Nutrition Education Clearinghouse
Society for Nutrition Education
2140 Shattuck Ave.
Suite 1110
Berkeley, CA 94704

National Safety Council
444 N. Michigan Ave.
Chicago, IL 60611

Office of Health Information, Health Promotion, Physical Fitness and Sports Medicine
Department of Health and Human Services
200 Independence Ave. S.W.
Washington, DC 20201

President's Council on Physical Fitness and Sports
400 Sixth St. S.W.
Washington, DC 20201

Wellness Resource Center
42 Miller Ave.
Mill Valley, CA 94941

Chapter 9

Children's Health

BOOKS

This chapter describes books on adolescent as well as child health. *See also Chapter 16, Alcoholism and Drug Abuse, for titles on juvenile alcoholism and smoking.*

General

Arena, Jay M., and Bachar, Miriam. *Child Safety Is No Accident: A Parents' Handbook of Emergencies.* Durham, NC: Duke Univ. Pr., 1978. 308 pp. $12.75.
Aimed at both professionals and lay people, this guide covers the treatment of accidents and other health crises, but also stresses preventive behavior and the creation of a life-style conducive to safety. Includes helpful illustrations and first-aid chart. Authoritative and comprehensible.

Boston Women's Health Book Collective. *Ourselves and Our Children: A Book by and for Parents.* New York: Random, 1978. 288 pp. $12.95; $6.95 (paper).
This sociologically significant work on parenting discusses a wide array of topics, including certain health-related issues. Among these are "health and safety regulations" and "family-based health care," which addresses environmental, nutritional, and exercise problems. Other concerns are the interface between parents and the medical community, stress, children with special needs, hospitalization, abuse, and sources of help. Excellent bibliography. Thorough, straightforward, and intriguing, this rather philosophical look at child rearing has limited value as health literature.

Brazelton, T. Berry. *Doctor and Child.* New York: Delacorte, 1976. 234 pp. $8.95; Dell. $4.95 (paper).
A physician offers advice on child rearing that includes such common concerns as the effect of childbirth drugs on the baby, colic, overstimulation, hyperactivity, discipline, toilet training, sibling rivalry, television, toys, and hospitalization. Using a low-keyed, commonsense approach, Brazelton assesses problems with remarkable objectivity and suggests tactics that are moderate yet practical. The passage on hyperactivity, for instance, mentions drugs and psychotherapy but recommends, for most, a combination of calm guidance and proper diet. A return to the instincts of parenting.

Diagram Group. *Child's Body: A Parent's Manual.* New York: Paddington, 1977. 300 pp. $6.95 (paper); Bantam. $2.95 (paper); London: Paddington. £3.50 (paper).
This ingenious handbook deals with child development and health from conception to adulthood. With exceptional comparative diagrams, the authors demonstrate the stage-by-stage changes that occur physically, emotionally, and intellectually. Covering almost all aspects of child care in great detail, this work outstrips similar guides in its chapters on the sick child, children with special needs, and first aid. Authoritative and most impressive. Highly recommended.

Howell, Mary. *Healing at Home: A Guide to Health Care for Children.* Boston: Beacon, 1978. 288 pp. $12.95; $5.95 (paper).
The author provides detailed information relating to the care of a wide variety of childhood ailments. She holds that most of the medical care provided by professionals for a fee does not require lengthy education or complicated technology. Parents can learn simple skills of examination, principles of healing, and substances for treatment. For example, the differential diagnosis of swollen lymph glands of the neck is discussed to teach parents to do this at home. Dr. Howell also describes how to examine the eye for a corneal scratch by means of a fluorescein dye strip, something probably best left to an ophthalmologist. This is a somewhat unorthodox book in that most physicians would recommend, for many of the conditions described, that the child be taken to a pediatrician or an emergency room. Stimulating and challenging.

Illingworth, Ronald S. *The Normal Child: Some Problems of the Early Years and Their Treatment,* 6th ed. New York: Churchill Livingstone, 1975. 326 pp. $18.50; Edinburgh: Churchill Livingstone. £6.50.
Written by a British pediatrician, this baby and child care book covers basically minor ailments and psychological difficulties that parents may confront. It includes sections on hospitalization and accident prevention and management. General and technical references appear after each chapter. The technical language and sophisticated tone will appeal more to the educated reader.

Ong, Beale H. *Doctor's Call Hour.* New York: Wyden, 1978. 249 pp. OP.
A pediatrician answers more than 500 questions about child development and illness. Among the topics discussed are the stages of childhood, infection, orthopedics, teeth, allergies, safety, emotional matters, and education. Comprehensive and readable.

Pantell, Robert H., Fries, James F., and Vickery, Donald M. *Taking Care of Your Child: A Parents' Guide to Medical Care.* Reading, MA: Addison-Wesley, 1977. 409 pp. $10.95.
Flow charts are the unique feature of this pediatric handbook by three physicians. Instructed by these "decision charts," parents will know whether to treat their child's health problem at home or to seek professional help. Besides addressing 91 common problems, the authors discuss growth and development, medical checkups and procedures, the "home pharmacy," and prevention of accidents, diseases, and dental problems. Special attention is given to auto and bike safety and immunization. Appended forms for family health records and growth charts. Highly recommended.

Pomeranz, Virginia E., and Schultz, Dodi. *The Mothers' and Fathers' Medical Encyclopedia,* rev. ed. Boston: Little, 1977. $17.50; New York: NAL, 1978. 689 pp. $2.50 (paper).
A pediatrician and a journalist provide a concise reference guide to 2,200 topics related to child health. The book is alphabetically arranged, with instructive illustrations. Five appendixes give advice on choosing a doctor, a glossary of medical root terms, recommended readings and addresses, poison control center phone numbers, forms for vital statistics and emergency phone numbers. An excellent, introductory reference aid.

Princeton Center for Infancy. *The Parenting Advisor,* ed. by Frank Caplan. New York: Anchor, 1977. 569 pp. $12.95.
A parent education group in collaboration with 12 pediatric specialists covers a wide variety of parenting concerns. Basic patterns and routines, nutritional issues, clothing and equipment needs, and toy safety are considered. Also explained are the stages and common problems of physical development, language acquisition, learning and playing, personality formation, and socialization. Especially noteworthy is the detailed medical information provided in chapters on healthy and sick babies. Includes a lengthy bibliography. An authoritative medical and developmental guide, this work is also a balanced and articulate review of numerous expert opinions.

Rothenberg, Robert E. *Disney's Growing Up Healthy: Avoiding Sickness and Accidents.* New York: Danbury, 1976. 141 pp. OP.
Illustrated with color pictures of Disney characters, this health book for children discusses such topics as accident prevention and first aid; bathing

and washing; care of the eyes, ears, teeth, hands, feet, skin, feelings; shots and vaccinations, including a detailed immunization table; posture; weight problems; dangerous insects and plants; and the future of medicine. Filled with simple anatomical drawings, step-by-step instructions, and health tips. Comprehensive and of value to parents as well as children.

Ryan, James H. *Pablum, Parents and Pandemonium: Glimpses of a Pediatrician's World.* New York: Crowell, 1975. 291 pp. $7.95. OP.
A pediatrician takes a candid, thoughtful look at his art, his patients, and numerous problems from the mundane to the extraordinary. Topics include genetic counseling, sudden infant death syndrome, polio, child abuse, hyperactivity, drug abuse, and brain death. Filling his pages with anecdotes, Ryan philosophizes about pediatricians and other doctors, peer review, unnecessary surgery, and the future. Of special note are his bill of rights and responsibilities of children. Touching and often humorous. A book to savor.

Shiller, Jack G. *Childhood Injury: A Common Sense Approach.* New York: Stein & Day, 1978. 256 pp. $8.95.
A pediatrician provides a detailed guide to avoiding or handling a vast array of injuries and medical emergencies. Organized by symptom group, the work advises parents on whether to get professional help or treat the child themselves. Appendixes on safe and unsafe toys; car safety, with references; and poisonous plants. An essential tool for homes and libraries.

Thurmond, Nancy Moore. *Mother's Medicine.* New York: Morrow, 1979. 383 pp. $9.95.
This work covers basic concerns and daily routines, feeding and nutrition from birth through age six, home remedies and basic health measures. A chapter on parental concerns includes advice on thumb sucking, tooth grinding, head banging, bed-wetting, obesity, choking, stuttering, the special child, and curiosity about sex. Other chapters discuss ways to ensure serenity and growth in the home and include such topics as hospitalization, dental care, going to the doctor, and child abuse. Some special features are lists of infant clothing and equipment, a laundry stain chart, recipes, a detailed table of essential nutrients, and recommended readings. A helpful handbook on living with children but not particularly enlightening on medical matters.

Trimmer, Eric, with Goldschmied, Elinor. *The First Seven Years.* New York: St. Martin's, 1979. 142 pp. $8.95; London: Heinemann. £4.95.
Written by a British medical writer, this colorful guide to the care and development of children includes distinct sections on early problems, teeth, speech and reading, learning through play, coping with twins, the handicapped child, and the child in hospital. Also provided are growth and development charts and a 20-page section on common health problems, with advice on

when to consult a doctor. Though superficial in parts, the work is concise and reliable.

Health Books for Children

Other health books for children and young adults are included under the various subject sections in this and other relevant chapters in Part III.

Allison, Linda. *Blood and Guts: A Working Guide to Your Own Insides.* Boston: Little, 1976. $7.95; $4.95 (paper).
Allison points out that the human being is a walking miracle, a creature who can move along perfectly upright with very little to stand on, whose heart can pump up to twelve gallons of blood per minute, whose eyes permit three-dimensional vision, whose brain is many times more complex than the most advanced computer. Recommended for children 10 and up.

Burstein, John. *Slim Goodbody: What Can Go Wrong and How to Be Strong.* New York: McGraw-Hill, 1978. 48 pp. $6.95. (Grades K–6).
This children's health advocate explains, with humorous and colorful illustrations, numerous ailments and injuries that youngsters may suffer. Topics include colds and flu, temperatures and thermometers, childhood diseases, medications, breaks and sprains, burns and cuts, poor vision, earaches, allergies, handicaps, dental problems, operations and hospitalization. Includes a section on miscellaneous facts, and excellent advice concerning headaches. Slick. Recommended.

Donahue, Parnell, and Capallaro, Helen. *Germs Make Me Sick: A Health Handbook for Kids.* New York: Knopf, 1975. 96 pp. $5.99, $2.95 (paper). (Grades 4 and up).
Concentrating on bacterial and viral diseases, this charming book acquaints children with ailments of the respiratory and gastrointestinal tracts and with various types of rashes and skin problems. The authors also inform and reassure about mononucleosis, meningitis, polio, urinary tract infections, kidney disorders, rheumatic fever, and rabies. In the final chapter, Donahue and Capallaro discuss fever, medication, hospitalization, immunization, and prevention. Highly recommended.

Gilbert, Sara. *Feeling Good: A Book about You and Your Body.* New York: Four Winds Pr., 1978. 181 pp. $6.95. (Grades 7 and up).
The physical, emotional, and mental changes of adolescence are the subject of this book for teenagers. Among the topics covered are growth and development; nutrition and exercise; overweight, acne, and other embarrassments; sexual impulses, pregnancy, and venereal disease; drug abuse, including

excessive drinking and cigarette smoking; suicide. Annotated reading list, with helpful addresses. Well-balanced and candid.

Nourse, Alan E. *Fractures, Dislocations, and Sprains.* A First Book. New York: Watts, 1978. 64 pp. $4.90. (Grades 4 and up).
A physician focuses on bones and joints and on the injuries affecting them. Includes excellent illustrations, a glossary, and a few additional readings that are suitable more for adults than for children.

Nourse, Alan E. *Lumps, Bumps, and Rashes: A Look at Kids' Diseases.* A First Book. New York: Watts, 1976. 66 pp. $4.90. (Grades 4 and up).
Measles, strep and staph infections, and common viral diseases are major topics. Dr. Nourse also devotes much attention to immunizations, explaining why they are needed and how they work. Glossary is included.

Winn, Marie. *The Sick Book.* New York: Four Winds Pr., 1976. 150 pp. $8.95. (Grades 3–7).
In terms that children can easily understand the author discusses many common, generally minor, health problems. Covered in Part One are germs; fever; cuts and bruises; digestive troubles; colds and flu; chicken pox and other "childhood illnesses"; pneumonia; tonsillitis, appendicitis, and their respective operations; breaks and sprains; asthma and other allergies. The second section explains how different body systems function, and in the last part medical jargon is simplified. Question and answer format does not detract from the book's effectiveness.

Infant and Preschool Care

Aukema, Susan, and Kostick, Marilyn. *The Curity Baby Book: A Common-Sense Guide to Baby Care.* New York: Dorison House, 1976. 143 pp. $7.95.
This baby-care book contains the usual advice on helping a child through its first few years. Especially worthwhile, however, are the sections on infant feeding and family nutrition, including meal plans for children and nursing mothers; common illnesses and child safety, including a detailed first-aid guide; dental hygiene; caring for the handicapped child; buying safe equipment and toys; and growth charts. Most reliable.

Caplan, Frank, and Caplan, Theresa. *The Second Twelve Months of Life: A Kaleidoscope of Growth.* New York: Grossett & Dunlap, 1979. 317 pp. $14.95; $9.95 (paper).
Focusing on one-year-olds, the founders of the Princeton Center for Infancy and Early Childhood begin with a "minicourse in infant and toddler development." For each month, they explore the changes in motor development, language acquisition, sensory powers and learning, social development, per-

sonality, self-help routines, play and playthings. Included are convenient growth charts, and a wealth of developmental exercises, games, rhymes and finger plays. Bibliography. Highly recommended.

Jones, Sandy. *Good Things for Babies*. Boston: Houghton, 1976. 115 pp. $8.95; $4.95 (paper).
This is described as "a catalog and source book of safety and consumer advice about products needed during the first 24 months of life." Included are recommended readings, backpacks, bathing and dental care, beds and accessories, children's books and music, breast-feeding aids, car and bicycle seats, carriages and walkers, chairs and playpens, toys, nursery decoration, shoes and booties, safety, and poison prevention. Each item has a brief description and mail-order information. Contains a directory of U.S. Consumer Product Safety Commission offices. With over 250 illustrations, this work responds well to a distinct need, but will require frequent revisions.

Leach, Penelope. *Babyhood*. New York: Knopf, 1976. 350 pp. $10.00; London: Lane. £5.75.
Concerned with the child's general development from birth to age two, this book covers the common questions and complaints of this period. Its only value as a source of health information rests in identifying the patterns of normal behavior and minor ailments. The author, a British psychologist, gives much attention to intellectual development and to problems of temperament. Written with ease and clarity.

Leach, Penelope. *Your Baby and Child: From Birth to Age Five*. New York: Knopf, 1978. 512 pp. $15.95.
Leach broadens the range of her previous book (*Babyhood*) with this health and development guide to the entire preschool period. Of particular value is her 57-page encyclopedia/index, with instructions regarding first aid, accidents, infectious diseases, nursing, safety, and diet. Appendixes include growth charts, numerous organizational addresses, and quick measures against clothing on fire, electric shock, arterial bleeding, choking, and drowning. Far superior to *Babyhood*. Highly recommended.

McDonald, Linda. *Everything You Need to Know about Babies*. Pasadena, CA: Oaklawn, 1978. 192 pp. $5.95 (paper).
Providing comprehensive information on infant and child care, this authoritative work is particularly valuable for alerting parents to developmental problems. Checklists, comparative drawings, and detailed descriptions all elaborate the material on vision, hearing, speech, nutrition, dental and foot care. Other topics of special interest are toys, accident prevention, regular and emergency medical care, and common disorders. An appendix suggests addresses and literature concerned with breast-feeding, development and edu-

cation, various physical problems, automotive and product safety, and day care. Exceptional; highly recommended.

Stoppard, Miriam. *Dr. Miriam Stoppard's Book of Baby Care.* New York: Atheneum, 1977. 193 pp. $10.95; London: Weidenfeld & Nicolson. £4.50.
In this rather general book on baby care, a British physician discusses the usual health and developmental concerns of early childhood. Short glossary. Clearly written but unexceptional.

Stoutt, Glenn R., Jr. *The First Month of Life: A Parent's Guide to Care of the Newborn.* Oradell, NJ: Medical Economics, 1977. 161 pp. $4.50 (paper).
Speaking to inexperienced parents, a pediatrician describes the needs, physical characteristics, behavior, and problems of the healthy newborn. The author also discusses shaking, child abuse, resuscitation steps, and auto safety. Stoutt's advice about breast-feeding and early solids is not altogether up-to-date; otherwise the work is acceptable.

Nutrition and Physical Fitness

Brewster, Dorothy Patricia. *You Can Breastfeed Your Baby . . . Even in Special Situations.* Emmaus, PA: Rodale, 1979. 596 pp. $14.95; $11.95 (paper).
An active member of the La Leche League answers a myriad of questions about breast-feeding and suggests proven methods of handling both common and rare problems. Using hundreds of case histories, Brewster explains how to nurse in spite of maternal or infant handicaps, illnesses, hospitalization, and several nonmedical dilemmas. Appends a list of helpful organizations and a substantial bibliography. Enthusiastic, but sensible about insurmountable obstacles.

Eden, Alvin N., with Heilman, Joan Rattner. *Growing Up Thin.* New York: McKay, 1975. 223 pp. $7.95; New York: Berkley. $1.50 (paper).
Suggesting a sane approach to weight control, a pediatrician emphasizes both proper nutrition and regular exercise for each age group of children. Topics include causes of fat, social consequences and health effects, poor and nutritious eating habits, the benefits of exercise, and ways to "fatproof" children. Among the book's special features are tables for scoring a child's risk of obesity, a chapter "for teenagers only," and caloric values of common activities. Reliable and most instructive: superior to similar guides.

Ellis, Audrey. *The Kid-Slimming Book.* Chicago: Regnery, 1976. 276 pp. OP.
Containing much more than recipes, this book establishes the nutritional foundation for sound eating patterns. Beginning with a general discussion of childhood obesity, the author includes optimum weight graphs, nutrient and

calorie charts, daily food plans and menus for different age and calorie groups. Ellis outlines several types of diets and provides information on fats and oils and artificial sweeteners. Recipes include those suitable for packed lunches. Authoritative and thorough.

Ewy, Donna, and Ewy, Rodger. *Preparation for Breast Feeding.* New York: Dolphin, 1975. 125 pp. $3.50.
The art of breast-feeding is put forth with step-by-step instructions on avoiding or overcoming problems and enhancing the benefits. Topics include pre-delivery preparation, early adjustment, process of lactation, emotional and social concerns, fallacies, common problems for the mother and for the infant. For easy reference the Ewys provide a summary of key ideas. Appendix has La Leche League addresses and excellent suggested readings. Authoritative and reassuring.

Gilbert, Sara. *Fat Free: Common Sense for Young Weight Worriers.* New York: Macmillan, 1975. 114 pp. $6.95; $1.95 (paper).
Aimed at teenagers, this work covers the emotional aspects of overweight, being fat vs. feeling fat, causes, positive and negative attitudes about reducing, healthy diets vs. dangerous methods, and helpful tips. Appendixes provide a calorie-carbohydrate chart and sources of additional information. Safe, practical, and appealing.

Lambert-Lagace, Louise. *Feeding Your Child.* Cambridge, ON: Habitex Books, 1976. 274 pp. $3.95 (paper).
In this nutritional guide, a Canadian dietitian discusses the poor diet of today's children and recommends specific measures to help develop healthy eating habits during the early years. Beginning with prenatal care, Lambert-Lagace outlines the proper diet for different ages, suggests tactful ways to overcome poor eating behavior, and advises on problems such as allergy, constipation, diarrhea, thinness, overweight. Menus, recipes, and nutrition charts are included. Despite some mention of cholesterol, the author fails to draw a connection with the dairy products she endorses. Otherwise, the work is most instructive.

Lorin, Martin I. *The Parents' Book of Physical Fitness for Children.* New York: Atheneum, 1979. 279 pp. $9.95.
A pediatrician offers advice on improving the physical fitness of children. Nutrition receives special emphasis, along with running and other exercise programs and sports. Topics include the major food components, vitamins and minerals, fiber, and food additives. Taking a holistic approach, the author devotes separate chapters to the infant, toddler, preschool, school-age, and adolescent child. The work ends with ten suggestions that encapsulate the book's major points.

McWilliams, Margaret. *Nutrition for the Growing Years,* 2nd ed. New York: Wiley, 1975. 452 pp. $14.95; Chichester: Wiley. £10.35.
In this elementary text, a nutritionist explains the functions of specific nutrients, their role in physical and mental development, and the nutritional needs of children from conception through adolescence. Also provided are a theoretical discussion of weight control, guidelines for feeding sick and handicapped youngsters, and answers to questions that parents frequently ask. Contains bibliographies, tables of weights and nutrient values, glossary. Although the work makes no mention of cholesterol and other current issues of childhood nutrition, it is recommended as a reference.

Mason, Gussie. *Help Your Child Lose Weight and Keep It Off.* New York: Grosset, 1975. 117 pp. OP.
The founder of two weight-loss camps explains her techniques for helping children reduce, and discusses motivation, shopping, nutrition, and exercise. In addition, she provides menus and recipes, including hamburger and lunch-box ideas. Also presented are 30 simple ways to foster good eating habits and self-esteem.

Mitchell, Ingrid. *Breastfeeding Together.* A Continuum Book. New York: Seabury, 1978. 146 pp. $7.95.
A midwife details the reasons why breast-feeding should be preferred to bottle-feeding. Included are several statements from parents, a chapter on the La Leche League, and a bibliography. Accurate and comprehensible, but with a rigid point of view.

Powers, Hugh, and Presley, James. *Food Power: Nutrition and Your Child's Behavior.* New York: St. Martin's, 1978. 230 pp. $8.95.
A pediatrician and a medical writer claim that many seemingly normal children suffer from "carbohydrate overload," with several physical and behavioral effects. As a remedy, they propose a diet combining strict carbohydrate control, high protein intake, vitamin supplements, and the absence of sugar and caffeine. Included are appendixes on foods high in essential nutrients and those with hidden sugars. The nutritional message is presented poorly but contains many sound arguments.

Dental Care

See also Dental Care in Chapter 8, Wellness, Physical Fitness, and Self-Health Care.

Doss, Helen, and Well, Richard L. *All the Better to Bite With.* New York: Messner, 1976. 64 pp. $7.29. (Grades 3–5).
A writer and a dentist collaborate to teach children about animal and human teeth and about proper dental hygiene. Included are such topics as the shed-

ding of primary teeth; the causes of tooth and gum disease; the value of flossing; dental exams; filling, replacing, straightening teeth; and good nutrition. The last chapter offers six ways to learn more about teeth. Excellent.

Moss, Stephen J. *Your Child's Teeth: A Parent's Guide to Making and Keeping Them Perfect.* Boston: Houghton, 1977. 143 pp. $8.95; $3.95 (paper).
Focusing on prevention, a dentist begins with conception and tooth development and continues with material on pacifiers, nursing, teething, stains, loose primaries, injuries, and numerous other concerns. Moss also discusses tooth anatomy; brushing and flossing; diet; fluoride; choosing a dentist; checkups; X rays and anesthesia; orthodontics, including choosing an orthodontist and cost considerations; and the role of dentistry today. Although a few topics are treated superficially, this remains a most useful handbook.

Schaleben-Lewis, Joy. *The Dentist and Me.* Milwaukee, WI: Raintree, 1977. 32 pp. $7.93. (Grades K–3).
This delightful book describes the dental checkups of two children, one with no cavities and one who needs a filling. Both are taught about dental procedures and caring for their teeth.

Silverstein, Alvin, and Silverstein, Virginia. *So You're Getting Braces.* Philadelphia: Lippincott, 1978. 112 pp. OP.
Parents as well as youngsters will appreciate this explanation of orthodontics, which includes a brief history and a look into the future. Also discussed are the anatomy of jaws and teeth, types of malocclusions, the mechanics of braces, and the need for cooperation with the dentist. Recommended reading list. Uncomplicated and clearly written.

Weiss, Joy. *Embraceable You: A Guide for Orthodontic Patients and Their Parents.* New York: Health Science Publg., 1975. 162 pp. $8.95.
An orthodontist and psychologist discusses the various reasons, possible results, and financial considerations of having teeth straightened. Whether answering technical questions or surveying the psychological side of orthodontia, Weiss's explanations are informative and witty—albeit sometimes rather involved. Glossary and scholarly references. Highly recommended for educated adults and clever kids.

Wilkin, Refna. *Dental Health.* A First Book. New York: Watts, 1976, 61 pp. $4.90 (Grades 4–6).
This children's work describes anatomy of the mouth, tooth structure, preventive and corrective dental care. Among the topics covered are tooth troubles like decay, plaque, and malocclusions; dental procedures such as X rays, fluoride treatments, extractions, braces, and other orthodontic measures; daily tooth hygiene and diet. Also discusses adult problems. A glossary is included. Entertaining with historical anecdotes and cartoons.

Asthma and Allergies

See also Asthma and Allergies in Chapter 17, Other Health Problems and Concerns.

Silverstein, Alvin, and Silverstein, Virginia B. *Allergies*. Philadelphia: Lippin-
    cott, 1977. 128 pp. $5.95; $3.50 (paper). (Grades 4 and up).
In this work for children, the authors explain the history, causes, and types of
allergy, as well as diagnosis and treatment methods. Separate chapters are
devoted to hay fever, asthma, food allergies, skin allergies, insect stings, drug
allergies, and allergic headaches. Addresses are given for obtaining further
information. Highly detailed but clearly presented.

Silverstein, Alvin, and Silverstein, Virginia B. *Itch, Sniffle & Sneeze: All About
    Asthma, Hay Fever and Other Allergies*. New York: Four Winds, 1978. 48 pp.
    $6.95. (Grades 1–5).
Thoroughly explaining allergies to young children, this work contains information on symptoms and the biological processes they signal, causes, common
allergens, diagnosis, treatments, and everyday methods of coping. A glossary
and colorful, instructive illustrations add to the work's appeal.

Somekh, Emile. *The Complete Guide to Children's Allergies: Care and Treatment of
    Your Allergic Child*. Los Angeles: Corwin, 1979. 207 pp. $10.
A pediatrician and allergist provides an authoritative work on this complex
subject. After answering several general questions, he reviews a wide variety
of allergens; skin testing; allergic diseases of the skin, nose, and lungs; and the
process of desensitization. Thirteen appendixes include information on medications and vaccines; pollen maps; avoiding hidden allergens; breathing exercises; allergy-free foods; institutes, camps, and organizations; and allergy
journals. Includes glossary. There is substantial material on asthma, but information in some other areas seems superficial.

Autism

Lovaas, O. Ivar. *The Autistic Child: Language Development through Behavior
    Modification*. New York: Halsted, 1977. 246 pp. $15.95; London: Halsted.
    £11.30.
Addressing a general readership, this noted authority on autistic children
explains the elements of a program by which such youngsters acquire language. Progressing from primitive expressions to high levels of verbal spontaneity and storytelling, Lovaas not only describes procedures but also supplies 13 short "training manuals" for helping a child in specific areas. He
pauses, moreover, to consider several theoretical questions on behavior
modification and language development. The terminology and professional
abbreviations of this sophisticated work will hinder many, but educated readers will welcome the systematic aids and enlightening case histories found
here.

Paluszny, Maria J., and others. *Autism: A Practical Guide for Parents and Professionals.* Syracuse, NY: Syracuse Univ. Pr., 1979. 179 pp. $9.95.
Five contributing specialists discuss the characteristics of autism, possible causes, and methods of diagnosis and treatment. Calling it an organic, developmental disorder, the authors suggest an interdisciplinary approach with therapy geared to changes in age and developmental level. A chapter on parent involvement reviews theories that blame parents and explores their current participation on the therapeutic team. Contains a bibliography of professional literature. The text itself is enlightening and sophisticated, without technical jargon. Recommended.

Rothenberg, Mira. *Children with Emerald Eyes: Histories of Extraordinary Boys & Girls.* New York: Dial, 1977. 294 pp. $10.95; London: Souvenir Pr. £5; £3 (paper).
A psychologist presents the case histories of several schizophrenic and autistic children with whom she has worked. More than dry, clinical reports, Rothenberg's accounts, and the dialogue with which they are threaded, draw the reader fully into the pain and poetry of their lives. The message is simple: to be with and accept these children, whether cured or lost. Eloquent.

Cancer

Baker, Lynn S., Roland, Charles G., and Gilchrist, Gerald S. *You and Leukemia: A Day at a Time,* rev. ed. Philadelphia: Saunders, 1978. 205 pp. $7.95 (paper); London: Saunders. £5 (paper). (Ages 8 and up).
In this superb handbook for leukemic children, three physicians thoroughly describe organ functions, blood components, and the various effects of this disease. They explain its nature, causes, and types; methods of diagnosis and treatment; remission-inducing and maintenance programs; complications and side effects; the support of clinical personnel; emotions and family responses; and thoughts about dying. Especially effective are the authors' honest but hopeful approach, their warnings about unconventional therapies, and their detailed examination of procedures, designed to prepare youngsters as much as possible. Further reading list, glossary. A treasure, combining highly technical material and a warm conversational style. Highly recommended.

Eys, Jan Van, ed. *The Truly Cured Child: The New Challenge in Pediatric Cancer Care.* Baltimore: University Park, 1977. 177 pp. $7.50; Lancaster: MTP Pr. £4.50 (paper).
An anthology of essays by professional contributors, this is a philosophical work that emphasizes the ethics of pediatric cancer treatment. Contents include such themes as "the conflicts between the patient and the demands imposed by institution and research" and "conflicts between the personal needs of the staff and the ideal of humane patient treatment." Although it

contains some medical terminology, the book is highly recommended for educated lay people as well as for professionals.

Johnson, F. Leonard, and Miller, Marc. *Shannon: A Book for Parents of Children with Leukemia*. New York: Hawthorn, 1975. 132 pp. $6.95.
A leukemic child's grandmother and a pediatric oncologist collaborate in a unique study of the disease's physical and social effects. Woven into the personal narrative is valuable information about the nature and diagnosis of leukemia, various therapies and their side effects, and cancer frauds. Acute lymphoblastic and acute myelogenous leukemias are well contrasted. Not entirely current.

Cerebral Palsy

Connor, Frances P., Williamson, Gordon G., and Siepp, John M., eds. *Program Guide for Infants and Toddlers with Neuromotor and Other Developmental Disabilities*. New York: Teachers College, 1978. 415 pp. $13.95.
Written in cooperation with the United Cerebral Palsy Association, this guide is aimed primarily at therapists and educators but is useful to parents as well. In nontechnical language the contributors discuss such topics as nutrition; daily hygiene; motor, language, cognitive, and psychosocial development; and specific activities designed to respond to a child's unique needs. Appendixes include descriptions of adaptive equipment. Highly recommended for parents involved in the child's therapy process.

Cruickshank, William M., ed. *Cerebral Palsy: A Developmental Disability*, 3rd rev. ed. Syracuse, NY: Syracuse Univ. Pr., 1976. 624 pp. $24.
Providing an impressive overview of cerebral palsy, 17 contributors consider the interrelationships between this central nervous system disorder and other developmental problems. Although most chapters are rather technical, the work is a necessary reference tool, which blends the different perspectives of medical, psychological, therapeutic, social work, and rehabilitation professionals. A substantial bibliography is included.

Finnie, Narcie R. *Handling the Young Cerebral Palsied Child at Home*, rev. ed. New York: Dutton, 1975. 224 pp. OP.; London: Heinemann, £2.80.
Covering a host of everyday problems, this illustrated guide for parents offers methods for managing the handicapped child and fostering healthful development. A highly praised, frequently cited work. Indispensable.

Joel, Gil F. *So Your Child Has Cerebral Palsy*. Albuquerque: Univ. of New Mexico Pr., 1975. 53 pp. $2.45 (paper).
Written by a victim of this disorder, this book discusses the emotional effects of cerebral palsy and suggests ways in which parents can strengthen the child's self-image. Insightful.

Chronic Illness and Handicaps

Ayrault, Evelyn West. *Growing Up Handicapped: A Guide for Parents and Professionals to Helping the Exceptional Child.* A Continuum Book. New York: Seabury, 1977. 216 pp. $9.95.
Herself a victim of cerebral palsy, a clinical psychologist examines the behavioral and social problems of physically handicapped children at different stages of development. Topics include parental reactions to handicaps, family relationships, self-image, behavioral problems of young children, discipline, adolescent concerns, learning disabilities, psychological evaluation, early schooling, play therapy suggestions, and the rehabilitation team. Appendixes contain 13 directories of various services, including rehabilitation centers, self-help devices, and local affiliates of national agencies. Illustrated with numerous case histories, this work provides a helpful view of the psychological aspects of a handicapped childhood. Recommended.

Baker, Bruce L., and others. *Steps to Independence: A Skills Training Series for Children with Special Needs.* Champaign, IL: Research, 1976. 4 manuals, 108 to 125 pp. $5.95 each (paper).
Addressing parents and teachers, this series offers step-by-step instructions for helping handicapped children acquire varying degrees of autonomy. The manuals also suggest methods of handling behavioral problems.

Bleck, Eugene E., and Nagel, Donald A., eds. *Physically Handicapped Children: A Medical Atlas for Teachers.* New York: Grune & Stratton, 1975. 304 pp. $19.75; London: Grune & Stratton. £13.50.
This valuable reference work begins with an explanation of anatomy, including a passage on medical terminology. Chapters contain discussions of amputation, asthma, cerebral palsy, communication disorders, epilepsy, cystic fibrosis, juvenile diabetes, heart disease, muscular dystrophy, spinal defects, traumatic paraplegia and quadriplegia, poliomyelitis, juvenile rheumatoid arthritis, sickle cell disease, spinal muscular atrophy, and visual disorders. All chapters contain subject bibliographies, and most give specific advice regarding teaching. There is also a section on normal motor development in infancy, with accompanying chart. In a chapter on emergencies, instruction is given for cardiopulmonary resuscitation, and for treatment of convulsions and fainting. A final chapter contains tables of literature for parents of handicapped children, with addresses of organizations and publishers. Glossary. Somewhat technical but clearly invaluable.

Burton, Lindy. *The Family Life of Sick Children.* Boston: Routledge, 1975. 264 pp. $18.75; $5.95 (paper); London: Routledge. £6.95; £2.95 (paper).
Focusing on cystic fibrosis, this sociological work addresses the physical, emotional, and financial problems of families so affected. The author discusses clearly symptoms and diagnosis, coping with an inherited disease, daily treatment, hospitalization, equipment and space needs, communication, changing

expectations of family members, and the loss of a child. Statistics and technical bibliography; list of organizations, chiefly British. Of limited but obvious value to concerned laypersons.

Forrai, Maria S., and Anders, Rebecca. *A Look at Mental Retardation.* Lerner Awareness Series. Minneapolis: Lerner, 1976. 36 pp. $4.95. (Grades 3–6).
This beautifully designed work explains to youngsters how the mentally handicapped are different from normal and gifted children. Topics include causes, intelligence tests, learning potential, and the retarded child's need for care and appreciation.

Forrai, Maria S., (photographs), and Pursell, Margaret Sanford (text). *A Look at Physical Handicaps.* Lerner Awareness Series. Minneapolis: Lerner, 1976. 36 pp. $4.95. (Grades 3–6).
Emphasizing permanent childhood disabilities, the authors cover such conditions as poliomyelitis, paralysis, blindness, deafness, and amputations. Also discussed are communication aids like braille and sign language.

Gordon, Sol. *Living Fully: A Guide for Young People with a Handicap, Their Parents, Their Teachers, and Professionals.* New York: John Day, 1975. 296 pp. OP.
The emotional, social, and vocational problems of handicapped youngsters are addressed in this work. Includes an excellent "Bill of Rights for Parents" and resource appendix. Most supportive.

Love, Harold D., and Walthall, Joe E. *A Handbook of Medical, Educational, and Psychological Information for Teachers of Physically Handicapped Children.* Springfield, IL: Charles C. Thomas, 1977. 219 pp. $13.75.
Aimed at parents as well as teachers, this work presents a historical view of handicaps, an introduction to anatomy, and a review of various health problems. Among these are cerebral palsy, allergies, diabetes, epilepsy, tuberculosis, rheumatic fever and congenital heart disease, hemophilia, burns, amputations, accidents, scoliosis (curvature of the spine), arthritis, leukemia, sickle cell anemia, and sensory disabilities. The last section focuses on the school environment, with chapters on psychological testing, architectural barriers, and vocational placement. End-of-chapter references; glossary. Rather uneven, with some topics receiving cursory treatment and others in-depth coverage.

McCollum, Audrey T. *Coping with Prolonged Health Impairment in Your Child.* Boston: Little, 1975. 240 pp. $11.50.
A professional counselor addresses families with chronically ill children. In successive chapters, she discusses health impairment in infants and toddlers, in early childhood, in mid-childhood, and in adolescence. McCollum's advice

to parents ranges from suggestions about practical concerns to psychological support against their own and their children's fears and grief. Special attention is given to facing the diagnosis, safeguarding relationships, adjusting to hospitalization, communicating effectively, and utilizing sources of assistance. McCollum places emphasis on maintaining the family and on permitting the children to grow and mature as naturally as possible. Sensitively done.

McNamara, Joan, and McNamara, Bernard. *The Special Child Handbook*. New York: Hawthorn, 1978. 330 pp. $12.50.
Concerned with a wide range of problems affecting physically or mentally handicapped children, the parents of five "special" children provide a guide to coping and making the system work. Topics include recognizing special needs; where to go for diagnosis; preparing the child for this process; emotional reactions; finding suitable schools and programs; parents groups, community agencies, play groups, day care, and other sources of support; financial problems and solutions; legal considerations. Each chapter concludes with a directory, and a final list of organizations, arranged by state, follows an annotated bibliography. An indispensable tool.

Petersen, Palle. *Sally Can't See*. New York: John Day, 1977. 24 pp. $5.79. (Grades K–4).
Despite her handicap, a 12-year-old blind girl is learning to play music, swim, ride, and read braille. This book attempts to stress her normality but offers, even for young children, a rather superficial introduction to this disability. Excellent photography.

Scott, Eileen P., Jan, James E., and Freeman, Roger D. *Can't Your Child See?* Baltimore: University Park, 1977. 201 pp. $8.95; Lancaster: MTP Pr. £4.95.
A social worker, a pediatrician, and a psychiatrist collaborate on this work about visually handicapped children. Topics include various eye disorders, diagnosis and its emotional impact on the family, care and development of infants and toddlers, everyday concerns of living with blind children, multiple handicaps, hospitalization, play activities and toys, schooling, and concerns about the future. A suggested reading list is provided. With numerous case histories, this work achieves the goal of reassuring parents and helping them cope with the child's disability.

Schulman, Jerome L. *Coping with Tragedy: Successfully Facing the Problem of a Seriously Ill Child*. Chicago: Follett, 1976. 335 pp. $9.95.
A pediatric psychiatrist uses conversations with children, parents, and doctors to explore the changing perspectives of families who cope with severe childhood illness. The book covers a variety of afflictions, including leukemia, mental retardation, hemophilia, muscular dystrophy, cystic fibrosis, and spina bifida. Filled with profound personal insights, these genuinely positive dialogues are highly recommended to anyone in similar circumstances.

Travis, Georgia. *Chronic Illness in Children: Its Impact on Child and Family.* Stanford: Stanford Univ. Pr., 1976. 556 pp. $19.50.
Intended primarily for social workers, this work is valuable for its overview of both the "medical realities" and the "psycholosocial implications" of several chronic illnesses. Among these are asthma, kidney disease, congenital heart disease, cystic fibrosis, head injuries, hemophilia, juvenile rheumatoid arthritis, juvenile diabetes, leukemia, muscular dystrophy, sickle cell anemia, spina bifida, and spinal cord injuries. A chapter on community resources includes general information on medical care, financial aid, public and social services, homemaker services, day care, foster home care, and adoption. Substantial, with 41 pages of notes. Written in lay terms; recommended for the reference needs of educated readers.

Weber, Leonard J. *Who Shall Live? The Dilemma of Severely Handicapped Children and Its Meaning for Other Moral Questions.* New York: Paulist Pr., 1976. 138 pp. $3.95 (paper).
This philosophical work explores such ethical concerns as the value and quality of life, euthanasia, letting die, and who shall decide. Believing that there *are* certain situations when treatment should be withheld, the author suggests specific guidelines for decision making. Weber presents a balanced study, however, with careful attention to several conflicting opinions. References included. Recommended.

Hospitalization

Elder, Barbara Schuyler Haas. *The Hospital Book,* 4th ed. Baltimore: John Street, 1975. 48 pp. $3. (Preschool–Grade 5).
With anatomical drawings, this coloring book introduces children to hospital routines and to such uncommon procedures as the use of oxygen tents, intravenous treatments, and traction. Both positive and negative aspects of hospitalization are shown. Highly recommended.

Hofmann, Adele D., Becker, R.D., and Gabriel, Paul H. *The Hospitalized Adolescent: A Guide to Managing the Ill and Injured Youth.* New York: Free Pr., 1976. 249 pp. $14.95.
Aimed at hospital personnel, this work also has value for the layperson. Emphasizing the psychological aspects of illness and hospitalization, the authors argue that the normal emotional forces of adolescence make the impact of illness especially traumatic. In addition to age, other factors are the chronicity of the problem and the degree of personal autonomy that remains. Much of the book is devoted to instructing care-givers on effective ways to respond to their patients. These sections can also prove helpful to parents. The last part addresses special problems. Some technical terminology; recommended for the educated reader.

Ludwick, Rebecca O., and Rogers, Donna G. *Your Children's Hospital Book.*
Nashville: The Children's Hospital of Vanderbilt Univ., 1976. 40 pp. $1.
(Grades 1–7).
In addition to explaining hospital procedures, this work is a coloring book for
children, including games and a crossword puzzle. Some anatomical drawings.

Odor, Ruth. *Brian's Trip to the Hospital.* Cincinnati: Standard Publg., 1977. 24
pp. $1 (paper). (Preschool–Grade 1).
The experiences of a boy undergoing tonsillectomy are described, including
his postoperative discomfort. Religious tone.

Singer, Marilyn. *It Can't Hurt Forever.* New York: Harper, 1978. 186 pp. $7.95.
(Ages 10–14).
Revealing both negative and positive aspects of hospitalization, this work
concerns the heart operation of an 11-year-old girl. Hospital routines are well
detailed. Rather grim in parts.

Sobol, Harriet Langsam. *Jeff's Hospital Book.* New York: Henry Z. Walck, 1975.
47 pp. $6.95. (Grades K–4).
The mother of a cross-eyed boy tells of his brief hospitalization for corrective
surgery. Although Jeff was initially anxious about the procedures, his questions were answered clearly and everything went as predicted. Recommended.

Watts, Marjorie-Ann. *Crocodile Medicine.* New York: Warne, 1978. 28 pp.
$6.95. (Preschool–Grade 1).
Concerning long-term hospitalization, this work reveals the wide range
of emotions that children may experience in such circumstances.
Recommended.

Ziegler, Sandra. *At the Hospital: A Surprise for Krissy.* Elgin, IL: Child's World,
1976. 32 pp. $4.50. (Preschool–Grade 2).
Several routine procedures are well described in the story of a child's tonsillectomy. In addition, the emotional support offered by Krissy's parents and the
hospital personnel is shown to be especially important.

Hyperactivity

Cratty, Bryant J. *Remedial Motor Activity for Children.* Philadelphia: Lea &
Febiger, 1975. 327 pp. $13.50; London: Lea & Febiger. £10.
A University of California at Los Angeles specialist in kinesiology surveys the
development of motor ability in children, various kinds of movement disorders, methods of evaluation, and remedial programs and exercises. Included
are chapters on sports, handwriting, and working with hyperactive young-

sters. Speaking primarily to professionals, Cratty writes in a conversational tone that makes for easy, pleasant reading by anyone concerned with children in motion.

Feingold, Ben F., and Feingold, Helene S. *The Feingold Cookbook for Hyperactive Children: And Others with Problems Associated with Food Additives and Salicylates.* New York: Random, 1979. 328 pp. $10; $5.95 (paper).
Written by an expert on nutritional treatment of hyperkinesis, this cookbook begins with an explanation of the diet and the effects of certain chemicals and nutrients, and provides a brief look at other conditions that may respond to the diet, advice from parents, and a four-week diet plan. The recipes cover a full range of food types with no separate section on special occasions or situations.

Roth, June. *Cooking for Your Hyperactive Child.* Chicago: Contemporary, 1977. 271 pp. $10.95; $4.95 (paper).
In addition to her menus and recipes, the author includes a general discussion of the problem and its dietary management, advice on eliminating food additives and suspected allergens, and warnings about fruits that are natural salicylates. Each recipe is marked to show whether it is free of dairy, egg, wheat, corn, or sugar. The subject remains complicated, necessitating some highly restrictive diets, but Roth succeeds in presenting her material as simply as possible.

Schrag, Peter, and Divoky, Diane. *The Myth of the Hyperactive Child: And Other Means of Child Control.* New York: Pantheon, 1975, 285 pp. $10.
Two journalists propose that the majority of hyperactive or learning-disabled children are victims of the "system's" demand for acceptable, homogenous behavior: "The issue is not the child's silent agony, but those things about him which . . . make him a nuisance." The child, considered "predelinquent," is treated for his individuality, which is labeled a syndrome. In this highly polemic work, the authors envision an Orwellian world, sustained by the efforts of doctors and educators. An appendix offers advice on "self-defense" for parents confronted with the hyperactivity question. Thought-provoking but extreme.

Stevens, Laura J., Stevens, George E., and Stoner, Rosemary B. *How to Feed Your Hyperactive Child.* New York: Doubleday, 1977. 240 pp. $7.95.
This cookbook contains 400 recipes free of salt and additives; a chapter on making staples from scratch to avoid hidden ingredients in commercial goods; and suggestions for special occasions. Appendixes present the diet plan, with permitted and prohibited foods; a list of safe brands for specific items; suggestions for evaluating the diet; a guide to basic nutrition; menus; and equivalents.

Walker, Sydney, III. *Help for the Hyperactive Child.* Boston: Houghton, 1978.
211 pp. $8.95; London: Houghton, £5.50.
Examining the problem of hyperactivity, a neuropsychiatrist asserts that it is
not itself a disease but rather a symptom of some underlying organic or
functional disorder. Behavior-altering drugs like Ritalin, he contends, not
only are dangerous but also mask symptoms without eliminating the cause.
Equally suspect are treatments ranging from coffee to psychosurgery. Believing that hyperactivity can arise from any of numerous causes, Walker criticizes
the popular dietary theories as too sweeping and urges a multidimensional
approach to diagnosis. Includes a chapter on parents' resources. An articulate, well-balanced analysis of a complex problem. Highly recommended.

Wender, Paul H., and Wender, Esther H. *The Hyperactive Child and the Learning
Disabled Child: A Handbook For Parents,* new ed. New York: Crown, 1978. 138
pp. $6.95.
A pediatrician and a child psychiatrist carefully examine the symptoms of
hyperactivity, its causes, patterns, and treatment. To avoid misinterpretation,
the doctors thoroughly discuss ten major characteristics and address the
problems of medications and psychological management. The Wenders delib-
erately play down popular dietary measures, especially regarding food
additives. Also covered are related learning disabilities, with suggestions for
lessening their effects. A sound, practical aid.

Juvenile Diabetes

See also Chapter 14, Diabetes.

Babington, Caroline Hastings. *Cooking Creatively for Your Diabetic Child.*
Garden City, NY: Doubleday, 1979. 224 pp. $8.95.
The author, the mother of a diabetic, is also a home economist with a nutrition
degree. After an initial chapter on diet and insulin therapy, Babington supplies recipes in 13 categories, including school lunches, desserts, condiments
and dressings, and festive occasions. Eight appendixes include the six food
exchanges of the American Diabetes Association, a daily exchange worksheet
and scoreboard, charts for equivalents and metric conversion, information on
herbs and spices, and peak seasons for fruits and vegetables. The recipes
themselves include exchange equations. An educational guide with attractive,
enjoyable dietary suggestions.

Briggs, Christy. *Dining with Your Diabetic Child.* Salt Lake City, UT: Kerry and
Christy Briggs, 1978. 79 pp. $4.95 (paper).
The mother of a diabetic child provides a cookbook designed to facilitate
dietary routines while appealing to the culinary tastes of the entire family.
Approved by the Utah affiliate of the American Diabetes Association, the

book includes recipes for soups, casseroles, salads, meat dishes, seafood, chicken, and breakfasts. Each recipe shows the number of food choices that are acceptable for a diabetic child's intake. There are also six weeks of dinner menus and one week of breakfast suggestions; miscellaneous recipes, canning instructions; and several tips for making the diabetic diet more appealing to a child. A valuable introduction to diabetic meal planning.

Court, John M. *Helping Your Diabetic Child.* New York: Taplinger, 1974. 223 pp. $8.95; $4.95 (paper).
A physician thoroughly explains the nature and treatment of juvenile diabetes. Among the topics covered are insulin and insulin reactions, diet, urinary tests, exercise, illnesses and diabetes, dental care, identification badges, summer camps, and instructions for teachers and other responsible adults. Court emphasizes the emotional impact of the disease, with chapters on parental and patient attitudes and a section devoted to answering their most frequent questions. Appended are nutrition guides and recipes, advice on emergency feeding, a list of summer camps, a glossary, and recommended reading. Indispensable.

Covelli, Pat. *Borrowing Time: Growing Up with Juvenile Diabetes.* New York: Crowell, 1979. 160 pp. $9.95.
Beginning with his diagnosis at age ten, a young writer recounts his 15-year struggle with diabetes. He paints a striking portrait of a child and adolescent, fiercely rebelling against the restrictions of his disease and eventually coming to terms with the severe anxieties of youth. He tells of daily injections, insulin reactions, eye and foot complications. More than an autobiography, the book is filled with factual information on juvenile diabetes and ends on a hopeful note. A highly emotional, rather melancholy work that forcefully presents the complex problems of diabetic youth.

Kipnis, Lynne, and Adler, Susan. *You Can't Catch Diabetes from a Friend.* Gainesville, FL: Triad, 1979. 64 pp. $9.95.
Aimed at children, this work about juvenile-onset diabetes describes the daily health routines of four youngsters between 7 and 14 years of age. Each receives insulin injections, follows a diabetic diet, and tests his urine for sugar. While all are presented as normal, active children, the book also addresses such problems as controlling blood glucose, experiencing insulin reactions, and explaining the disease and its restrictions to friends. An uncomplicated, enlightening work that focuses on the common components of treatment rather than examining unusual therapies. Essential.

Sandler, Richard, and Sandler, Michael. *Daily Management of Youth-Onset Diabetes Mellitus.* Springfield, IL: Charles C. Thomas, 1977. 92 pp. $10.25.
Two endocrinologists discuss diabetic routines, and the chronic and acute problems associated with the disease. Among the broad topics covered are

diet, insulin, exercise, urine testing, hypoglycemia, checkups, and emotional aspects of childhood diabetes. Subtitled "an integrated guide for patients and physicians," the work has sections for patients and their parents, in addition to those aimed specifically at doctors. A highly detailed aid to patient involvement in diabetes management, marred only by some undefined medical jargon and a wholly technical bibliography.

Mental Health and Emotional Well-Being

Brehm, Sharon S. *Help for Your Child: A Parent's Guide to Mental Health Services.*
    Englewood Cliffs, NJ: Prentice-Hall, 1978. 170 pp. $9.95; $4.95 (paper).
A psychologist provides information on recognizing when a child needs professional help, overcoming emotional and practical barriers, and utilizing available services. After surveying the various types of facilities, Brehm discusses personnel, tests and diagnostic procedures, specific treatment methods, the advantages and disadvantages of each, family communication and support, financial considerations, rights and responsibilities of the parties involved. An extremely practical, informative handbook.

Gallagher, A. Roswell, and Harris, Herbert I. *Emotional Problems of Adolescents,*
    3rd ed. New York: Oxford Univ. Pr., 1976. 203 pp. $10.95.
In nontechnical language, two physicians examine such problems as adolescent sexuality, anxiety states, psychosomatic conditions, and severe disorders. Excellent advice on helping teens includes examples of active listening, but the line between minor and serious problems remains obscure. Bibliography.

Klagsbrun, Francine. *Too Young to Die: Youth and Suicide.* Boston: Houghton,
    1976. 201 pp. $6.95; Pocket Bks. $1.75 (paper). (Grades 7 and up).
In this study of suicide, the author uses taped interviews to examine the motives and messages of young suicides, the effects of their acts on others, and the societal factors that either provoke or prevent self-destruction. Klagsbrun dispels several misconceptions and urges parents and others to take suicide threats seriously. Appends statistical tables, directory of suicide-prevention agencies by state, and recommendations of popular and technical literature. Well done.

Madison, Arnold. *Suicide and Young People.* A Clarion Book. New York: Seabury, 1978. 146 pp. $6.95.
Directed at children, this work reviews historical attitudes about self-destruction, its occurrence in certain ethnic groups, and its increase among youth as young as ten years of age. Madison looks at suicide equivalents, such as drug abuse, and various preventive measures, such as suicide-prevention centers. Includes selected list of these centers, by state, and a short bibliography. Adequate but uninspiring.

Marks, Jane. *Help: A Guide to Counseling and Therapy without a Hassle.* New York: Messner, 1976. 191 pp. $7.79; Dell. $1.75 (paper). (Grades 7 and up).
Teenagers are advised concerning seeking emotional help for themselves. Among the topics covered are the benefits of therapy; positive and negative aspects of individual and group sessions; different kinds of counselors, therapists, and services; handling parents; special problems of pregnancy and suicide; and how teenagers can determine their own progress. The material includes specific advice and sources for finding a good therapist and suggested readings. Written in colloquial language, this is a unique and much-needed aid. Recommended.

Mason, Robert L., Jr., Richmond, Bert O., and Fleurant, Lucien B. *The Emotionally Troubled Child: A Guide for Parents and Teachers in the Early Recognition of Mental and Nervous Disorders in Children.* Springfield, IL: Charles C. Thomas, 1976. 176 pp. $13.25.
By three specialists in child psychology, this work provides lay readers with a manageable guide to emotional disturbance in youngsters. With case histories and discussions, the authors explore problems from preschool through adolescence, provide a checklist of symptoms, arranged by age groups, and discuss finding help and fostering mental health. An excellent, long-overdue aid to nonprofessionals, written entirely in a conversational style.

Ramos, Suzanne. *Teaching Your Child to Cope with Crisis.* New York: McKay, 1975. 238 pp. $9.95.
Although this guide includes many problems that are not directly health related, it is worthwhile for its sections on hospitalization, coping with death, sexual concerns, and emotionally disturbed children. Includes a chart discussing certain "myths" about children and documents theories that disprove them. Clearly written, with emphasis on preventing severe psychological damage.

Rutter, Michael. *Helping Troubled Children.* New York: Plenum, 1976. 376 pp. $17.50; London: Penguin. £1.25 (paper).
An eminent specialist in child psychiatry provides an overview of emotional development and difficulties during the middle years of childhood. Concerned more with typical conditions than with extreme cases, Rutter examines a variety of child-care practices and their effects. He discusses the influence of family, community, school, and peer group; kinds and degree of psychological disturbance; and various methods of treatment. References and further reading lists are provided. Objective and conversational in tone, this excellent reference work helps both parents and professionals gain an essential perspective.

Sahler, Olle Jane Z., ed. *The Child and Death.* St. Louis: Mosby, 1978. 300 pp. $10.95 (paper).
The product of 29 contributors from diverse backgrounds, this philosophical

work is divided into four sections: the family and the fatally ill child; the responses of care-givers; survivorship; ethical and educational considerations. Especially relevant is the first section, which discusses such topics as family emotions; communication; genetics; and the effects of hospital, hospice, and home on the dying child. Also noteworthy is the annotated bibliography in section four. A perfect blending of objective and subjective perspectives.

Smith, Lendon H. *Improving Your Child's Behavior Chemistry.* Englewood Cliffs, NJ: Prentice-Hall, 1976. 228 pp. $7.95; Pocket Bks., $2.50 (paper).
The work discusses possible causes and characteristics of behavioral problems and explores a variety of remedies including diet therapy, medications, and counseling. Believing that in stressful situations chemical disruptions often provoke destructive responses, "the Children's Doctor" examines the role of several factors, such as genetics, intrauterine influences on the unborn child, the blood-sugar cycle, allergies, and adrenaline. While not discounting psychological causes, Smith argues that a well-nourished brain is essential to successful functioning. Included are a series of checklists to help examine a child's emotional makeup and a bibliography. The work is cluttered with anecdotes and case material, but is thought provoking.

Winnicott, D. W. *The Piggle: An Account of the Psychoanalytic Treatment of a Little Girl.* New York: International Universities Pr., 1977. 201 pp. $12.
This work is a verbatim account of the three-year treatment of an emotionally disturbed child. Beginning at age two, her sessions with an eminent psychoanalyst concerned the girl's bizarre reaction to the birth of a sister. Poignant and insightful.

Speech Disorders and Hearing

Adler, Sol. *The Non-Verbal Child: An Introduction to Pediatric Language Pathology,* 2nd ed. Springfield, IL: Charles C. Thomas, 1975. 262 pp. $15.75.
Written by a specialist in pediatric speech disorders, this multidisciplinary text surveys the growth and development of communicative behavior; the brain mechanisms involved; the nature, symptoms, and causes of various dysfunctions; the diagnostic tests and treatments available. Despite some technical language and subject matter, this comprehensive work is a valuable reference tool for concerned parents as well as professionals.

Agranowitz, Aileen, and McKeown, Milfred Riddle. *Aphasia Handbook for Adults and Children.* Springfield, IL: Charles C. Thomas, 1975. 336 pp. $16.
In the second part of this worthwhile aid, numerous step-by-step lessons are presented and explained. Although the authors direct their material to professional therapists, many of these detailed exercises will prove manageable enough for willing parents to attempt with their children. Suitable for work on a variety of speech and hearing problems.

Eisenson, Jon. *Is Your Child's Speech Normal?* Reading, MA: Addison-Wesley,
    1976. 163 pp. $7.95; $3.95 (paper).
A psychologist and speech specialist discusses normal language development
and various speech disorders in children, such as stuttering, cluttering, voice
problems, hearing loss, brain damage, and delayed speech. Included are
suggestions for getting professional assistance and an annotated list of readings on specific problems. Thorough and reassuring.

Litchfield, Ada B. *A Button in Her Ear*. Concept Books. Chicago: Whitman,
    1976. 32 pp. $5.75. (Grades 2–4).
This entertaining book describes the misunderstandings that result from a
young girl's hearing loss, her visit to an audiologist, and her improvement with
a hearing aid. A satisfactory introduction to the subject.

Peter, Diana. *Claire and Emma*. New York: John Day, 1977. 32 pp. $5.79;
    London: A. C. Black, £1.95. (Grades K–4).
Appealing color photographs and sparse text characterize this story about two
small sisters, deaf from birth. Topics include the disability's effect on their
relationships, balance problems, hearing aids, and lipreading. Not especially
informative.

Simmons-Martin, Audrey Ann. *Chats with Johnny's Parents*. Washington, DC:
    Alexander Graham Bell Assn. for the Deaf, 1975. 82 pp. $4.50 (paper).
Addressing parents of hearing-impaired children, this work offers practical
advice on helping children acquire speech, daily language use, lipreading,
hearing aid care, and behavioral concerns. The author also covers the fundamentals of hearing and speech development.

Teenage Sexuality

See also Chapter 10, Women's Health, for books on teenage pregnancy.

Hamilton, Eleanor. *Sex, with Love: A Guide for Young People*. Boston: Beacon,
    1978. 179 pp. $3.95 (paper); London: Beacon, £5.95.
Aimed at teenagers, this work by a certified sex therapist discusses sexual
development, male and female anatomy, intercourse, autoeroticism and petting, the pressures of dating, homosexuality, sex language, deviant sex, birth
control, wanted and unwanted pregnancy, sex myths, and love. Advice on
finding professional help, a list of community resources, and an annotated
bibliography are appended. Candid and recommended for the uninhibited.

Johnson, Eric W. *V.D.*, new, rev. ed. Philadelphia: Lippincott, 1978. 129 pp.
    $6.95. (Grades 5–12).
An educator warns adolescents about venereal diseases by discussing their
critical incidence, their spread, and the major types. Diagnosis, treatment, and

prevention are topics of major concern, and a hotline service, "Operation Venus," is described in detail. Frank and comprehensive.

Kaplan, Helen Singer. *Making Sense of Sex: The New Facts about Sex and Love for Young People.* New York: Simon & Schuster, 1979. 154 pp. $10.95.
The author is head of the Human Sexuality Program of the Payne Whitney Psychiatric Clinic at New York Hospital–Cornell Medical Center. The book, although somewhat academic in tone, is written primarily for adolescents who need the facts and also the reassurance that their sexual feelings are normal. In a very clear manner, Dr. Kaplan provides frank, explicit, comprehensive, and up-to-date information about the biology and psychology of the sexual experience. Major topics discussed are making love—reality and myth; biology of sex; sexual response; sexual problems—dysfunctions, variations and gender disturbances; what normal sex is; reproduction; birth control; sexually transmitted diseases; stages of human sexuality; love and sex. Emphasis is placed on the connections between human sexuality and the development of caring and loving relationships with others. Contains excellent illustrations. Recommended.

Lieberman, E. James, and Peck, Ellen. *Sex and Birth Control: A Guide for the Young.* New York: Schocken, 1975. 299 pp. $2.95 (paper); London: Wildwood House. £1.35 (paper).
This manual for young adults provides comprehensive, frank, and non-moralizing information and advice on sex and sexual relationships. Contraceptive methods are detailed.

Tensen, Gordon. *Youth and Sex: Pleasure and Responsibility,* 2nd ed. Chicago: Nelson-Hall, 1979. 173 pp. $9.95; $5.95 (paper).
An update of a book originally published in 1973. The author, a child psychiatrist, has produced a frank discussion for adolescents of the major topics of concern—masturbation, petting, contraception, intercourse, venereal disease, pregnancy, abortion, and sexual variations. Tensen avoids any attempt at moralizing but he does inject his own values and leaves room for parents and other readers to discuss the material from their own value system or religious viewpoint. The style is readable and will appeal to the teenage audience for whom it is intended. Informative and reassuring. Highly recommended.

Personal Narratives

Bell, David. *A Time to Be Born.* New York: Morrow, 1975. 192 pp. $5.95.
Through four case histories, a pediatrician describes his experiences in an intensive-care nursery. The narrative confronts the issues and emotions stirred by the brain-damaged victim of a traumatic birth, a newborn heroin addict, a premature baby, and a home-delivered infant. Sensitive and suspenseful.

Bittinger, Marvin L., ed. *Living with Our Hyperactive Children.* New York: Two
    Continents, 1977. 199 pp. $8.95.
Seven families with hyperactive children describe their experiences and frustrations and their ways of coping. Showing the disorder in its many manifestations, the contributors round out their accounts with advice to other parents.
Glossary is included. Composed almost entirely of personal narratives, this
work would be more illuminating if each section were followed by explanatory
commentary.

Cobb, Mary Ann. *Lorie: A Story of Hope.* Nashville, TN: Nelson, 1979. 181 pp.
    $3.95 (paper).
In this personal narrative, the mother of a child with Down's Syndrome
describes her own acceptance of the disorder and the religious conversion that
helped her appreciate her daughter. Includes some recommended readings.

Craig, Eleanor. *One, Two, Three: The Story of Matt, A Feral Child.* New York:
    McGraw-Hill, 1978. 294 pp. $10.95; New York: NAL. $2.50 (paper); London: McGraw-Hill. £8.20.
A social worker relates the story of a nonverbal, abusive boy of six, whose
dependent mother kept him at the level of a baby. Despite pessimistic predictions they both manage to improve, with help from the author and other
professionals. Realistic yet poignant.

Franks, Hugh. *Will to Live.* Boston, MA: Routledge, 1979. 147 pp. $11.50;
    $2.95 (paper).
A devastatingly honest account of Robby, who at the age of six was diagnosed
as suffering from Duchenne muscular dystrophy, a disorder for which there is
no known cure. Franks describes Robby's school experiences, the psychological pain of his relationship with his first father, and tribulations, travels, and
problems arising from their efforts to come to grips with the disease. A very
literate book that focuses attention on feelings rather than medical detail.
However, more description of the latter would have made the former more
real and meaningful.

Greenfeld, Josh. *A Place for Noah.* New York: Holt, 1978. 311 pp. $10.
In a spontaneous and introspective journal, the author of *A Child Called Noah*
continues the story of his brain-damaged son, from age 5 to 11. Greenfeld
speaks of the meager hopes and continual frustrations of their family life since
essentially giving up the search for a cure. Although the specter of Noah's
dismal future haunts its pages, the work is a poignant testimony to survival and
love. Recommended.

Kaufman, Barry Neil. *Son-Rise.* New York: Harper, 1976. 154 pp. $8.95;
    Warner. $2.25 (paper).
Faced with the knowledge that their only son is autistic, Barry and Suzi

Kaufman overcome their initial grief and enter the private world of Raun, celebrating his uniqueness and ultimately bringing him into their family circle. Criticizing professional methods, the author eloquently demonstrates how his family's efforts canceled a bleak prognosis. Although it remains uncertain whether the Kaufmans' success could be duplicated by other parents, the work is superb.

MacCracken, Mary. *Lovey: A Very Special Child.* Philadelphia: Lippincott, 1976. 189 pp. $9.95; New York: NAL. $1.95 (paper); London: Deutsch. £3.95; Sphere. £0.85 (paper).
A teacher of emotionally disturbed and learning-disabled children relates the case of an abused, withdrawn girl of eight. Initially nonverbal, Hannah eventually responds to MacCracken's compassionate treatment with speech and an eagerness to learn. Well done.

Massie, Robert, and Massie, Suzanne. *Journey.* New York: Knopf, 1975. 363 pp. $10; New York: Warner. $1.95 (paper); London: Gollancz. £6.00.
The parents of a hemophiliac describe their struggle to keep their son alive and give him as normal a childhood as possible. Though hopeful and inspiring, the work also criticizes hospitals, insurance companies, and even the Red Cross for neglecting their responsibilities. More than a moving testimony to the perseverance of one hemophiliac, this personal narrative clears away many misconceptions about the disease. Includes an appendix on the genetic transmission of hemophilia.

Schaefer, Nicola. *Does She Know She's There?* New York: Doubleday, 1978. 235 pp. $7.95.
In this personal narrative about a brain-damaged girl, the child's mother tells of the family's adjustment over the years and of the parents group that offered support. Electing to keep her spastic, retarded daughter at home, Schaefer emphasizes the rights of children who must be institutionalized.

Siegel, Dorothy Schainman. *Winners: Eight Special Young People.* New York: Messner, 1978. 191 pp. $7.79. (Grades 7 and up).
Emphasizing the value of willpower and a positive attitude, the author describes the experiences of young people with leukemia, deafness, juvenile rheumatoid arthritis, paralysis, drug addiction, blindness, hemophilia, and limb deformity. Aimed at teenagers, the narrative also provides specific information about the disorders themselves. Recommended.

Trachtenberg, Irene. *My Daughter, My Son.* New York: Summit, 1978. 271 pp. $10.
In this personal narrative, a mother describes the physical and emotional effects of ulcerative colitis on her family. Without a genetic link, this devastating disease struck two of her three children and ultimately required drastic

surgery for both. Filled with introspective passages, this sensitive work recounts the various treatments that failed before ileostomy was elected. Includes the address of the National Foundation for Ileitis and Colitis.

Woodson, Meg. *Following Joey Home.* Grand Rapids, MI: Zondervan, 1978. 160 pp. $6.95.
In this deeply religious narrative, the mother of two children with cystic fibrosis tells of her son's hospitalization during the final three weeks of his life. Emotionally charged, but with scant information on the disease itself.

Other Health Problems and Concerns

Anorexia Nervosa

Bruch, Hilde. *The Golden Cage: The Enigma of Anorexia Nervosa.* Cambridge, MA: Harvard Univ. Pr., 1978. 168 pp. $8.95; Random. $2.50 (paper); London: Open Bks. £5.50.
Citing numerous case histories, a psychiatrist specializing in eating disorders discusses this hunger disease of the privileged. With precision and sensitivity, the author introduces the victims and their perspectives and describes the affliction's dire effects. In examining possible causes and treatments, Dr. Bruch reveals both the failures and the successes of professional intervention. The book offers hope for recovery through early diagnosis and psychotherapy. Recommended.

Bed-wetting

Baller, Warren R. *Bed-Wetting: Origins and Treatment,* rev. ed. New York: Pergamon, 1976. 124 pp. $14.75; Oxford: Pergamon. £8.25; £3.75 (paper).
This thorough study covers the nature and causes of the problem, the numbers and types of bed wetters, various treatments, and long-range effects. Using a nonpunitive approach, Baller argues for conditioning treatments and family empathy. He also discusses the evidence of improved self-concept with successful control. Includes a chapter on helping handicapped persons, appended information on services, bibliography. Although technical terms are few, the overall flavor is rather clinical.

Down's Syndrome

Pueschel, Siegfried, ed. *Down's Syndrome: Growing and Learning.* Human Potential for Children Series. Kansas City: Andrews and McMeel, 1978. 175 pp. $8.95; $4.95 (paper).
This work is the product of four contributors: a pediatrician, the mother of a child with Down's Syndrome, a social worker, and a physical therapist. They present a historical view of Down's Syndrome; discuss its causes, characteristics, expectations; examine the available resources, methods of motor development stimulation, schooling and vocational training; and consider its

emotional impact and such concerns as feeding, adolescent changes, and leaving home. Photographs; bibliography. A compassionate, enlightening overview.

Dyslexia

Simpson, Eileen. *Reversals: A Personal Account of Victory over Dyslexia.* Boston: Houghton, 1979. 246 pp. $8.95.
A personal narrative detailing the author's school-days experience of being unable to read and spell and write a simple sentence without error, of being considered stupid and lazy and even retarded by her family and teachers. Simpson explains what it is like to be afflicted with a neurophysiological disorder that makes an otherwise normal child reverse numbers, letters, syllables, and words. An excellent insight into an affliction that affects some 20 million Americans.

Epilepsy

Silverstein, Alvin, and Silverstein, Virginia B. *Epilepsy.* Philadelphia: Lippincott, 1975. 64 pp. $5.95; $1.95 (paper). (Grades 4–7).
Adults as well as young people are introduced to this enigmatic disease. Among the topics discussed are the problem of misunderstanding and prejudice, historical perspectives, and various kinds of seizures, causes, and research areas. Especially valuable is the chapter on living with the disease, including information on drugs and other control methods and suggestions for dealing with a seizure in progress. Includes the addresses of the Epilepsy Foundation of America and the National Institute of Neurological Diseases and Stroke.

Phenylketonuria

Schuett, Virginia, and others. *Low Protein Cookery for Phenylketonuria.* Madison, WI: Univ. of Wisconsin Pr., 1977. 378 pp. $19.50.
A nutritionist and five mothers of phenylketonuria (PKU) victims are responsible for this valuable cookbook. In addition to the recipes, they discuss PKU, an inherited metabolic disease, and provide material designed to facilitate meal preparation, including information on special ingredients and recipe adaptation. Helpful hints include advice on special occasions, traveling, camping, eating out, and planning for a baby-sitter. Some recipes are designated suitable for the whole family or for camping; all supply phenylalanine, protein, and calorie values.

Skin Care

Nourse, Alan E. *Clear Skin, Healthy Skin.* A Concise Guide. New York: Watts, 1976. 63 pp. $4.90; London: Watts. £1.95. (Grades 7 and up).
Written by a retired physician, this work discusses the causes of acne, home treatment measures, medical treatments, basic hygiene and good grooming. A few suggested readings. Reliable.

Spina Bifida

Reid, Robert. *My Children, My Children.* New York: Harcourt, 1977. 186 pp.
$8.95; London: BBC Pubns. £3.50.
In a popular study of spina bifida, a British science writer examines the moral
and physical dilemmas associated with this major birth defect of the spinal
column and with the hydrocephalus that can follow. Also described are various theories regarding the cause of the defect. With vivid portraits of the
individuals involved, Reid transforms history into spellbinding narration.

Sudden Infant Death Syndrome

Bergman, Abraham B., and Choate, Judith. *Why Did My Baby Die?* New York:
Okpaku Communications, 1975. 152 pp. $6.95.
A pediatrician and the mother of a sudden infant death syndrome (SIDS)
victim collaborate to explore the physical, emotional, and sociological effects
of the syndrome, commonly know as "crib death." With personal narratives
and letters, the authors review SIDS history and recent research; discuss the
findings of studies and the efforts of parents' groups like the National Foundation for Sudden Infant Death Syndrome; and evaluate political progress
and current management of crib-death cases. Well documented, with statistical graphs and bibliography appended. Wonderfully supportive.

PAMPHLETS

Administration for Children, Youth and Families, Office of Human Development Services, 200 Independence Ave. S.W., Washington, DC 20201.

Auto Safety and Your Child, 1978, DHEW Publn. No. (OHDS) 78-30123, 12
pp.
Child Development in the Home, 1974, DHEW Publn. No. (OHDS) 77-30042,
20 pp.
*Children with Emotional Disturbances: A Guide for Teachers, Parents and Others
Who Work with Emotionally Impaired Preschoolers,* 1978, DHEW Publn. No.
(OHDS) 78-311115, 145 pp.
*Children with Health Impairments: A Guide for Teachers, Parents and Others Who
Work with Health Impaired Preschoolers,* 1978, DHEW Publn. No. (OHDS)
78-31111, 130 pp.
*Children with Hearing Impairment: A Guide for Teachers, Parents and Others Who
Work with Hearing Impaired Preschoolers,* 1978, DHEW Publn. No. (OHDS)
78-31116, 170 pp.
*Children with Speech and Language Impairments: A Guide for Teachers, Parents
and Others Who Work with Speech and Language Impaired Preschoolers,* 1978,
DHEW Publn. No. (OHDS) 78-31113, 165 pp.
*Children with Visual Handicaps: A Guide for Teachers, Parents and Others Who
Work with Visually Handicapped Preschoolers,* 1978, DHEW Publn. No.
(OHDS) 78-311112, 125 pp.
Head Start Can Help Communities Fight Childhood Diseases with Immunizations,
1978, flyer.

Responding to Individual Needs In Head Start. Part I. Working with the Individual Child, 1975, DHEW Publn No. (OHD) 75-1075, 93 pp.

When Your Child Goes to the Hospital, 1976, DHEW Publn. No. (OHD) 76-30092, 36 pp.

Alcohol, Drug Abuse and Mental Health Administration, 5600 Fishers La., Parklawn Bldg., Rockville, MD 20857.

Caring about Kids: Dyslexia, 1978, DHEW Publn. No. (ADM) 78-616, 9 pp.

Caring about Kids: Helping the Hyperactive Child, 1978, DHEW Publn. No. (ADM) 78-561, 9 pp.

Caring about Kids: Stimulating Baby Senses, 1977, DHEW Publn. No. (ADM) 77-481, 10 pp.

Causes, Detection and Treatment of Childhood Depression, 1978, DHEW Publn. No. (ADM) 78-612, 7 pp.

The Child's Emotions: How Physical Illness Can Affect Them, 1978, DHEW Publn. No. (ADM) 78-497, 6 pp.

Childhood Environment and Mental Health: A Conversation with Dr. Jerome Kagan, 1978, DHEW Publn. No. (ADM) 78-611, 5 pp.

Children at Risk, 1978, DHEW Publn. No. (ADM) 78-724, 21 pp.

Detection and Prevention of Learning Disorders, 1976, DHEW Publn. No. (ADM) 76-337, 31 pp.

Emotions in the Lives of Children, 1978, DHEW Publn. No. (ADM) 78-644, 17 pp.

Mental Health at School, 1974, DHEW Publn. No. (ADM) 74-105, 23 pp.

New Light on Autism and Other Puzzling Disorders of Childhood, 1978, DHEW Publn. No. (ADM) 78-612, 7 pp.

"Psychosomatic" Diabetic Children and their Families, 1978, DHEW Publn. No. (ADM) 78-477, 9 pp.

Q's and A's on Child Mental Health: An Interview with Dr. Burton L. White, 1977, DHEW Publn. No. (ADM) 77-413, 11 pp.

The Tie between Physical and Behavioral Irregularities of Children, 1978, DHEW Publn. No. (ADM) 78-605, 9 pp.

Why Young People Become Antisocial, 1978, DHEW Publn. No. (ADM) 78-642, 10 pp.

American Academy of Pediatrics, Box 1034, Evanston, IL 60204.

Common Childhood Problems, HE-11, 1976.

Immunization Recommendation, HE-12, 1978.

Institutions and Camps for Asthmatic Children, HE-13, 1976.

Other pamphlets are available on adolescence, adoption, child abuse, drugs, neonatal care, nutrition, physical fitness, and sports.

Blue Cross Association, 840 N. Lake Shore Dr., Chicago, IL 60611.

Childhood, 1976, 92 pp.

Mental Health Association, 1800 N. Kent St., Arlington, VA 22209.

A Child Alone in Need of Help, 1978, 5 pp.
What Every Child Needs for Better Mental Health, 6 pp.

Physicians' Art Service, Patient Information Library, 343-B Serramonte Plaza Office Ctr., Daly City, CA 94015.

Cast Care, 16 pp.

Prudential Insurance Company, Public Relations Department, Box 36, Newark, NJ 07101.

Childhood Diseases: Now You Can Help to Prevent or Treat Them, 18 pp.
Childhood Safety Is No Accident, 14 pp.

Public Affairs Committee, Inc., 381 Park Ave. S., New York, NY 10016.

Asthma—How to Live with It, No. 437.
Health Care for the Adolescent, No. 403.
Immunization—Protection against Childhood Diseases, No. 565.
New Hope for the Retarded Child, No. 210A.
Serious Mental Illness in Children, No. 352.
Talking to Preteeners about Sex, No. 476.
When Your Child Is Sick, No. 441.

Public Health Service, Health Services Administration, 5600 Fishers La., Parklawn Bldg., Rockville, MD 20857.

Books That Help Children Deal with a Hospital Experience, 1978, DHEW Publn. No. (HSA) 78-5224.
Facts about Sudden Infant Death Syndrome, 1979, DHEW Publn. No. (HSA) 79-5259, 11 pp.
Feeding the Child with a Handicap, 1975, DHEW Publn. No. (HSA) 75-5009, 19 pp.
Lead Poisoning in Children, 1978, DHEW Publn. No. (HSA) 78-5142, 25 pp.
Rubella, 1975, DHEW Publn. No. (HSA) 75-5107, 12 pp.
Services for Crippled Children, 1977, DHEW Publn. No. (HSA) 77-5216, 20 pp.
The Sudden Infant Death Syndrome, 1979, DHEW Publn. No. (HSA) 78-5251.
What Do You Know about PKU? DHEW Publn. No. (HSA) 75-5703, flyer.

AUDIOVISUAL PRODUCERS AND DISTRIBUTORS

Concept Media
Box 19542
Irvine, CA 92714
Human development; physical growth; importance of play; cognitive development; role of parents; adolescence; teenage pregnancy and alcoholism; teenage obesity; handicapped children; intelligence in children.

**Encyclopaedia Britannica
Educational Corporation**
425 N. Michigan Ave.
Chicago, IL 60611
Self awareness and importance in
children; identity.

McGraw-Hill Films
110 15 St.
Del Mar, CA 92014
Emotional development; parenting;
teenage behavior; infant growth;
language development; shyness.

Parents' Magazine Films
Distibuted by PMF Films Inc.
Box 1000
Elmsford, NY 10523
Caring for children; child
development, emotional growth in
children; illness; death;
encouraging healthy development;
behavioral, emotional, and physical
disabilities; handicapped children;
family relationships, play and self-
expression; feelings in children.

Perennial Education, Inc.
477 Roger Williams
Box 855, Ravinia
Highland Park, IL 60035
Sex education; menstrual hygiene;
adolescent pregnancy; human
growth.

Professional Research, Inc.
12960 Coral Tree Pl.
Los Angeles, CA 90066
Parenting; feeding; accident
prevention; toilet training; allergies;
respiratory problems;
immunization; temperature;
digestive tract.

Ross Laboratories
625 Cleveland Ave.
Columbus, OH 43216
Infant nutrition; toilet habits.

Single Concept Films
2 Terrain Dr.
Rochester, NY 14618
Colds in babies; upset stomach;
immunization; children and
accidents in the home; measles,
mumps, and chicken pox; allergies;
the well baby checkup; the newborn;
early development.

Trainex Corporation
Box 116
Garden Grove, CA 92642
Infant care; breast-feeding; health
care of the normal infant; accidents
and poisoning; allergy; care of the
sick child; immunization; preventive
dental care; growth and
development.

RESOURCE ORGANIZATIONS

**American Academy of Child
Psychiatry**
1800 R St.
Washington, DC 20009

American Academy of Pediatrics
1801 Hinman Ave.
Evanston, IL 60204

**American Speech and Hearing
Association**
4030 Old Georgetown Rd.
Bethesda, MD 20014

**Association for Children with
Hearing Disabilities**
5225 Grace St.
Pittsburgh, PA 15236

Child Welfare League of America
67 Irving Pl.
New York, NY 10003

Children's Bureau
Office of Child Development
330 Independence Ave. S.W.
Washington, DC 20201

Council for Exceptional Children
1920 Association Dr.
Reston, VA 22091

Down's Syndrome Congress
529 S. Kenilworth
Oak Park, IL 60304

Epilepsy Foundation of America
1828 L St. N.W.
Washington, DC 20036

**Muscular Dystrophy Association of
   America**
810 Seventh Ave.
New York, NY 10019

**National Association of Private
   Schools for Exceptional Children**
Box 928
Lake Wales, FL 33853

**National Cystic Fibrosis Research
   Foundation**
3379 Peachtree St. N.E.
Atlanta, GA 30326

National Foundation/March of Dimes
Box 2000
White Plains, NY 10602

**National Institute of Child Health
   and Human Development**
Landow Bldg.
Bethesda, MD 20014

**National Society for Autistic
   Children**
169 Tampa Ave.
Albany, NY 12208

**National Sudden Infant Death
   Syndrome Foundation**
310 S. Michigan Ave.
Chicago, IL 60604

**Sex Information and Education
   Council of the United States
   (SIECUS)**
84 Fifth Ave.
New York, NY 10011

**Spina Bifida Association of
   America**
Box G-1974
Elmhurst, IL 60126

Chapter 10

Women's Health

BOOKS

See also Chapter 17, Other Health Problems and Concerns, for books on Birth Control and Family Planning, Genetics, Human Sexuality, and Infertility.

General

Boston Women's Health Book Collective. *Our Bodies, Ourselves.* New York: Random, 1978. 383 pp. $12.95; $6.95 (paper); Harmondsworth, Middlesex: Penguin. £3.50 (paper).
This is a comprehensive source book of feminist readings covering a broad range of subjects related to women's health. Topics include sexual relationships, health and nutrition, rape, self-defense, venereal disease, birth control, abortion, childbearing, menopause, and health care. An essential, landmark work.

Cherry, Sheldon H. *For Women of All Ages: A Gynecological Guide to Modern Female Health Care.* New York: Macmillan, 1979. 235 pp. $12.95.
Organized into seven stages of a woman's life, this gynecological guide thoroughly covers the physical and emotional changes that occur naturally and the various disorders that can arise. Topics include normal and abnormal development of the reproductive organs from infancy through prepuberty; misconceptions, problems, and hygiene of adolescence; health care in the young childbearing years and such concerns as infections, venereal disease, contraceptive methods, and abortion, fertility, and sexual function; the numerous concerns of pregnancy and childbirth; the later reproductive years, including cancer and other specific disorders, emotional problems, physical

fitness and diet; health and sexuality in the premenopausal, menopausal, and later years. Superbly illustrated, this is a sensitive and authoritative work.

Cooke, Cynthia W., and Dworkin, Susan. *The MS. Guide to a Woman's Health: The Most Up-to-Date Guide to a Woman's Health and Well Being.* New York: Anchor, 1979. 443 pp. $14.95; $7.95 (paper).
Written by a physician and a contributing editor of *Ms.* Magazine, this handbook covers strategies both for maintaining health and for managing illness. Among the topics discussed are the reproductive organs over a lifetime; contraception, abortion, and sterilization; genetics; infertility and pregnancy; orgasm, sexual dysfunction, rape; and various benign and malignant disorders. The authors address such general health concerns as diet; drugs, including over-the-counter drugs, caffeine, and tranquilizers; stress and vitality, and so on. Also included is a health appraisal checklist.

Corea, Gena. *The Hidden Malpractice: How American Medicine Treats Women as Patients and Professionals.* New York: Morrow, 1977. 309 pp. $10.
In this well-documented exposé a feminist reporter discusses first "how women have been barred from healing" and then "how the male domination of medicine affects the health care women receive." Among the topics covered here are the patient-doctor relationship, the treatment of venereal disease, birth control and male contraception, abortion, sterilization, childbirth, and other health concerns of women. Historical and sociological in approach, this once radical work is rather outdated now.

Diagram Group. *Woman's Body: An Owner's Manual.* New York: Paddington, 1977. 256 pp. $6.95 (paper); New York: Bantam. $2.75 (paper); London: Corgi. £1.35 (paper).
Profusely illustrated with more than 1,000 drawings, diagrams, and charts, this book provides simple explanations of major concerns such as growth and development, sexuality, contraception, pregnancy, abortion, menopause, food, illness, aging, mind and body. Individual panels, numbered for cross-reference, and a comprehensive index enable the reader to find answers to particular questions quickly and easily. Particularly valuable is coverage of events in pregnancy, contraception, fertilization and implantation, labor, childbirth, problem births, postnatal care. The textual description is terse and linked with illustrations of the highest quality. Indispensable.

Dreifus, Claudia, ed. *Seizing Our Bodies: The Politics of Women's Health Care.* New York: Vintage, 1978. 321 pp. $4.95 (paper).
Twenty-four feminist contributors with diverse backgrounds review the history of women's health care and comment on such controversial topics as oral contraception, the Dalkon Shield, sterilizing the poor, male contraception, abortion, childbirth methods, sex hormones, diethylstilbestrol (DES)

and other gynecological drugs, breast cancer, unnecessary hysterectomy, menopause, women workers in the health services industry, self-help, and the women's health movement today. Bibliography included. A militant anthology, often outrageous but undeniably thought provoking.

Edelstein, Barbara. *The Woman Doctor's Diet for Women.* New York: Ballantine, 1979. 182 pp. $2.25 (paper).
A physician specializing in weight control discusses the difference between male and female metabolism; fat formation with puberty, pregnancy, and oral contraceptives; the best and worst times in life for dieting; different types of diets; and male attitudes. Threading her text with numerous tips for dieting women, Dr. Edelstein offers several diets for specific situations and heartily endorses the use of diet pills. Overtly chauvinistic toward male doctors; intriguing and blatantly commercial.

Ehrenreich, Barbara, and English, Deirdre. *For Her Own Good: 150 Years of the Expert's Advice to Women.* New York: Anchor, 1979. 325 pp. $3.95 (paper).
A biologist and a sociologist contend that generations of expert advice have clouded the basic instincts of women and undermined their self-confidence. Despite its sociological orientation, the work covers such medical topics as the role of midwives and women doctors, past and present; the attitudes of male physicians toward the gynecological and psychological problems of women; the mothering role. More than a heavily documented history of attitudes, this is a feminist declaration of independence; polemic but thought provoking.

Llewellyn-Jones, Derek. *Everywoman: A Gynecological Guide for Life,* 2nd ed. Salem NH: Faber (dist. by Merrimack Bk. Serv.), 1978. 382 pp. $10.95; $4.95 (paper); London: Faber. £4.25; £1.50 (paper).
An Australian physician provides a comprehensive handbook on gynecological health and illness. Topics include puberty, sexuality, birth control and abortion, pregnancy and fetal development, childbirth, anesthesia, the Rh factor and other pregnancy complications, breast development and nursing, common gynecological disorders, cancer, hysterectomy, menopause. Glossary and further reading list included. A balanced, enlightened presentation.

Scott, Joseph W. *Woman, Know Thyself.* Thorofare, NJ: Charles B. Slack, 1976. 399 pp. $12.50.
Believing that women need and deserve to be informed about their state of health, an obstetrician provides a detailed gynecological manual that discusses female reproductive and sex organs; menstruation; menopause; normal and abnormal pregnancy states; venereal disease; bladder and bowel dysfunctions; cancer; sex and family planning; hormone-related conditions and therapy; fatigue, diet, and weight control; skin problems; the gynecologist and the hospital; numerous surgical procedures and their complications; and

miscellaneous problems. Recommended reading section and glossary included. A balanced, encyclopedic aid. Absolutely essential.

Seaman, Barbara, and Seaman, Gideon. *Women and the Crisis in Sex Hormones.* New York: Rawson, Wade, 1977. 426 pp. $12.95; New York: Bantam. $3.50 (paper); Brighton: Harvester. £12.50.
A science writer and a physician alert layreaders to the hazards of synthetic estrogens and certain other contraceptive aids. Included are sections on diethylstilbestrol (DES); oral contraceptives; alternatives such as the intrauterine device (IUD), the diaphragm, "natural" methods, sterilization, and abortion; male contraception; estrogen replacement therapy and the cancer controversy; and other, more mundane remedies to menopausal discomforts. Organizational addresses are appended. A heavily documented exposé, slanted but thought provoking.

Sims, Naomi. *All about Health and Beauty for the Black Woman.* New York: Doubleday, 1976. 296 pp. OP.
This well-written book by a black model contains a 50-page chapter on the reproductive system. This includes such topics as personal hygiene; menstruation; pregnancy; menopause; cancer, venereal disease, and other diseases; birth control; the internal examination; instructions for a childbirth emergency; advice on rape. Supportive and up-to-date.

Stewart, Felicia Hance and others. *My Body, My Health: The Concerned Woman's Guide to Gynecology.* New York: Wiley, 1979. 566 pp. $13.95; $5.95 (paper).
A vast compendium of information intended to satisfy most health information needs of women. Coverage is extensive and includes methods of birth control, natural family planning, sterilization, Pap smears, abortion, pelvic examination, common reproductive-tract infections, ovarian cysts, menstrual problems, infertility, menopause, dilatation and curettage (D & C) and hysterectomy. This cooperative effort is a first-class publication with excellent illustrations. The textual material is clear and concise. Will doubtless become a classic lay work on health concerns of women. Recommended.

Menstruation

Dalton, Katharina. *Once a Month.* Pomona, CA: Hunter, 1979. 206 pp. $5.95 (paper); London: Harvester. £10.50; Fontana. £1 (paper).
A British authority on premenstrual syndrome describes the myriad of physical and emotional problems that she identifies as symptoms. Suggested treatments range from merely warning family and associates about the disorder to receiving progesterone therapy from a physician. Also discussed briefly are hysterectomy and menopause. Glossary is included. A rather simplistic work in which premenstrual syndrome appears to be a convenient cause of too many problems.

Delaney, Janice, and others. *The Curse: A Cultural History of Menstruation.* New York: Dutton, 1976. 276 pp. $9.95; New York: NAL, 1977. $1.95 (paper). Although this work has limited medical value it is a scholarly and often amusing study of menstruation. Divided into seven parts, the work discusses historical and current "taboos"; the menstrual process, menarche, and pre-menstrual syndrome; the menstruating woman in the popular imagination, including chapters on "red humor"; advertising and menstrual products; menstrual images in literature; menopause; miscellaneous matters such as the cessation of menstruation; male cycles and simulated menstruation. Fascinating.

Maddux, Hilary C. *Menstruation.* Villanova, PA: Tobey, 1975. 210 pp. $5.95; $2.95 (paper).
This sensible work on menstruation debunks many common myths; reviews anatomy and physiology; discusses attitudes and education; and advises on menstrual problems and preventive nutrition, exercise, and checkups. In a final section, birth, birth control, and menopause are touched on. Includes glossary, bibliography, menstrual charts, and a nationwide directory of women's centers, health care clinics, and referral services. Candid and practical.

Shuttle, Penelope, and Redgrove, Peter. *The Wise Wound: Eve's Curse and Everywoman.* New York: Marek, 1978. 335 pp. $9.95; London: Gollancz. £7.95.
Two British poets present an analysis of the psychological and mystic significance of menstruation. Abounding in archetypal imagery, the work proposes that this phase of woman's cycle is not a curse but a source of creativity and power. A most imaginative but poorly written work, of limited value as a health book.

Voelckers, Ellen. *Girls' Guide to Menstruation.* MS Series. New York: Rosen, 1975. 128 pp. $4.98. (Ages 12–18).
Written by a 23-year-old woman, this work introduces teenage girls to the menstrual cycle. Especially helpful are the sections on early and irregular menses, cramps, and methods of protection. Responds well to the uneasiness and embarrassment that many girls feel. Bibliography.

Weideger, Paula. *Menstruation and Menopause: The Physiology and Psychology, The Myth and the Reality.* New York: Knopf, 1976. 285 pp. $10.
Focusing on the cultural aspects of menstruation and menopause, a psychologist discusses the menstrual cycle from puberty, fertility control, "complaints" and syndromes, cultural taboos, the sexual cycle, shamans and gynecologists, the menarche, the behavioral aspects of menstruation and menopause and changing attitudes. Appended are a questionnaire used in compiling the book, notes, and bibliography. A mildly feminist, intriguing investigation, though not especially informative on medical matters.

Female Sexuality

Bode, Janet. *Fighting Back: How to Cope with the Medical, Emotional, and Legal Consequences of Rape.* New York: Macmillan, 1978. 279 pp. $8.95.
Written by a rape victim, this work is a keen and articulate examination that considers every aspect of the crime. As health literature, the work is filled with psychological insights and contains a chapter on "medical mismanagement" that suggests specific treatments and alerts women to the callous attitudes and humiliating procedures they may encounter. Bibliography is included. Highly recommended.

Hite, Shere. *The Hite Report: A Nationwide Study of Female Sexuality.* New York: Macmillan, 1976. 438 pp. $12.50; New York: Dell. $2.75 (paper); Leicester: Summit Bks, Australia. £1.75 (paper).
This controversial work examines the responses to a five-part questionnaire on female sexuality, distributed nationally between 1972 and 1974. Topics considered include masturbation, orgasm, intercourse, clitoral stimulation, lesbianism, sexual slavery, the sexual revolution, and the sexuality of older women. Interesting but statistically lopsided.

Horos, Carol V. *Vaginal Health.* Villanova, PA: Tobey, 1975. 186 pp. $5.95; $2.95 (paper).
Although vaginal infections occur relatively often, few women are adequately equipped to avoid or identify them. This aid to preventive medicine instructs women about reproductive anatomy; the gynecological examination; normal changes in vaginal discharge; daily hygiene; the effects of douches and vaginal sprays; the causes, transmission, symptoms, diagnosis, and treatment of venereal disease and other vaginal infections. Horos also provides material on the complications of certain infections, preventive measures, breast examination, and choosing a gynecologist. Included are a glossary and a directory of resources for women's health care.

Kline-Graber, Georgia, and Graber, Benjamin. *Woman's Orgasm: A Guide to Sexual Satisfaction.* Indianapolis: Bobbs-Merrill, 1975. 184 pp. $7.95.
A physician and a registered nurse, both specializing in sex therapy, offer a scholarly guide to female orgasm that includes a discussion of its physiology and a review of past and current theories. The body of the work contains detailed programs for achieving orgasm with self-stimulation and with intercourse. A final chapter concerns sex education of children. Included are notes and bibliography. Clearly and tastefully presented.

Abortion

Barr, Samuel J., and Abelow, Dan. *A Woman's Choice: The New Dimensions in Abortions.* New York: Rawson, Wade, 1978. 254 pp. $10.95.

Using case histories, a physician examines the various reasons women have for choosing abortion. A compassionate, introspective work.

Denes, Magda. *In Necessity and Sorrow: Life and Death in an Abortion Hospital.* New York: Basic, 1976. 247 pp. $13.50; New York: Penguin. $2.95 (paper).
A clinical psychologist looks at legalized abortion through the eyes of patients, relatives, physicians, and staff at an abortion hospital. Denes's interviews reveal a complexity of motivations and feelings, set in counterpoint to her own deeply personal reactions. Objective yet stirring.

Nathanson, Bernard N., and Ostling, Richard. *Aborting America.* New York: Doubleday, 1979. 321 pp. $10.
A well-known obstetrician and gynecologist, at one time the most prominent doctor in the fight to repeal abortion laws, now believes that abortion on request is wrong. In 1974, Dr. Nathanson admitted that he had "presided over 60,000 deaths." The book offers a rare insight into the abortion movement and the organization of the abortion industry. Although the author skillfully analyzes the arguments for and against abortion and presents the views of the major religious groups in the United States, he does not account for his own change of opinion.

Wilkie, Jack, and Wilkie, Barbara. *Handbook on Abortion.* Cincinnati, OH: Hayes, 1979. 210 pp. $1.75.
This is not a guide to abortion as the title may suggest. Instead, it may be considered as the "bible" of the prolife movement. The authors argue that the major ploy of the proponents of abortions is to dehumanize the living human in the uterus since "it is easier to destroy a 'fetus,' an 'embryo' or the 'product of conception' than to destroy an unborn 'baby.' " The book describes how abortions are performed and contains vivid, color photographs of the products of abortion. By a question and answer technique, the authors develop the arguments of the Right to Life Movement. A most controversial book that should be useful to those who wish to understand the viewpoint of those opposed to abortion.

Pregnancy

Ashdown-Sharp, Patricia. *A Guide to Pregnancy and Parenthood for Women on Their Own.* New York: Random, 1977. 201 pp. $3.95 (paper).
A British journalist provides women with a manual for single parenthood, both chosen and unplanned. Primarily concerned with the latter, Ashdown-Sharp covers diagnosing pregnancy; deciding what to do; abortion or single pregnancy; marrying, rearing a child alone, or choosing adoption or foster care; and contraception. A practical, objective guide, this work discusses financial concerns, conflicting opinions, and helpful resources and literature.

Brewer, Gail, ed. *The Pregnancy-after-30 Workbook: A Program for Safe Childbearing—No Matter What Your Age.* Emmaus, PA: Rodale, 1978. 233 pp. $8.95 (paper).
This detailed guide for older pregnant women is the product of nine contributors. Broad topics include the risks of late childbearing, a "no-risk" pregnancy diet, recommended exercises, preparation for childbirth and breast-feeding, the advantages and techniques of breast-feeding, the emotional adjustment to parenthood, postpartum crisis, and sex during and after pregnancy. Contains end-of-chapter references and appended information directory. Especially valuable are the many illustrations, quizzes, and charts that provide both statistics and practical advice. Highly recommended.

Brewer, Gail Sforza, and Brewer, Tom. *What Every Pregnant Mother Should Know: The Truth about Diet and Drugs in Pregnancy.* New York: Random, 1977. 244 pp. $8.95; New York: Penguin. $2.95 (paper).
A childbirth instructor and an obstetrician collaborate on this controversial work about nutrition in pregnancy. Asserting that toxemia is a disease of malnutrition, the authors advocate a high-protein diet, salted to taste, and no diuretics. They also argue that nutrition is poorly covered in medical schools. Concerned with preventing low birth weight, the Brewers devote extensive space to diet plans, recipes, and menus. Included are a protein counter, information directory, and bibliography. Contains little material on drugs, other than diuretics.

Dilfer, Carol. *Your Baby, Your Body: Fitness during Pregnancy.* New York: Crown, 1977. 149 pp. $8.95; $5.95 (paper).
Exercise during pregnancy not only is possible but clearly promotes an easier labor and delivery and a faster postpartum recovery. The author, who conducts a prenatal/postpartum fitness program, discusses the physical changes pregnancy causes in a woman's body, posture, calisthenics, aerobics, individualizing routines, exercises for specific body areas, exercises especially for childbirth, relaxation, and pain relief. Organizational addresses and bibliography are included. Simple and reliable.

Elkins, Valmai Howe. *The Rights of the Pregnant Parent.* New York: Two Continents, 1977. 290 pp. $4.95 (paper).
A Canadian childbirth instructor explains the rationale behind prepared childbirth and contrasts it with earlier practices. Sharing the experiences of numerous mothers, the author emphasizes the right to a supportive doctor, the right to a healthy baby, the right to childbirth education, the right to a shared birth experience with husband or coach, the right to childbirth with dignity, and the right to family-centered maternity care that promotes bonding. Elkin discusses related topics such as nutrition and drugs, choosing a childbirth class and a hospital, unnecessary procedures, midwives, home births, and birth centers. Includes glossary, notes, and bibliography. Both reasonable and exciting.

Gillespie, Clark. *Your Pregnancy Month by Month*. New York: Harper, 1977. 226
pp. $10.
In clear, often witty, language, an obstetrician presents an attractive guide to
pregnancy. The numerous topics include selecting a doctor, pregnancy tests,
dangerous substances, physical and emotional changes, spontaneous abortion, nutrition and weight, illnesses and infections, accidents, multiple births,
toxemia, varicose veins, adolescent or late pregnancies, precautions about
pets, cesarean section, Rh blood factor, prematurity, the hospital stay, labor,
including the Lamaze method, postpartum concerns, and birth control. Each
chapter, representing a separate month, begins with a drawing of the fetus at
that stage and ends with a blank memo page. Includes a glossary and three
diets; regular, bland, and low-sodium.

Hartman, Rhonda Evans. *Exercises for True Natural Childbirth*. New York:
Harper, 1975. 139 pp. $10.95.
An excellent preparation for labor and delivery, this work explains and illustrates fundamental exercises. Hartman also suggests ways to relieve such
discomforts as leg cramps, heartburn, varicose veins. Breast and nipple care,
nutrition, the stages of labor, breast-feeding, postpartum exercises and adjustment are all covered. Intimate and informative.

Isbister, Clair. *Birth of a Family: A Preparation for Parenthood*. New York:
Hawthorn, 1978. 252 pp. $8.95.
In this handbook for prospective parents, an Australian pediatrician discusses
pregnancy and fetal development, labor, and various methods of childbirth.
Emphasis throughout is on promoting healthful relationships, as reflected in
chapters on family types, mothers and fathers, adjusting to the child, family
planning, and the working mother. Appendixes provide detailed prenatal and
postnatal exercises; glossary and bibliography are included. More philosophical than practical, this introduction to parenting is sensible and clearly written.

McCauley, Carole Spearin. *Pregnancy after 35*. New York: Pocket Bks., 1978.
215 pp. $1.95.
In addition to the common concerns of pregnancy, the older expectant
mother faces unique problems. The reversal of infertility, the risks that late
pregnancy may pose to both mother and child, and the altering of long-
established life-styles are all covered here. Rounding out McCauley's handbook are such general topics as diet and drugs, emotions, fathering, single
parenting, childbirth methods, and insurance. Appendixes provide a nutrition chart, a glossary, a bibliography, and organizational addresses. A sound,
enjoyable aid.

Marzollo, Jean, comp. *9 Months 1 Day 1 Year: A Guide to Pregnancy, Birth and
Baby Care*. New York: Harper, 1976. 191 pp. $4.95 (paper).
This unique work is largely a collection of parents' impressions about preg-
nancy, labor and delivery, and the first year of a baby's life. Topics include the

advantages and disadvantages of different birth methods, doctors and midwives, hospital and home births, old wives' tales, checkups, minor complaints in pregnancy, nutrition, hygiene, emotions, preparation for labor, breast- or bottle-feeding, rooming-in, circumcision, the hospital stay, the first week home, breast-feeding problems, bottle sterilization, infant bathing and hygiene, postpartum depression, infant illnesses, weaning, teething, parenting problems, the rights of parents. Appendixes suggest infant paraphernalia and books about pregnancy, birth, and baby care. Enjoyable and succinct.

Noble, Elizabeth. *Essential Exercises for the Childbearing Years: A Guide to Health and Comfort Before and After Your Baby Is Born.* Boston: Houghton, 1976. $12.95; $5.95 (paper); London: Murray, £2.95.
Another excellent guide to fitness during and after pregnancy, this work emphasizes the value that some exercises have in preventing later gynecological and urinary problems. Also provided are exercises for women with cesareans. Lists of organizations and literature. Recommended.

Oettinger, Katherine B., with Mooney, Elizabeth C. *Not My Daughter: Facing Up to Adolescent Pregnancy.* New York: Prentice-Hall, 1979. 184 pp. $8.95.
A well-written, readable book on a major social problem. Each year more than one million teenage girls in the United States become pregnant. Of these, about one third seek abortions. The authors wish to help parents and adolescents understand, cope with, and prevent teenage pregnancy. They discuss healthy sexuality in the home and how to communicate with teenagers. They attempt to guide parents and teenagers through the decisions that must be made with respect to abortion choices and financial and educational realities, and in coping with anger and dismay. A comprehensive, up-to-date guide to community resources, services and organizations, and innovative programs currently available is especially valuable. While the book is warm and sensitive, encouraging frank and healthy discussion, it may offend those who are not inclined to accept the abortion alternative.

Patterson, Janet, and Patterson, R. C., Jr. *How To Life with a Pregnant Wife.* New York: Nelson, 1976. 163 pp. $3.95 (paper).
An obstetrician and his wife collaborated on this guide for expectant fathers. Topics include symptoms of pregnancy, heredity, month-by-month developments, myths, the pregnant husband, "crisis great and small," labor and natural childbirth, postpartum care, birth control methods, and breast- vs. bottle-feeding. Glossary is appended. A clearly written but undistinctive work.

Robe, Lucy B. *Just So It's Healthy.* Minneapolis: CompCare, 1979. 96 pp. $3.95 (paper).
This book has a terse message: "If you are pregnant, don't drink alcohol." It suggests that heavy drinkers stand a 93 percent chance of having babies with some form of abnormality. One out of every 2,000 newborns has severe fetal

alcohol syndrome. Robe discusses the effects of heavy, moderate "social," and binge drinking during pregnancy. Also covered are the effects on the unborn baby of various classes of drugs—antibiotics, anticoagulants, antidiabetics, antihistamines, antihypertensives, corticosteroids, diuretics, hormones. Although one may quibble with the validity of some of the pharmacological data presented, the use of alcohol and drugs during pregnancy is clearly hazardous. Recommended by the National Clearinghouse for Alcohol Information and by the American Association for Maternal and Child Health.

Russell, Keith P. *Eastman's Expectant Motherhood,* 6th rev. ed. Boston: Little, 1977. 239 pp. $3.95.
First published in 1940, this work discusses the symptoms of pregnancy, fetal growth and development, nutrition and weight gain, common discomforts and their treatment, more serious conditions, labor and delivery, childbirth methods and procedures, breast-feeding, and other postpartum concerns. Appendixes suggest personal names and provide dietary guidelines. An adequate but conservative work, offering very little encouragement for prepared childbirth and totally ignoring the father's potential role.

Thompson, Judi. *Healthy Pregnancy the Yoga Way.* New York: Doubleday, 1977. 148 pp. $3.95.
An instructor of Yoga provides a unique work designed to enhance pregnancy, facilitate childbirth, and alleviate postpartum difficulties. In addition to the breathing techniques and numerous illustrated exercises, the author gives sensible dietary suggestions that admit the need for meat and other basic foods. Also included are several do's and don'ts for expectant mothers and warnings about smoking, aspirin dependency, and alcohol.

Zackler, Jack, and Brandstadt, Wayne, eds. *The Teenage Pregnant Girl.* Springfield, IL: Charles C. Thomas, 1975. 323 pp. $15.
Nineteen contributors with diverse professional credentials discuss the incidence and special problems of teenage pregnancy. Topics include obstetrical and medical concerns, psychological effects, diet and pregnancy, programs for pregnant teens, and adolescent contraception. Despite its professional orientation and a few technical sections, the work provides a valuable overview of the peculiar problems of the pregnant adolescent.

The Unborn Child

Annis, Linda Ferrill. *The Child before Birth.* Ithaca, NY: Cornell Univ. Pr., 1978. 197 pp. $12.50; $4.95 (paper); Hemel Hempstead, Herts: International Book Dist. £8.75; £3.50 (paper).
This excellent work details the stages of prenatal development; sensory development and prenatal learning; the effects of nutrition; maternal characteristics and experiences, including smoking and drinking; medications and

drug abuse; prematurity and postmaturity. Material is also provided on preventing birth defects through genetic counseling and amniocentesis, sex determination, and abortion. Glossary and references are included. Comprehensive; elegantly presented.

Montagu, Ashley. *Life before Birth,* rev. and updated. New York: NAL, 1977.
   248 pp. $1.95 (paper).
An eminent anthropologist describes fetal development and the various factors influencing it. These include nutrition and oxygen; mother's age; drugs; smoking and alcohol; noninfectious and infectious disorders; allergies and blood incompatibilities; emotions and fatigue; radiation; noise and other physical influences; prematurity, cesarean section, postmaturity, multiple births; and delivery. Glossary is included. A reliable guide that both explains the hazards and suggests preventive measures.

Nilsson, Lennart. *A Child Is Born,* rev. ed. New York: Delacorate, 1977. 160 pp.
   $11.95; London: Faber. £2.95. (paper).
This work contains Nilsson's exquisite photographs of the developing child, from conception to birth. In addition it shows the male and female reproductive organs and the process of fertilization, skillfully magnified, and contains sections on chromosomes, pregnancy tests, prenatal exercises and childbirth education, labor and delivery, breast-feeding, and postnatal concerns. A splendid book.

Rorvik, David M., and Shettles, Landrum B. *Choose Your Baby's Sex: The One Sex-Selection Method That Works.* New York: Dodd, Mead, 1977. 177 pp.
   $7.95.
A science writer and an obstetrician describe historical efforts at sex determination and review recent discoveries about "boy" and "girl" sperm and its reponse to acid and alkaline environments. Also discussed are the use of sperm banks and amniocentesis. Included are letters from satisfied parents, a question-and-answer chapter, an appended list of acid/alkaline foods, and a bibliography. Faddish.

Rosen, Mortimer G., and Rosen, Lynn. *In the Beginning: Your Baby's Brain before Birth.* New York: NAL, 1975. 143 pp. $3.95 (paper).
An obstetrician and an educator discuss heredity, fetal brain development, the effects of drugs and nutrition, fetal response to various sensations and stimuli, psychiatric concerns, the effects of labor and delivery on the fetus, various insults and fetal distress, and adjustments of the brain after birth. A detailed, clearly written work with a unique perspective.

Smith, David W. *Mothering Your Unborn Baby.* Philadelphia: Saunders, 1979.
   97 pp. $6.95 (paper).
A pediatrician and expert on human malformation thoroughly reviews nor-

mal fetal development, pregnancy and childbirth, and the components of a healthy diet. A chapter on hazards to the fetus details the malformations or deficiences caused by cigarettes, alcohol, anticonvulsive medicines, and many other drugs, conditions, and environmental factors. Also discussed are amniocentesis and abortion. A graphic yet urgently needed presentation. Highly recommended.

Childbirth and Cesarean Delivery

Arms, Suzanne. *Immaculate Deception: A New Look at Childbirth in America.* Boston: Houghton, 1975. 318 pp. $11.95; New York: Bantam. $2.50 (paper).
A photo-journalist criticizes the American way of birth, in sterile hospitals with anesthesia, handcuffs, and forceps, separated from the nurturing and support of family and friends. Finding fault even with "natural" childbirth methods, Arms favors home or maternity-center deliveries, with midwives in attendance. Includes many expressive pictures and personal accounts. Flawed by its romantic image of primitive childbirth, the work nevertheless presents a calm, articulate argument for change.

Bean, Constance. *Labor and Delivery: An Observer's Diary.* New York: Doubleday, 1977. 203 pp. OP.
In this fascinating narration, a childbirth instructor reports on several labors and deliveries, observed in both hospitals and homes. Described are a premature birth, deliveries where the mothers are totally or partially anesthetized, cesareans, Lamaze births, emergency births, and dilation and curettages. Particularly worthwhile is Bean's humorous picture of one home birth. Warm and revealing; totally objective.

Bing, Elizabeth. *Six Practical Lessons for an Easier Childbirth,* rev. ed. New York: Bantam, 1977. 139 pp. $2.25 (paper); London: Bantam £0.75 (paper).
The teacher who pioneered Lamaze birth in this country offers step-by-step instructions in the method. With many helpful photographs and anatomical drawings, Bing discusses the control of pain, bodily changes during pregnancy, neuromuscular control, exercises and birthing techniques, stages of labor, the husband's role, medication, and many other concerns. Birth reports are included. Thorough and reliable.

Brezin, Nancy. *The Gentle Birth Book: A Practical Guide to Leboyer Family-Centered Delivery.* New York: Simon & Schuster, 1980. 157 pp. $9.95.
The author maintains that the gentle birth method can be accomplished with no sacrifice of safety. Brezin explains each element of a gentle birth delivery and emphasizes the psychological, emotional, and social advantages as well as the physical and medical benefits. The writing is sparkling and lyrical: "Numb from the battering they receive in the birth canal, senses swamped by bright

lights and din of the operating room in which they are delivered, these infants resort to the only means available to them to express their misery. They cry—and cry—and cry. And in crying, they seal themselves off from contact with their parent, who becomes defensive and perhaps a little angry as well." A well-written American version of Leboyer's *Birth without Violence*. Recommended.

Chock, Judy, and Miner, Margaret. *Birth*. New York: Crowell, 1978. 168 pp. $14.95; London: Harper. £7.95.
Over 50 photographs vividly present the moment of birth. Among the topics covered in the accompanying text are the types of delivery, including Lamaze and cesarean, childbirth drugs, and the Leboyer method. Well done.

Donovan, Bonnie. *The Cesarean Birth Experience: A Practical, Comprehensive and Reassuring Guide for Parents and Professionals*. Boston: Beacon, 1977. 240 pp. $4.95 (paper); London: Beacon. £5.50; £2.50 (paper).
Having undergone two cesareans, the author provides an informative and progressive guide to this mode of delivery. She discusses the possible reasons for a cesarean, the pregnancy, emotional stress caused by the procedure, tests to determine fetal maturity and well-being, signs of labor, hospital routines, the controversy over fathers in the cesarean delivery room, the recovery room and postpartum stay, human bonding and breast-feeding, the history of cesareans, a list of choices for cesarean mothers, sources of emotional support. Appendix includes birth accounts, suggested readings, and organizations. Recommended.

Ewy, Donna, and Ewy, Rodger. *Preparation for Childbirth: A Lamaze Guide*, 2nd ed. Boulder, CO: Pruett, 1976. 116 pp. $5.95; New York: NAL. $1.95 (paper).
This superb Lamaze handbook discusses the rationale and advantages of the method and its modifications, reproductive anatomy, exercises, contractions in labor and delivery, neuromuscular control and breathing techniques, the father's role, the stages of birth, different kinds of births, and minor problems. Four birth reports by parents are presented, and suggestions for further reading. Most reliable, with excellent diagrams and photographs.

Feldman, Silvia. *Choices in Childbirth*. New York: Grossett & Dunlap, 1978. 269 pp. $14.95; $7.95 (paper).
In this highly acclaimed guide, a psychotherapist and family counselor thoroughly reviews various methods of childbirth, advocating none in particular but stressing the need for informed individuals to make their own choices. Topics include prenatal medical care, diet, and exercise; the cesarean birth and its effects; the pros and cons of childbirth drugs; several "natural" methods; possible participants; various settings, including out-of-hospital;

rooming-in; breast- and bottle-feeding; aids to postpartum adjustment. Includes addresses of childbirth organizations; bibliography. Both authoritative and sensitive. Highly recommended.

Galinsky, Ellen. *Beginnings: A Young Mother's Personal Account of Two Premature Births.* Boston: Houghton, 1976. 147 pp. OP.
In this eloquent narrative, the author describes her two pregnancies and the premature births of her children. Born eight weeks early, her first son weighed less than three pounds but survived and thrived. Her second died of hyaline membrane disease after arriving 11 weeks early. Highly recommended for Galinsky's sensitive style and insights.

Hale, Nathan Cabot. *Birth of a Family: The New Role of the Father in Childbirth.* New York: Anchor, 1979. 197 pp. $7.95.
Celebrating the instincts of fatherhood, this work describes the childbirth experiences of four couples in eloquent prose and photography. Hale closes by comparing mechanical approaches to childbirth with more natural, nonviolent methods. Although this latter discussion is not completely relevant, the book retains its value, having touched the roots of the father-child relationship.

Hathaway, Margie, and Hathaway, Jay. *Children at Birth.* Sherman Oaks, CA: Academy Pubns., 1978. 178 pp. $5.95.
A compendium of information and opinion to justify the presence of children at the birth of a baby. The authors believe that natural childbirth is the only way to have a baby and that medication should be used only for true medical problems, as a last resort. The authors rely heavily on the Bradley Method of the American Academy of Husband-Coached Childbirth. A good insight into alternative attitudes toward childbirth.

Hausknecht, Richard, and Heilman, Joan Rattner. *Having a Cesarean Baby.* New York: Dutton, 1978. 201 pp. OP.
The authors believe that the trend is toward a dignified, shared, informed, family-oriented childbirth experience. Cesarean birth need not be a merely biological procedure but can be as meaningful and joyful as other methods of childbirth. Some 400,000 babies (16 percent of all births) are now delivered annually by cesarean section. A simple, clear explanation is provided of the reasons for cesarean birth, tests for fetal maturity and health, types of anesthesia, surgical procedures in the delivery room, postoperative recovery and baby care, feeding, and home care. Also discussed are the risks of cesarean birth, the father in the delivery room, selection of an obstetrician and hospital, and "the Pregnant Patient's Bill of Rights." An explicit, informative book that is both well written and supportive. Highly recommended.

Hazell, Lester. *Commonsense Childbirth.* New York: Berkley, 1976. 281 pp. $2.25 (paper).
Written by the president of the International Childbirth Education Association, this work covers such topics as choosing an obstetrician, nutrition and exercise in pregnancy, labor, anesthesia, three types of delivery, husband's participation, breast-feeding, coping with unexpected problems, and sexual considerations. Appendixes include frequent questions about childbirth and breast-feeding, a step-by-step outline of labor, instructions for delivery in unplanned places, organizational addresses. Especially noteworthy are Hazell's contrasting depictions of anesthetized, "natural," and home deliveries, the last of which she enthusiastically details.

Kitzinger, Sheila. *Giving Birth: The Parent's Emotions in Childbirth.* New York: Schocken, 1978. 206 pp. $3.95 (paper); London: Sphere £0.05.
Compiled by a childbirth educator, this work consists primarily of parents' accounts of labor and delivery. Together with the author's own reflections, these personal testimonies reveal diverse physical and emotional responses to childbirth. Glossary is included.

Lamaze, Fernand. *Painless Childbirth.* New York: Pocket Bks., 1977. $1.95.
The doctor who developed the psychoprophylactic method of labor and delivery explains his concept of childbirth without pain and presents the rationale behind his now-famous teachings. Rather dryly presented but illuminating.

Leboyer, Frederick. *Birth without Violence.* New York: Knopf, 1975. 115 pp. $8.95; London: Fontana. £1.95 (paper).
Writing from the newborn's point of view, a French obstetrician describes insensitive practices that may heighten the terror of childbirth. Leboyer suggests, instead, the establishment of a calm, dimly lit setting; and poetically describes the positive effect of infant massage and bathing just after birth. Simple yet stirring; essential reading.

Parfitt, Rebecca Rowe. *The Birth Primer: A Source Book of Traditional and Alternative Methods in Labor and Delivery.* Philadelphia: Running Pr., 1977. 259 pp. $9.80; $5.95 (paper).
As an aid to decision making, this work presents the full range of childbirth alternatives. It begins with a detailed description of labor and delivery, including possible complications and postpartum concerns. Parfitt reviews the various theories and techniques of natural childbirth, including the Leboyer method; and the drugs, devices, surgeries, and procedures of more complicated births. Also discussed are the roles of midwives, fathers, and other participants; hospital births, home births, and those at maternity centers. Includes resources for childbirth education, glossary, annotated bibliography. Balanced and comprehensive.

Tucker, Tarvez, with Bing, Elizabeth. *Prepared Childbirth*. Villanova, PA: Tobey, 1975. 143 pp. $5.95; $2.95 (paper).
With an introduction by Elizabeth Bing, this work provides a step-by-step explanation of prepared childbirth as developed by Dick-Read and Lamaze. Tucker describes the stages of labor and the phenomenon of pain and mechanisms for its control; reviews historical attitudes and practices; examines the question of drugs; and details the rationale and tools of prepared childbirth. Also discussed are the controversial forceps delivery and episiotomy, choosing supportive participants and environment, breast-feeding, and rooming-in. A practical, balanced presentation. Recommended.

Walker, Morton, and others. *The Whole Birth Catalog*. New York: Simon & Schuster, 1979. $10.95.
An objective review of the major birth methods, this guide includes material on prenatal care; the ideas of Dick-Read, Lamaze, Bradley, and Leboyer; the benefits of yoga; and even acupuncture and hypnosis. Provides addresses of groups involved in natural childbirth.

Walton, Vicki E. *Have It Your Way*. New York: Bantam, 1978. 403 pp. $2.50 (paper); London: Bantam. £0.95 (paper).
This work is subtitled "an overview of pregnancy, labor and postpartum, including alternatives available in the hospital childbirth experience." Walton discusses the American way of childbirth; childbirth methods; choosing classes, health care, hospital, and pediatrician; the pregnancy; stages of labor; medications; special situations; the role of the labor coach; the newborn; breast-feeding; and postpartum concerns. Included are birth stories, glossary, and resource directory. Well done.

Wertz, Richard W., and Wertz, Dorothy C. *Lying-In: A History of Childbirth in America*. New York: Free Pr., 1977. 260 pp. $10; New York: Schocken, 1979. $4.95 (paper); London: Collier. £7.50.
In this flowing account, the authors cover the role of midwives and neighbors in colonial childbirths, the rise of medical interest, modesty and morality, childbirth as illness, the role of hospitals, natural childbirth revisited, and government involvement. They end with a review of current issues in childbirth. Bibliography. A scholarly work, enlivened by excerpts from historical sources.

Home Birth and Midwifery

Baldwin, Rahima. *Special Delivery: The Complete Guide to Informed Birth*. Millbrae, CA: Les Femmes, 1979. 170 pp. $9.95 (paper).
Introduced by David and Lee Stewart, authors of *Safe Alternatives in Childbirth*,

this well-illustrated work covers pregnancy, labor and delivery, and postpartum concerns. Although the author strongly favors home childbirth, her insights into the emotional and spiritual benefits of informed birth have universal value.

Brennan, Barbara, and Heilman, Joan Rattner. *The Complete Book of Midwifery.* New York: Dutton, 1977. 144 pp. $4.95 (paper).
Threaded with anecdotes and favorable comments from patients, this work describes the motivations and responsibilities of midwives and the enlightened policies of certain hospitals. Brennan, a certified nurse-midwife, advises seeking out such facilities rather than risking complications in a home birth. She provides a step-by-step outline of midwife-managed childbirth, a directory of nurse-midwifery services in the United States, and selected readings. Recommended.

Donegan, Jane B. *Women and Men Midwives: Medicine, Morality and Misogyny in Early America.* Contributions to Medical History. Westport, CT: Greenwood, 1978. 316 pp. $17.95; London: Greenwood. £12.75.
Using primary sources from the sixteenth to the nineteenth centuries, a historian constructs a vivid account of role, duties, and skills of midwives. Bibliography is included. Valuable for exposing the historical roots of modern feminist protests against male-dominated obstetrics.

Gaskin, Ina May. *Spiritual Midwifery.* Summertown, TN: Book Publg. Co., 1978. 480 pp. $8.50 (paper).
The product of a "spiritual community of eleven hundred long-haired vegetarians," this work reports numerous natural deliveries attended by community midwives. In addition the author presents physical and "spiritual" advice to parents and detailed instructions to midwives. Appendixes include a book list, needed equipment, required nursing skills, instructions about breast self-examination and Pap smears, and community statistics. An offbeat but fascinating work.

Gilgoff, Alice. *Home Birth.* New York: Coward, McCann, 1978. 223 pp. $8.95.
In an indictment of American hospitals, the author urges a return to home birth. "At their most life-giving moment women [in the hospital] are subject to a barrage of mistreatment that can cause emotional degradation and present serious risks to the well-being of both mother and baby." Gilgoff sees the development of a new generation of professional birth attendants, midwives who understand the desire to experience childbirth in a comfortable, secure family setting. Organizational addresses are appended. Marred by unwarranted invective against doctors, the work nevertheless presents a contemporary option that is increasingly practical.

Kitzinger, Sheila. *Birth at Home.* New York: Oxford Univ. Pr., 1979. 154 pp. $11.95.

A British childbirth educator explains the advantages of home birth and the risk factors that should be considered. Kitzinger lists addresses that may be helpful in locating medical participants and reviews the equipment that should be on hand. Especially noteworthy are the chapters on drugs and diet in pregnancy, the needs of siblings, and the father's role during labor. Includes detailed outline of labor, photographs, bibliography.

Kitzinger, Sheila, and Davis, John A., eds. *The Place of Birth: A Study of the Environment in Which Birth Takes Place with Special Reference to Home Confinements.* New York: Oxford Univ. Pr., 1978. 265 pp. $19.50; London: Oxford Univ. Pr. £7.50.

In this scholarly work, 22 professional contributors examine the controversial option of home deliveries. Topics include the relationship of prenatal care to choosing a birth setting, British policies for maternity care, statistical evidence against hospital deliveries, home births in Holland and in the United States, the role of the primary health care team in pregnancy, fatherhood, mother-infant interaction, the family and neonatal intensive care. Offers intelligent, responsible arguments for home-delivery systems; well documented.

Litoff, Judy Barrett. *American Midwives: 1860 to the Present.* Contributions in Medical History. Westport, CT: Greenwood, 1978. 199 pp. $15.95; London: Greenwood. £12.25.

Heavily documented work by a historian traces the midwife controversy from the beginnings of obstetric specialization through the shaky rise of nurse-midwifery in recent decades. A most realistic study that refrains from romanticizing the midwife.

Sousa, Marion. *Childbirth at Home.* Englewood Cliffs, NJ: Prentice-Hall, 1976. 208 pp. $7.95.

This work discusses the reasons why home birth may be superior to hospital deliveries, the risks involved, likely birth attendants, securing good prenatal care and classes, necessary birth equipment and procedures, postnatal medical care, and breast-feeding. Included are a physician's report on the incidence and management of home birth complications; end-of-chapter references; bibliography. Practical and articulate.

Stewart, David, and Stewart, Lee, eds. *Safe Alternatives in Childbirth,* 2nd ed. Chapel Hill, NC: Natl. Assn. of Parents & Prof. for Safe Alternatives in Childbirth, 1978. 187 pp. $5. (paper).

Written for both lay people and professionals, this is an impressive collection of articles by 22 contributors who favor a return to home births. Offering numerous references and statistical tables, the work presents convincing arguments for the safety of home births in normal circumstances. Recommended.

Ward, Charlotte, and Ward, Fred. *The Home Birth Book.* Garden City, NY: Doubleday, 1977. 149 pp. $5.95.
Several contributors professionally involved in obstetrics and pediatrics present a favorable view of home childbirth. Parents' accounts emphasize its value as a family-centered experience. Introduced by Ashley Montagu (*Life before Birth*), the work is recommended for its multidisciplinary approach.

Postpartum Care

DelliQuadri, Lyn, and Breckenridge, Kati. *Mother Care: Helping Yourself through the Physical and Emotional Transitions of New Motherhood.* Los Angeles: Tarcher, 1978. 206 pp. $8.95.
To help women cope with postpartum changes, the authors discuss physical problems, tension, fatigue, nutrition, mothering, depression, and redefined family roles. Topics range from infant care to sex after birth. In endeavoring to advise on these numerous concerns, the book lacks focus and bogs down in psychological jargon.

Jaffe, Sandra Sohn, and Viertel, Jack. *Becoming Parents: Preparing for the Emotional Changes of First-Time Parenthood.* New York: Atheneum, 1979. 329 pp. $11.95.
The authors focus their attention on the emotional health of the parents during the crucial first year of the first child. They deal with sexual, behavioral, and emotional changes experienced together with guilt, distrust, and frustration. Good advice is given on dividing household duties, parental jealousy, house-bound frustration, the no-sleep blues, the willing and unwilling parent, breast-feeding, careers and guilt, postpartum reactions, and sex after childbirth. Composite pictures are presented of six families. Informative and readable. Highly recommended.

Panter, Gideon G., and Linde, Shirley M. *Now That You've Had Your Baby: How to Feel Better and Happier Than Ever after Childbirth.* New York: McKay, 1976. 241 pp. $9.95; Englewood Cliffs, NJ: Prentice-Hall. $3.95 (paper); London: Prentice-Hall. £2.90.
An obstetrician and a medical writer collaborate on this excellent postpartum guide for new mothers. Among the topics covered are the hospital stay, going home, fatigue and emotional problems, adjusting to and caring for the baby, other relationships, getting help around the house, physical changes and problems after delivery, breast-feeding, nutrition and exercise, resumption of sex, the postpartum checkup, family planning, financial concerns. Glossary is appended. A needed, easily readable work.

Menopause

Anderson, Barrie, and others. *The Menopause Book.* New York: Hawthorn, 1977. 288 pp. $12.50.
Seven professional contributors address the physical and psychological problems of menopause, discussing both medical therapies and simpler methods of coping. Especially fine is the chapter "Estrogen: What to Do Until the Results Are In."

Cherry, Sheldon H. *The Menopause Myth.* New York: Ballantine, 1976. 109 pp. $1.50 (paper).
Using a question-and-answer format, a gynecologist discusses the physiology and symptoms of menopause, its psychological and sexual aspects, hormonal treatment, heart disease and menopause, osteoporosis (loss and weakening of bone), breast diseases, common gynecological problems, physical fitness and weight control, male menopause. While noting that estrogen has not been proven carcinogenic, Cherry cautions against its widespread or excessive use. Includes case histories, instructions for breast examination, exercises, nutritional material. A cautious, authoritative work, aimed at dispelling common misconceptions. Highly recommended.

Cooper, Wendy. *Don't Change: A Biological Revolution for Women.* New York: Stein & Day, 1975. 185 pp. $25; London: Hutchinson. £3.25; Arrow £0.75 (paper).
Contending that most change-of-life symptoms result from estrogen deficiency, a British journalist promotes the benefits of hormone-replacement therapy. The author discusses the diverse problems of menopause, including osteoporosis; reviews female biology; and confronts the questions of heart disease and cancer. Estrogen, Cooper asserts, does not induce cancer in middle-aged women but actually delays its onset. She substantiates her arguments with extensive medical references, with testimonies of women, and with the mixed opinions of several specialists. A balanced, comprehensible presentation.

Nachtigall, Lila, and Heilman, Joan. *The Lila Nachtigall Report: The Intelligent Woman's Guide to Menopause, Estrogen, and Her Body.* New York: Putnam, 1977. 245 pp. $7.95.
A woman gynecologist examines menopause, including extensive material on the role and effects of estrogen. Considerable attention is devoted to the cancer controversy. Written for intelligent readers, this work is a balanced analysis of some highly controversial issues.

Newman, Jo Hynes. *Our Own Harms: The Facts behind Menopause and Estrogen Therapy.* Newport Beach, CA: Quail Street, 1976. 176 pp. OP.
Filled with anatomical figures and witty line drawings, this work describes the

physiology of menstruation and menopause; considers the feminine situation, premenstrual tension, and the psychological significance of menopause; and examines common disorders and medical therapies of menopause. Newman urges a most conservative use of estrogen. In ending, she covers sex and birth control in the middle years.

Page, Jane. *The Other Awkward Age: Menopause.* Berkeley, CA: Ten Speed Pr., 1977. 168 pp. $8.95; $4.95 (paper).
Prompted by a Young Women's Christian Association study group in Seattle, this work characterizes menopause as a period "when the body's hormone balance gets out of kilter." Page thoroughly examines the issue of hormone therapy; reviews historical attitudes about menopause; explains when surgery may be necessary; and discusses continued sexual activity, other middle-age tensions, the difference between concerned and callous doctors. Appendix includes list of medications with hormones, suggested readings, and glossary. Highly informative and balanced; rather dry presentation.

Parrish, Louis. *No Pause at All.* New York: Reader's Digest, 1976. 216 pp. OP.
A physician specializing in endocrinology and psychiatry addresses various problems associated with the climacteric experienced by both men and women. With numerous examples from his practice, the author attempts to reassure the middle-aged that physical changes need not threaten their sense of emotional and sexual fulfillment. A proponent of hormone therapy for certain conditions, Parrish nevertheless stresses the need for a general treatment program involving diet, exercise, skin care, posture, and mental attitude. An adequate overview, offering few details.

Reitz, Rosetta. *Menopause: A Positive Approach.* Radnor, PA: Chilton, 1977. 276 pp. $9.95; New York: Penguin. $2.95 (paper).
Attempting to dispel misconceptions and negative attitudes, a feminist writer discusses the menopausal process; symptoms such as hot flashes, weight gain, depression, and other complaints; emotions; exercise; self-examination; negative terminology; masturbation; sexual satisfaction; hormones and the dangers of estrogen-replacement therapy; cancer, nutrition in middle age; and male menopause. Bibliography is appended. Includes many candid comments from menopause workshop participants. A defiant, rather revealing work.

Hysterectomy

Gifford-Jones, W. *What Every Woman Should Know about Hysterectomy.* New York: Funk & Wagnalls, 1977. 229 pp. $8.95.
A gynecologist provides facts to help women avoid unnecessary hysterectomy. Among the areas covered are the reasons for and against the procedure; advice on choosing a doctor; descriptions of related procedures, including

dilatation and curettage; help in dealing with the psychological effects; and hysterectomy as cancer treatment. Recommended.

Huneycutt, Harry C., and Davis, Judith L. *All about Hysterectomy.* New York: Reader's Digest, 1977. 384 pp. OP.
This guide offers extensive information on hospital procedures, but does not cover other aspects of hysterectomy as thoroughly as do similar works. Unnessential.

Jameson, DeeDee, and Schwalb, Roberta. *Every Woman's Guide to Hysterectomy: Taking Charge of Your Own Body.* Englewood Cliffs, NJ: Prentice-Hall, 1978. 157 pp. $8.95; $3.95 (paper); London: Prentice-Hall. £6.55; £2.90 (paper).
Written by a hysterectomy patient and a professor of nursing, this unique work contains the introspective journal that Jameson wrote while facing the procedure. Schwalb explores the decision-making process, urging patient involvement; the hospital stay; and postoperative feelings. Especially interesting is the discussion of consumer involvement in health care. Appends lists of organizations, literature, and audiovisual materials; patient's bill of rights; and glossary. Philosophical and feminist. Recommended.

Nugent, Nancy. *Hysterectomy: A Complete Up-to-Date Guide to Everything about It and Why It May Be Needed.* New York: Doubleday, 1976. 181 pp. OP.
A medical reporter provides an excellent consumer's guide that includes detailed information on the various reasons for this procedure, and the types, methods, and emotional effects of hysterectomy.

Breast Care and Breast Cancer

See also Chapter 13, Cancer.

Cope, Oliver. *The Breast: Its Problems—Benign and Malignant.* Boston: Houghton, 1978. 240 pp. $8.95; $3.95 (paper).
Aimed at the educated consumer, this work is meant to inform and aid the patient in decision making. Dr. Cope presents his material thoroughly and in clear, sophisticated language. He explains the biology of the normal breast; benign and malignant tumors; the demographics of breast cancer; treatment, including hormone therapy and immunotherapy; diagnosis and symptoms; emotional aspects; and general breast care. Appended are several consumer references and instructions for self–breast examination.

Cowles, Jane K. *Informed Consent.* New York: Coward, McCann, 1976. 224 pp. $8.95.
This excellent work stresses the need for women to have a choice regarding breast cancer surgery. In addition to discussing the six points involved in

"informed consent" (as defined by the Department of Health, Education and Welfare in 1975), Cowles supplies 22 suggestions on "how to get the system to give you better care." Five appendixes cover the nature of cancer, breast function, untreated cancer, types and stages of breast cancer. Includes breast examination diagrams, glossary, bibliography.

Fredericks, Carlton. *Breast Cancer: A Nutritional Approach.* New York: Grossett & Dunlap, 1979. 196 pp. $4.95 (paper).
A nutrition expert contends that estrogen is responsible for much breast cancer. Claiming that proper nutrition can break down the hormone into a harmless substance, Fredericks urges a diet low in refined sugar and other processed carbohydrates, supplemented by specific vitamins and minerals. Includes several nutritional charts. An extreme point of view.

Greenfield, Natalee S. *First Do No Harm . . . A Dying Woman's Battle against the Physicians and Drug Companies Who Misled Her about the Hazards of the Pill.* New York: Two Continents, 1976. 164 pp. $7.95.
Written by the patient's mother, this journal details how estrogen in an oral contraceptive accelerated the spread of a young woman's breast cancer. Something of a muckraker, the book also describes her legal battle to expose medical and pharmaceutical negligence. Includes dialogue from depositions and an epilogue on the suit's outcome.

Kushner, Rose. *Breast Cancer: A Personal History and an Investigative Report.* New York: Harcourt, 1975. 400 pp. $10. Updated and revised as *Why Me? What Every Woman Should Know about Breast Cancer to Save Her Life.* New York: NAL, 1977. 376 pp. $2.50 (paper).
This controversial work contains discussions of myths, quackery, oral contraceptives, surgical biopsy and other procedures, psychological effects, male chauvinism, and the "economic incentive" for surgery. Against mastectomy performed immediately after a positive biopsy, Kushner calls for more compassionate and studied treatment of breast cancer. Includes statistical charts, bibliography and notes. A landmark work. Highly recommended.

McCauley, Carole Spearin. *Surviving Breast Cancer.* New York: Dutton, 1979. 240 pp. $10.95.
Called "an in-depth report on the latest theories of causation and alternative treatments," this work attempts to review a wide range of questions concerning breast cancer. Among the areas covered are heredity, estrogens, diet, psychological makeup, viruses, diagnostic and treatment methods, coping emotionally, and rehabilitation and aftercare. Both conventional and unconventional viewpoints are considered, although the author leans toward the latter. This compassionately written book includes case studies of 15 women who have survived from 5 to 40 years after detection. In addition, there are

three appendixes on terminology, books, and concerned organizations. Highly informative and readable.

National Cancer Institute. Office of Cancer Communications, *The Breast Cancer Digest: A Guide to Medical Care, Emotional Support, Educational Programs and Resources.* DHEW Pubn. No. (NIH) 79-1691. Bethesda, MD: Natl. Cancer Inst., 1979.
Intended for health professionals, this comprehensive and clearly presented work is also an excellent reference for laypersons. It offers a straightforward overview of the rates, risks, and development of breast cancer; tests, treatments, and rehabilitation; recurrent, metastatic, and advanced breast cancer; the financial impact of this disease; its psychosocial impact; programs and services. Includes glossary. Essential.

Nethery, Susan. *One Year and Counting: Breast Cancer, My World, and Me.* Grand Rapids, MI: Baker, 1978. 240 pp. $3.95 (paper).
In this personal narrative the author tells of her two mastectomies and her anxious wait to see if the cancer has metastasized. An unexceptional but optimistic journal, with a deeply religious orientation.

Rothenberg, Robert E. *The Complete Book of Breast Care.* New York: Ballantine, 1976. 244 pp. $1.95 (paper).
Directed at the layperson, this comprehensive handbook covers such topics as breast anatomy and function, size differences, brassieres, pregnancy and breast-feeding, sex, menopause, disease and its various treatments. Includes a section on breast examination. Much of the text is the question-and-answer format. Simply written, with encyclopedic coverage. Recommended.

Winkler, Win Ann. *Post-Mastectomy: A Personal Guide to Physical and Emotional Recovery.* New York: Hawthorn, 1976. 197 pp. $7.95.
A mastectomy patient provides several practical aids for postsurgical recovery. Appendixes include approved cancer-detection centers; comprehensive cancer centers; shopping for clothing, prostheses, and other items. Suggested readings, tapes, and records. An essential handbook.

Zalon, Jean, with Block, Jean Libman. *I Am Whole Again: The Case for Breast Reconstruction after Mastectomy.* New York: Random, 1978. 151 pp. $8.95.
This work details the author's radical mastectomy, the emotional turmoil she experienced, and her search for a surgeon to reconstruct her breast. In more than a personal narrative, Zalon informs women about what to expect, ways to seek help, family reactions, and the actual surgical procedures involved. Explicit photographs and discussions with other mastectomees are included. Most encouraging.

PAMPHLETS

The American College of Obstetricians and Gynecologists, One E. Wacker Dr., Chicago, IL 60601.

More than 50 booklets are available including:
Anemia During Pregnancy.
Bleeding in Pregnancy.
Breast Problems in Women.
Cancer and Women.
Cancer of the Cervix: Must So Many Women Die?
Changes during Pregnancy.
Fetal Monitoring.
Food, Pregnancy and Family Health.
High Blood Pressure during Pregnancy.
How Can I Tell I'm Pregnant?
Hysterectomy.
Important Facts about Abortion.
Important Facts about Post-Partum Sterilization.
Important Facts about the Pill.
Is It Safe to Have Surgery during Pregnancy?
Obstetrician-Gynecologist: The Woman's Physician.
Painful Intercourse.
Pregnancy and Daily Living.
Pregnancy Tests.
Should a Woman Work during Pregnancy?
Sterilization by Laparoscopy.
Uterine Tumors.
What Happens during Labor?
What Hormones Have to Do with Pregnancy.
Vulvular Physiology and Disorders.

Bureau of Community Health Services, Health Services Administration, 5600 Fishers La., Rockville, MD 20857.

Female Physical Examination for Contraception: A Self-Instructional Booklet, 1976, DHEW Pubn. No. (HSA) 76-10023, 19 pp.
Food for the Teenager during Pregnancy, 1978, DHEW Pubn. No. (HSA) 78-16024, 29 pp.
The Hassles of Becoming a Teenage Parent, 1978, DHEW Pubn. No. (HSA) 78-5624, 9 pp.
Teenage Pregnancy: Everybody's Problem, 1979, DHEW Pubn. No. (HSA) 79-5619, 9 pp.
Understanding Female Sterilization: A Self-Instructional Booklet, 1976, DHEW Pubn. No. (HSA) 76-16025, 13 pp.

Cesarean Birth Council International, Box 4331, Mountain View, CA 94040.
Cesarean Birth Recovery Exercises.
Family-Centered Cesarean Birth Options.

Father Attended Cesarean Births—Opinions by an Obstetrician, Pediatrician and Anesthesiologist.
Typical Hospital Protocol—Allowing Fathers to Attend Cesarean Births.

C/SEC, Inc. (Cesareans/Support, Education and Concern), 15 Maynard Rd., Dedham, MA 02026.

Frankly Speaking.
Guide for Cesarean Birth at Boston Hospital for Women.
Guidelines of Childbirth Educators.
Manual for Setting Up Prepared Childbirth Classes for Cesarean Parents.
Once a Cesarean, Always a Cesarean.

C-Section Experience, Box 65, Glencoe, IL 60022.

Father's Fact Sheet for Unexpected Cesarean Deliveries.
Newsletters.
Parents' Guide to Cesarean Birth.
Reading Souce List.

DES Action, Box 1977, Plainview, NY 11803.

DES—Exposed Offspring: How You Can Help.
DES—The Facts.
From One DES Teenager to Another.

Food and Drug Administration, Office of Consumer Inquiries, 5600 Fishers La., Parklawn Bldg., Rockville, MD 20857.

Women and Estrogens, 1976, DHEW Publication No. (FDA) 76-3022.

HealthRight, Women's Health Forum, 41 Union Sq., Rm. 106, New York, NY 10003.

Breast Cancer.
The Gynecological Checkup.
Hysterectomy.
Infections of the Vagina.
Menopause.
Saline Abortion.
Sterilization.
Vacuum Aspiration Abortion.
What Can One Woman Do?

La Leche League International, Inc., 9616 Minneapolis Ave., Franklin Park, IL 60131.
Booklets and pamphlets are available on a wide variety of topics relating to breast-feeding, childbirth, child care, and nutrition. Booklets include:

A Child Is Born.
Emergency Childbirth.
Family Book of Childcare.
The Home Birth Book.
Husband-Coached Childbirth.
Methods of Childbirth.
Nourishing Your Unborn Child.
Nursing Your Baby.
The Womanly Art of Breastfeeding.

Pamphlets include:

Does Your Baby Need a Pacifier?
Father-to-Father: On Breastfeeding.
How a Baby Learns to Love.
Nipple Care.
Shall I Breastfeed My Baby?
Why Breastfeed Your Baby?

Maternity Center Association, 48 E. 92 St., New York, NY 10028.
Available publications and teaching aids include:

A Baby Is Born.
Birth Atlas.
Comfort during Pregnancy.
The Female Pelvis.
For the Expectant Father.
Newborn Baby.
Nutrition and Birth.
Organs of Human Reproduction.
Preparation for Childbearing.
Preventive Maternity Care.
Relaxation and Breathing.

National Women's Health Network, 2025 I Street N.W., Suite 105, Washington, DC 20006.
A series of resource guides is available that brings together readings, bibliography, key resource people, and the latest medical information from the woman's point of view. *Health Resource Guides,* which are described in detail in Chapter 4, are available on the following topics:

Abortion
Birth Control
Breast Cancer
Childbirth
DES
Hysterectomy

Menopause
Self-Help
Sterilization

Cost: $3.00 per copy; $20.00 for complete set.

Office of Cancer Communications, National Cancer Institute, Bethesda, MD 20014.

Breast Self-Examination, 1976, DHEW Pubn. No. (NIH) 76-649.
Progress against Cancer of the Breast, 1978, DHEW Pubn. No. (NIH) 78-328.
Progress against Cancer of the Uterus, 1978, DHEW Pubn. No. (NIH) 78-171.
Questions and Answers about DES Exposure before Birth, 1976, DHEW Pubn. No. (NIH) 76-1118.
Were You or Your Daughter Born after 1949? 1977, DHEW Pubn. No. (NIH) 77-1226.
What You Need to Know about Cancer of the Breast, 1979, DHEW Pubn. No. (NIH) 79-1556.

Ortho Pharmaceutical Corporation, Professional Services Department, Rte. 202, Raritan, NJ 08869.
Simple, pocket-size booklets available are:

The Bond of Love: A Guide for the Nursing Mother.
For Your Information . . . Vaginitis.
Lippes Loop: Your Intrauterine Contraceptive.
The Rh Negative Woman Asks about Rhogam.
VD: A Fact of Life.

Personal Products Company, Milltown, NJ 08850.
Pamphlets are available on topics relating to female reproductive anatomy, menarche and menstrual cycle, and personal hygiene. Typical titles are:

For Boys: A Book about Girls.
Growing Up and Liking It.
How Shall I Tell My Daughter?

Physicians' Art Service, Patient Information Library, 343-B Serramonte Plaza Office Center, Daly City, CA 94105.
Several excellent, well-illustrated booklets are available:

Breast Lumps: A Guide to Understand Your Breasts, Breast Problems, Biopsies and Surgeries.
Contraception: Facts on Birth Control.
A Guide to Understanding Hysterectomy and Related Surgeries.
Menopause.

Public Affairs Committee, Inc., 381 Park Ave. S., New York, NY 10016. Relevant booklets are:

Abortion: Public Issue, Private Decision, No. 527.
Pregnancy and You, No. 482.
The Woman Alcoholic, No. 529.
Women and Smoking, No. 475.
Your Menopause, No. 447.

Sex Information and Education Council of the United States (SIECUS), 84 Fifth Ave., New York, NY 10011. SIECUS Study Guides:

Sexual Relations during Pregnancy and the Post Delivery Period. by S. Leon Israel and Isadore Rubin.
Teenage Pregnancy: Prevention and Treatment. by Philip Sarrell.

AUDIOVISUAL PRODUCERS AND DISTRIBUTORS

American College of Obstetricians and Gynecologists
Film Service
Box 299
Wheaton, IL 60187
Contraception; infertility; breast self-examination; hysterectomy; urinary problems; Pap smear; uterine bleeding; menopause; pregnancy; abortion; breast-feeding.

Robert J. Brady Co.
A Prentice-Hall Company
Bowie, MD 20715
Breast self-examination; prenatal care; contraception; recurrent cystitis; hysterectomy; mastectomy.

Churchill Films
662 North Robertson Blvd.
Los Angeles, CA 90069
Birth control; pregnancy; labor and delivery.

La Leche League International, Inc.
9616 Minneapolis Ave.
Franklin Park, IL 60131
Mothering; breast-feeding.

Medfact, Inc.
1112 Andrew Ave. N.E.
Massillon, OH 44646
Family planning; birth control; intrauterine devices; the rhythm method; the 21-day pill; the 28-day pill; tubal ligation; contraceptive foam; pregnancy; pelvic examination; menstruation; douching; abortion; self–breast examination; vaginal and abdominal hysterectomy.

Medi-Cine Sales Corporation
8201 Pendleton Pike
Indianapolis, IN 46226
OB/GYN Series.

Milner Fenwick, Inc.
2125 Green Spring Dr.
Timonium, MD 21093
Contraceptive methods; including oral contraceptives, intrauterine devices, and diaphragms; tubal ligation; abortion; prenatal care; cesarean birth; natural childbirth; nutrition and fitness in pregnancy; fetal monitoring; Leboyer technique; obstetrical anesthesia; hysterectomy; infertility; endometriosis; lower

urinary tract infections; abnormal vaginal bleeding; colposcopy; common female dysfunctions.

National Foundation/March of Dimes
Box 2000
White Plains, NY 10602
Pregnancy and prenatal care; genetic counseling; birth defects.

Parents' Magazine Films
Distributed by PMF Films Inc.
Box 1000
Elmsford, NY 10523
Prenatal care; nutrition; parenting; child development.

Perennial Education, Inc.
477 Roger Williams
Box 855, Ravinia
Highland Park, IL 60035
Family living; sex education; menstrual hygiene; teenage sexuality; teenage pregnancy; abortion; family planning; sexually transmitted diseases; venereal disease; vaginitis; pelvic and breast examination; rape; pregnancy and nutrition; childbirth; breast-feeding; parenting.

Professional Research, Inc.
12960 Coral Tree Pl.
Los Angeles, CA 90066
Anatomy and physiology of pregnancy; prenatal management; weight control and exercise in pregnancy; labor; delivery in the hospital; postpartum concerns; breast-feeding; new baby care; natural childbirth; family planning.

Jeppersen Sanderson
8025 E. 40 Ave.
Denver, CO 80207
Understanding pregnancy; guidelines for healthy pregnancy; understanding labor and delivery;

premature infant; cesarean birth; breast-feeding; amniocentesis; breast examination and biopsy; dilatation and curettage; laparotomy; obstetrical anesthesia; birth control techniques; abortion; hysterectomy.

Single Concept Films
2 Tennison Dr.
Rochester, NY 14618
Sex education; after your baby; false labor; minor discomforts of pregnancy; preparation for motherhood; questions about pregnancy; family planning.

Soundwords, Inc.
56-11 217 St.
Bayside, NY 11364
Vaginal hygiene; pregnancy; childbirth; menstration; infertility; breast cancer; cancer of the uterus.

Sterling Educational Films
241 E. 34 St.
New York, NY 10016
The new baby; baby's first four months; ladies in waiting; teenage pregnancy.

Trainex Corporation
Box 116
Garden Grove, CA 92642
Postpartum care, infant care; breast-feeding; bottle-feeding; fetal development; labor, delivery; human reproductive system; breast cancer; cancer detection; disorders of the female reproductive system; birth control; oral contraceptives; intrauterine devices; diaphragm; condom; self-examination of the breast and Pap smear; venereal disease; uterine malignancy; breast diseases; syphilis and gonorrhea.

RESOURCE ORGANIZATIONS

American College of Nurse-Midwives
1012 14 St. N.W.
Washington, DC 20005

American College of Obstetricians
and Gynecologists
One E. Wacker Dr.
Chicago, IL 60601

American Foundation for Maternal
and Child Health
30 Beekman Pl.
New York, NY 10022

American Society for
Psychoprophylaxis in Obstetrics
(ASPO)
1411 K St. N.W.
Washington, DC 20005

Association for Childbirth
International
16705 Monte Cristo
Cerritos, CA 90701

Birthright
2800 Otis St. N.E.
Washington, DC 10003

Boston Women's Health Book
Collective
332 Charles River Rd.
Watertown, MA 02172

C/Sec, Inc. (Cesareans/Support,
Education and Concern)
15 Maynard Rd.
Dedham, MA 02026

Cesarean Birth Association of
America
125 N. 12 St.
New Hyde Park, NY 11040

Coalition for the Medical Rights of
Women
4079 A 24 St.
San Francisco, CA 94114

HealthRight
175 Fifth Ave.
New York, NY 10010

Home Oriented Maternity
Experience (HOME)
511 New York Ave.
Takoma Pk.
Washington, DC 20012

Homebirth
89 Franklin St.
Suite 200
Boston, MA 02110

The International Childbirth
Education Association
Box 5852
Milwaukee, WI 53220

La Leche League International, Inc.
9616 Minneapolis Ave.
Franklin Park, IL 60131

National Midwives Association
Box 163
Princeton, NJ 08540

National Women's Health Network
2025 I St. N.W.
Suite 105
Washington, DC 20006

New Moon Publications
Box 3488
Ridgeway Sta.
Stamford, CT 06905

Planned Parenthood Federation of America, Inc.
810 Seventh Ave.
New York, NY 10019

Sex Information and Education Council of the United States (SIECUS)
84 Fifth Ave.
New York, NY 10011

Women's Health and Abortion Project
30 W. 22 St.
New York, NY 10010

Women's Health Forum
175 Fifth Ave.
New York, NY 10010

Zero Population Growth, Inc.
1346 Connecticut Ave. N.W.
Washington, DC 20036

Chapter 11

Health of the Elderly

BOOKS

General

Anderson, Barbara Gallatin. *The Aging Game: Success, Sanity, and Sex after 60*. New York: McGraw-Hill, 1979. 240 pp. $12.95.
A professor of medical anthropology at Southern Methodist University in Dallas proposes tactics to maintain vitality and avoid the effects of aging. After introductory vignettes that illustrate the dark side of aging, Anderson delineates her strategy, urging the aging reader to accept himself as old, develop a clear perspective on late life, replace lost satisfactions, and develop the resources and alliances that count. Several options and guidelines are suggested to accommodate the varying circumstances in which older people may find themselves. Among the topics covered are money and work, love and sexuality, and social relationships with spouse, children, siblings, friends, and groups. In a chapter on physical and mental health, the author acknowledges the problems and emphasizes her attitudinal strategy but offers little concrete advice. The appendix of annotated readings and organizations is more specific. A realistic yet upbeat work, despite its surface treatment of health concerns.

Butler, Robert N. *Why Survive? Being Old in America*. New York: Harper, 1975. 496 pp. $17.50; $5.95 (paper).
A 1976 Pulitzer Prize winner, now the director of the National Institute of Aging, exposes and condemns the gross inequities confronting America's aged population. He discusses poverty and finances, work, employment, needed services, various forms of victimization, the politics of aging, death and dying, social relationships, and virtually every aspect of aging. Regarding

health concerns, Butler examines the medical needs of the aging, set against the apathy and inaccessibility of many health-care providers; the problems attending hospital care; drug safety; pacification through medication; medical research on aging; prevention of illness; medicare and medicaid; the need for a geriatric specialty; emotional problems and mental illness; senility; the deficiencies in mental health care; patients rights; nursing-home practices and reforms. Five appendixes on resource organizations and programs, notes, and a bibliography enhance the effectiveness of this incisive, sweeping indictment of policy and attitudes. Indisputably, a landmark work.

Butler, Robert N., and Lewis, Myrna I. *Sex after Sixty.* New York and London: Harper, 1976. 165 pp. $8.95. £5.20; Boston: Hall, 1977. $9.95 (large print); London: Prior, 1978. £4.95. Entitled *Love and Sex after Sixty.* New York and London: Harper, 1977. $1.95; £1.25.
Written by a famed psychiatrist and gerontologist, this guide to sexuality in the older years discusses the myth and reality of sexual desire and capacity after sixty. Dr. Butler also provides explicit yet tactful instructions on technique. Sensitive and constructive.

Cohen, Stephen Z., and Gans, Bruce Michael. *The Other Generation Gap: The Middle-Aged and Their Aging Parents.* Chicago: Follett, 1978. 290 pp. $10.95.
Viewing the aging process from a sociological perspective, a therapist–social worker and a writer focus on the relationships between the middle-aged and their elderly parents. Two sections in particular address the physical and psychological effects of aging: changes in physical appearance, sexuality, eyesight, hearing, and the other senses; overall stamina, accidents, mobility problems, and driving difficulties; arthritis, incontinence, and senility; emotional problems such as depression, adjustment to retirement, bereavement. Also covered are nursing homes, hospitals, and death. The authors advise on choosing a physician and provide a checklist for evaluating nursing homes. Suggested readings are appended. Striking a balance between sociological and health concerns, the authors suggest methods whereby both generations can interact responsibly yet maintain independence. Recommended.

Comfort, Alex. *A Good Age.* Illus. by Michael Leonard. New York: Crown, 1976. 224 pp. $9.95; Simon & Schuster, 1978. $5.95 (paper).
In a montage of topics related to aging, a physician and gerontologist accentuates the positive aspects of growing older. Among the 80 areas covered are alcohol, arthritis, blood pressure, depression, diabetes, disengagement, drop attacks (falls attributed to improper blood circulation), exercise, hearing, hypothermia, masturbation, nursing homes, prostate, quackery, rejuvenation research, sex, sight, smoking, and so on. Interwoven throughout the book are Michael Leonard's many sensitive portraits of notables and others whose older years were a period of challenge and creativity. Guidelines for "a prudent

diet" and a bibliography close the work. Although Dr. Comfort eschews an in-depth analysis of his topics, this uplifting volume can act as the springboard to further exploration. Recommended.

Cottin, Lou. *Elders in Rebellion: A Guide to Senior Activism.* Garden City, NY: Anchor, 1979. 224 pp. $8.95.
Though largely political and relatively militant, this work by a widely read columnist approaches the subject of health as a prime concern. Among the topics covered are the doctor-patient relationship, medical attitudes toward the health complaints of the aged, the need for geriatrics as a medical specialty, nursing homes and "adult homes," the absence of penal sanctions for neglect, recommended standards and accomplishments in home health care, handicapped elders in the community. A well-documented and vigorous work, but one that offers few practical strategies; of marginal value as consumer health literature.

Davis, Richard H., ed. *Aging: Prospects And Issues,* rev. Los Angeles: Univ. of Southern California, Andrus Gerontology Center, 1976. 211 pp. $4 (paper).
Divided into two major sections, this multidisciplinary anthology relies on the expertise of 13 health and social science professionals. Among the topics covered are physiological changes and mental health in aging, the elderly and the drug culture, the effect of changing legislation, and the personal space and psychosocial needs of older people. Especially useful is a pharmacologist's article on drug use and misuse, both individually and in long-term care facilities. Scientific references accompany each article, and an extensive bibliography in ten divisions includes material on such additional concerns as nutrition and dying. Highly recommended despite some specialized terminology.

Ellison, Jerome. *Life's Second Half: The Pleasures of Aging.* Old Greenwich, CT: Devin-Adair, 1978. 178 pp. $8.95.
In the author's rather mystical view of aging, the emphasis is on reawakening and transition rather than on confusion and deterioration. Death is seen not as something final, to be dreaded, but as a welcome threshold. Supplemental readings appended. An unusual but intriguing work.

Finkelhor, Dorothy C. *The Triumph of Age: How to Feel Young and Happy in Retirement.* Chicago: Follett, 1979. 264 pp. $10.95.
Viewing retirement as just another life stage, the author asserts that its problems cannot be handled with the same approaches that worked in other periods. A new set of attitudes is required. Offering specific alternatives to counterproductive emotions and attitudes, Finkelhor discusses relinquishing middle-aged responsibility, strengthening self-appreciation, relating to other people, combating loneliness, and handling other social concerns. Especially

useful are the chapters on sex and fear of death. The work is well structured and includes numerous checklists and other learning tools. The topic of health, however, is conspicuous by its absence, despite its critical importance to retired persons.

Freese, Arthur S. *The End of Senility.* New York: Arbor, 1978. 178 pp. $8.95. Providing a broad sweep of the causes and mimics of senility, a physician proclaims the obsolescence of old age. Among the topics covered are aging and longevity themes; forms of senility and pseudosenility; memory changes and methods of improving; sexuality; symptoms and countermeasures of mental health problems, including depression and suicide; proper nutrition; careful use of drugs and alcohol; choosing the right doctor; treating chronic, organic brain syndrome when it does occur; residental alternatives; preventing the worst through "reality orientation." Appended are resource suggestions in an annotated directory and a bibliography. Most enlightening and encouraging.

Galton, Lawrence. *Don't Give Up on an Aging Parent.* New York: Crown, 1975. 246 pp. $6.95.
A medical writer criticizes the attitudes of many doctors toward their elderly patients. Condescension and often neglect obstruct the treatment to which older patients are entitled. The author attempts to dispel the myths regarding the aging process and to emphasize the realities and the positive aspects. Considerable space is devoted to senility and its counterfiets, including "water on the brain" and depression; and to psychiatric aids to old-age fulfillment. Also discussed are thyroid difficulties, arthritis, chronic obstructive lung disease, cardiovascular disorders, eye and ear problems. Galton also urges that all necessary surgery be performed, not dismissed on the grounds of age; that diet be nutritious and balanced; that medications be handled cautiously. The final chapters focus on the nursing-home controversy, residential alternatives, and current geriatric research. A thoroughly documented, thought-provoking endeavor.

Gerontological Society. *Working with Older People: A Guide to Practice.* Vol. I: *The Knowledge Base,* rev. ed. Rockville, MD: Health Care Financing Administration, Health Standards and Quality Bureau, 1978. GPO No. 726-835/1606, 1-3. 191 pp.
Following a review of the objectives outlined in the Older American Act (1965), this study group examines the biological changes, health aspects, psychological and social aspects, and cultural-anthropological aspects of aging. Regarding physical and psychological concerns, the authors identify structural and functional changes and chronic problems. Oral health and preventive medicine are covered. Also examined are changes in intelligence, learning capacity, memory, information processing, personality. Bibliographies are included. Especially valuable regarding behavior and personality.

Gore, Irene. *Add Years to Your Life and Life to Your Years.* New York: Stein & Day, 1975. 132 pp. $1.95 (paper).
Contending that inactivity accelerates the aging process, the author emphasizes vitality as the key to healthy aging. She presents her view in three major sections: the causes of, factors affecting, and attitudes toward the aging process; the mental and physical components of sustained vitality; practical suggestions for aging well by controlling depression, safeguarding eyesight and hearing, caring for feet, eating properly, exercising regularly and maintaining activities, practicing safety measures, attending to the mind and emotions, and promoting social reforms. A practical, surprisingly thorough handbook that works against the unfortunate metaphor of the body as a machine, worn out from overuse.

Gross, Ronald, Gross, Beatrice, and Seidman, Sylvia, eds. *The New Old: Struggling for Decent Aging.* Garden City, NY: Anchor, 1978. 510 pp. $5.95 (paper).
This is a collection of articles by a heterogeneous group of individuals and groups concerned about aging. Divided into nine sections, the anthology covers such broad areas as living conditions, demographics, aging, death, joys of aging, activism, retirement, programs, and projects. The last section is a roster of organizations, services, networks, and literature. An all-embracing, highly acclaimed work. Recommended.

Harris and Associates, Inc. *The Myth and Reality of Aging in America.* Washington, DC: Natl. Council on Aging, 1975. 245 pp. OP.
Surveying the public's attitudes toward aging and providing a realistic base for future programs, this study conducted by Harris and Associates explores old age largely from a sociological perspective. Among the sections developed are the public image of most people over 65, social and economic contributions of the elderly, preparations for old age, the actual experience of being older, accessibility and use of community facilities, the media's portrayal of people over 65, the politics of old age. Appendixes include demographic information on the samples and an explanation of the survey design and process. Despite only peripheral relevance to health literature, this study has landmark significance and is a necessary reference tool in any geriatric library.

Hooker, Susan. *Caring for Elderly People: Understanding and Practical Help.* Boston: Routledge, 1976. 165 pp. $10.25; 1978, $4.25 (paper); London Routledge. £3.95; £1.95 (paper).
In this problem-oriented guide to attending the elderly, a British physiotherapist offers detailed advice for both health-care personnel and family members. Among the problems covered are normal and abnormal changes during aging, arthritis, stroke, fractures, Parkinson's Disease, falls and loss of balance, bronchitis, care of the feet and legs, obesity and diet, incontinence and constipation, bed care, behavioral changes, daily routines

and mobility, and exercises. Included is material on the causes and symptoms of each disorder, dangers and precautions. There are also chapters on outside services and financial help and on aids and gadgets with manufacturers' addresses. Glossary, resource directory, and bibliography are appended. Exceptional in its scope and readability.

Jury, Mark, and Jury, Dan. *Gramp.* New York: Penguin, 1978. 152 pp. $6.95 (paper).
In this rare and sensitive photographic journal, two young men trace their grandfather's gradual mental deterioration. Frank Tugend's senility progressed until he refused all nourishment and later died, about three years after he began to "fail." An exceptional work that focuses on an old man's right to live and die in dignity. Recommended.

Kalish, Richard A. *Late Adulthood: Perspectives on Human Development.* Monterey, CA: Brooks/Cole Publg., 1975. 133 pp. $4.95 (paper).
Directed at the "not-yet-old," this work is meant to promote knowledge and empathy in their dealings with the aged. The author explores aging from a psychosocial perspective, emphasizing such considerations as changing self-concepts, patterns of successful aging, mental illness, social attitudes toward aging and the aged, family relationships, independence and dependence, friends, ethnicity. Community involvement is also covered in sections on housing, transportation, religion, work and retirement, and interventions that place the aged in a passive life role. This latter topic includes a discussion of residential nursing facilities. Resource organizations are listed in text; references. A sensitive appraisal of value to readers with some knowledge of psychology.

Keddie, Kenneth M.G. *Action with the Elderly: A Handbook for Relatives and Friends.* New York: Pergamon, 1978. 163 pp $15; $7.50 (paper); Oxford: Pergamon. £7.50; £3.50 (paper).
A British psychiatrist discusses sociological and medical problems of the elderly, and their possible solutions. Among the topics covered are safety measures; medicine; sleep; sexuality; care of the eyes, ears, teeth, and feet; stroke rehabilitation; aids for the disabled; problems with elimination; psychological changes; and mental disturbances, including senility. There are chapter notes, suggestions for further reading; an appendix on American services for the elderly; and organizational addresses. Somewhat informative, but disjointed and poorly illustrated.

Luce, Gay Gaer. *Your Second Life: Vitality and Growth in Maturity and Later Years from the Experiences of the SAGE Program.* New York: Delacorte, 1979. 466 pp. $10.95.
In 1974 the author, a psychologist and science writer, founded the program Senior Actualization and Growth Exploration (SAGE). This sensitive and

inspiring book is an outgrowth of that program. In the first part, Dr. Luce explores attitudes toward age and longevity, relaxation and optimum health, breathing, self-image, massage, sexuality in later life, dreams and sleep, healing, meditation, and dying. The second section provides exercises and techniques designed to promote wellness. Covered here are stress and relaxation, autogenic training, massage, "numerous exercises for vitality and flexibility, participative listening," art and music as self-expression, food awareness and nutrition. The epilogue discusses the "ground rules" of SAGE, beginning with the directive to simply pay attention to your body. Extensive bibliography is included. A much-needed, sensible work. Highly recommended.

National Council on Aging, Research and Evaluation Department. *Fact Book on Aging: A Profile of America's Older Population.* Washington, DC: The Council, 1978. 263 pp. OP.
Regarding health matters, the authors cover life expectancy and mortality, acute and chronic conditions, visual and auditory impairments, dental disease, limited activity and mobility, disability days, medical manpower, utilization of outpatient and dental visits, brief and long-term inpatient care, economic considerations, life-crises reactions, psychiatric and organic brain disorders, factors affecting mental health services. Numerous charts and tables, references. Though hardly an in-depth treatment, the work is remarkably informative and readable.

Otten, Jane, and Shelley, Florence D. *When Your Parents Grow Old.* New York: Funk & Wagnalls, 1976. 298 pp. $9.95; New York: NAL, 1978. $2.25 (paper).
Health concerns are the major emphasis in this information guide. Among the topics covered are health maintenance and safety in the home, choosing a nursing home, the doctor-patient relationship, prevalent diseases of the elderly, behavioral changes, death and dying. Tension between the generations, guilt, communications, and the limits of responsibility are also discussed. Especially helpful is the supplementary material on community services, government benefits and insurance, and the appended listings of program information, organizations and agencies, and literature. Balanced and well structured. Recommended.

Sanders-Brown Research Center of Aging. *Your Health after 60,* ed. by M. M. Blacker, and D. R. Wekstein. New York: Dutton, 1979. 180 pp. $9.95; $4.95 (paper).
In 12 chapters written by medical experts, this guide for laypersons covers such common concerns as choosing a physician, the "miracle and menace of medication," arthritis and bone problems, dental health, vision and hearing problems, loss of memory, speech and language, stroke, low-back pain, physical exercise, and the experience of grief. The book's highlights include sections on osteoporosis, oral cancer, cataracts and glaucoma, depression, and self-help for back pain. In several chapters, the authors provide advice on

seeking help from medical centers and organizations. Certain warning signs are not emphasized enough, such as transient ischemic attacks, which require immediate medical attention; and the work lacks a supplementary bibliography. It excels, however, as an elementary, highly readable guide to common health concerns. Indispensable.

Schwartz, Arthur N. *Survival Handbook for Children of Aging Parents.* Chicago: Follett, 1977. 160 pp. $6.95.
In this practical and perceptive guide for children of the elderly, the director of adult counseling at Ethel Percy Andrus Gerontology Center focuses on the need to promote self-esteem in the aged. Although the work approaches aging from the child's perspective, it is valuable reading for the elderly themselves. In the chapter on senility, Dr. Schwartz demonstrates how easily other, minor problems may be mistaken for this catchall disorder; and how easily, in many cases, offending behavior can be alleviated. Also excellent are the chapters on nursing-home care and its alternatives, and on death and dying. The work closes with advice on enlisting the support of various organizations and services, many of which are listed. A sane and candid manual. Highly recommended.

Silverstone, Barbara, and Hyman, Helen Kandel. *You and Your Aging Parent.* New York: Pantheon, 1976. $10; $3.95 (paper).
A social worker and a medical writer collaborate on this guide to the emotional, physical, and financial problems that affect the aging and their families. They bring to light the myriad of feelings involved in the parent-child relationship during aging, several unhealthy modes of interaction flowing from these emotions, physical and mental disorders, as well as changes in sexual and social relationships. An especially insightful chapter concerns the final crisis of death and the ways in which the elderly and their families might respond. The second half of the book explores various types of action that can be taken when dealing with aged parents who are independent, physically or mentally impaired, or in need of long-term care. The final chapter concerns activism for and by the aged. Six appendixes list resource and service agencies, readings and directories; provide checklists for evaluating nursing homes and health-aide services, and describe common diseases and symptoms. A practical, comprehensive work that offers comfort and answers to all concerned parties.

Solnick, Robert L., ed. *Sexuality and Aging,* rev. Los Angeles: Univ. of Southern California, Andrus Gerontology Center, 1978. 195 pp. $4.50 (paper).
Composed of articles by 16 respected professionals, this work begins with a broad perspective on sexuality and aging and proceeds to an exploration of physiological, psychological, and sociological issues. Sexual problems, liberation, and learning are considered and set against the backdrop of the institution. Finally, the concept of love is introduced into the study and inspires

appreciation for the shared expression of life. A sensitive and realistic review of sexual frustration and fulfillment among the elderly. Highly recommended.

Services for the Elderly

Biegel, Leonard. *The Best Years Catalogue: A Sourcebook for Older Americans: Solving Problems & Living Fully.* New York: Putnam's, 1978. 224 pp. $12.95; $6.95 (paper).
In 11 well-illustrated sections, this work responds to the chief concerns of older people. Supplementing his material with numerous references and addresses for products or services, the author explores attitudes toward aging; nutrition and special diets; shelter, including nursing homes; general and special health matters, medical care, fitness, and sex; safety; leisure activities, including sports; transportation concerns, such as medical emergencies on the road, travel by the handicapped; finances; social and professional organizations; special communications aids for handicapped elders; legal rights. Although psychology and dying are among the topics neglected, the work is excellent within its scope. Recommended.

Butcher, Lee. *Retirement without Fear.* Princeton, NJ: Dow Jones, 1978. 159 pp. $8.95.
Devoting considerable space to the financial and legal aspects of aging, the author offers advice on retirement budgets, social security, pensions and other financial resources, medicare, aging, swindlers, programs and laws protecting the elderly. Also covered are such major concerns as the national nutrition program, the emotional pitfalls of aging and retirement, employment and other activities, senior activism. Regarding health, Butcher discusses nutrition, weight control, stress, and exercise. He provides tables on the leading causes of death among the aging, ideal weights, and stress-causing events. Much more needs to be said about coping with such problems as debilitating illness, medical attitudes toward the aging, and dying; but as far as it goes, the book is clearly relevant.

Consumer Guide, Editors of. *Getting Your Share: Social Security, Medicare, Government Benefits.* New York: Simon & Schuster, 1977. 162 pp. $2.95 (paper).
Offering comprehensive and highly specific instruction on claiming Social Security and other government benefits, an expert in retirement planning provides an essential handbook for the aging. Among the topics covered are the framework and deficiences of the Social Security system, eligibility, applying for benefits, preretirement benefits, working while collecting benefits, changes in status, appeal and benefit reinstatement, medicare coverage and exclusions, medicaid, programs that tie into Social Security, other financial resources, tax advantages after age 65. Especially valuable are the directory of

organizations and agencies, sample forms, and supplemental literature. The book includes a warning that Social Security rules are subject to periodic change. Highly recommended.

Gerontological Society. *Working with Older People: A Guide to Practice.* Vol. II: *Human Services,* rev. ed. Rockville, MD: Health Care Financing Administration, Health Standards and Quality Bureau, 1978. GPO No. 726-836/1607 1-3. 207 pp.

Lamenting the absence of an integrated service continuum, the authors begin this volume with a review of manpower opportunities, expanding resources, and remaining problems. Extensive space is devoted to defining and describing both target groups and services answering the peculiar needs of the well aged, minimally-to-severely impaired, and the dying. Ideal programs are outlined and existing services that approach the ideal are presented. A resource appendix provides bibliography, reference sources, and a directory of organizations. An excellent appraisal of the problem with highly reasonable proposals for change.

Holmes, Douglas, and Holmes, Monica Bychowski. *Handbook of Human Services for Older People.* New York: Human Sciences Pr., 1979. 288 pp. $16.95.

Eight kinds of services are profiled for professionals working with the elderly: multipurpose senior centers, legal counseling, employment services, homemaker and home health services, residential renovation and repair, day-care facilities, information and referral services, and nursing-home advocacy. Agencies and legislation on all levels of government are also detailed. Although it has limited application to medical concerns and less value as a lay tool, this work is recommended as a basic reference tool for consumer health librarians.

Nutrition and Physical Fitness

Bender, Ruth. *Be Young and Flexible after 30, 40, 50, 60 . . . .* Avon, CT: Ruben, 1976. 98 pp. $3.95 (paper; spiral binding).

Involved in federal, state, and private programs promoting fitness activities for the aging, the author is also an instructor of physical education and yoga. In this slim book, she illustrates over 60 exercises designed to foster total fitness. Among the varieties presented are foot and toe exercises, three levels of breathing, balancing and squatting, wake-up exercises, eye exercises, stretching, crawling, relaxation, and endurance exercises. Photographs and step-by-step instructions are included. This is a remarkably concise and practical book, with relatively large print. Recommended.

Caplow-Lindner, Erna, Harpaz, Leah, and Samberg, Sonya. *Therapeutic Dance/Movement: Expressive Activities for Older Adults.* New York: Human Sciences Pr., 1979. 283 pp. $15.95; $6.95 (paper).

More than a collection of movements for the elderly, this work presents a broad view of aging that includes considerations of the sociological and physical implications of aging. The history, meaning, and purposes of therapeutic dance are discussed; the needs and characteristics of the geriatric population are acknowledged; and the various components of the program are enumerated. The authors describe a session step-by-step, suggesting sequences of exercises and explaining their view of breathing, relaxation, and massage. The exercises themselves, music, and equipment are detailed. Especially valuable are suggestions for facilitating daily routines and the closing references to literature and organizations. An unusual, exciting approach.

Frankel, Lawrence J., and Richard, Betty Byrd. *Be Alive as Long as You Live.* Charleston, WV: Preventicare Pubns., 1977. 254 pp. OP.
In this large, well-illustrated manual, the authors present mobility exercises for older persons, whether they are ambulatory or chairbound. Includes almost 30 in-bed or bedside exercises; advice on interval training; a series of reflections on diet and nutrition, breathing, and attitude. Two appendixes include instruction in meditation and in initiating a group program. A rather dated bibliography follows. Useful and not overly strenuous techniques.

Harlow, Jan, Liggett, Irene, Mandel, Evelyn. *The Good Age Cookbook: Recipes from the Institute for Creative Aging.* Boston: Houghton, 1979. 221 pp. $10.95.
Low-cholesterol, low-salt and sugar, low-fat, and low-calorie dishes geared to the aging who are living alone or in couples. The recipes fall into 15 categories, including casseroles and one-dish meals, leftovers, vegetarian cookery, breads and quick breads, desserts, and nutritionally "indefensible" recipes referred to as "lapses." In addition, the authors cover shopping and storage, staples and flavoring ingredients, metric conversion tables, literature on both nutrition and aging. A remarkable, long-overdue book of practical and appealing recipes. Highly recommended.

Harris, Raymond, and others, eds. *Guide to Fitness after Fifty.* New York: Plenum, 1977. 374 pp. OP.
A scholarly presentation of research data and professional advice on fitness programs for the aging, this work contains contributions by 27 authorities in medicine, cardiology, physiology, rehabilitation, psychology, physical therapy, and gerontology. Among the topics covered are the effects of exercise on the aging process, cardiovascular fitness, motivation and life-style transformation, program development, suggested exercises for specific target areas, tension control techniques. Includes end-of-chapter references, numerous charts, and a glossary. Aimed primarily at professionals, this work is nevertheless a valuable reference aid for anyone concerned with fitness in later years.

Higdon, Hal. *Fitness after Forty.* Mountain View, CA: World Pubns., 1977. 262 pp. $4.95 (paper).
The benefits and hazards of exercise during and after middle age are dis-

cussed. Topics of interest are changes during the aging process, cardiovascular risk factors, exercise in cardiac rehabilitation, athletic slowdown with age, exercise in weight control, food for athletes, the roots of exercise aversion, the fitness rating of specific "sports," physical exams and athletic doctors, the importance of regularity and continuity, and 20 factors that determine life span. The author's anecdotal style is most appealing, although it limits the amount of factual information supplied.

Kordel, LeLord. *You're Younger Than You Think: The Mature Person's Guide to Vibrant Health.* New York: Putnam's, 1976. 311 pp. $8.95; New York: Popular Library, 1979. $2.25 (paper).
Emphasizing dietary strategies, the author offers advice on easing the aging process and achieving optimum health. Topics of interest are nutritional deficiencies; refined carbohydrates and other "killer foods"; promoting good digestion, and vitamins for healthy bones; diet and arthritis; kidney and bladder health; food and exercise for healthy skin; weight-control tips; foods to eliminate from the diet and foods to substitute; inexpensive marketing; home gardening; sleeping; and sexual activity in later years. Though most concerned with nutrition, Kordel also recognizes the importance of exercise, breathing, posture, and other factors. Especially valuable are chapters on habit control, heart health, relaxation, avoiding senility and premature aging, choosing a doctor. Clear, positive advice.

Rosenberg, Magda. *Sixty-Plus & Fit Again: Exercises for Older Men and Women.* New York: Evans, 1977. 142 pp. $6.95; $3.95 (paper); Boston: Hall, 1978. $10.95 (large print); London: Prior. £5.50 (large print).
The author, who conducts exercise programs for the elderly, provides a thorough handbook for initiating and developing physical activity after years of sedentary living. Covered are the health effects of exercise, common excuses, gradual conditioning and other precautions, everyday activities, warm-ups, walking, coordination and posture, individual stamina, breathing, chair and standing exercises, neck and tension exercises, aids to sleeping, facial exercises, muscle toning and weight control, advanced exercises and routines, jogging, yoga, isometric exercises, helpful equipment, and group programs. A most worthwhile book, despite the scarcity of illustrations.

Hearing and Vision

See also Hearing Impairment in Chapter 17, Other Health Problems and Concerns.

Brooks, Dennis L., and Henley, Arthur. *Don't be Afraid of Cataracts.* Secaucus, NJ: Stuart, 1978. 123 pp. $8.95. Dist. in U.K. by LSP Books, Godalming. £6.76.
An ophthalomologist and a medical writer collaborate on this general guide to

a major eye disorder. Among the topics covered are the warning signs of cataracts, demographics, types of cataracts, choosing a doctor, current treatment modalities, the healing process, and financial considerations. Although the authors stress that cataracts can occur at any age, they differentiate clearly between the special treatment needs of the elderly and those of younger patients. Especially informative is the material on the new ultrasound procedure, for which the aged are usually candidates. A highly comprehensible work, enhanced by relatively large print. Recommended.

Eden, John. *The Eye Book*. New York: Viking, 1978. 218 pp. $12.50; New York: Penguin, $3.95 (paper).
Although this is a general work on eye hygiene and disorders, it contains several chapters that are useful to the aging individual. Among the relevant topics covered are such problems as presbyopia, cataracts, and glaucoma. In addition there are chapters on eye anatomy and function, glasses and first aid. A glossary and resource directory are appended. Clear and down-to-earth.

Esterman, Ben. *The Eye Book: A Specialist's Guide to Your Eyes and Their Care*. Arlington, VA: Great Ocean Pubs., 1977. 264 pp. $10.95; $5.95 (paper).
Aimed at the general reader, this work covers concerns such as glaucoma, cataract, unsuspected illnesses revealed in eye exams, choosing an ophthalmologist, eye anatomy and function. Space is also devoted to prevention of blindness through injury and advances in ophthalmology. A valuable reference guide enhanced by large print.

Freese, Arthur S. *You and Your Hearing: How to Protect It, Preserve It, and Restore It*. New York: Scribner's, 1979. 184 pp. $9.95.
A prolific medical writer and contributing editor to *Modern Maturity* provides an explanation of ear anatomy and hearing function, the causes and types of hearing problems, and remedies ranging from hearing devices and surgery to such experimental approaches as transplants and implants. Although the work is general in scope, it contains a valuable section on the special hearing problems of the elderly, including a list of five warning signs for the individual who may not recognize his or her problem. In closing, the author provides an annotated directory of resource organizations and a rather scientific bibliography. Recommended.

Helleberg, Marilyn M. *Your Hearing Loss; How to Break the Sound Barrier*. Chicago: Nelson-Hall, 1979. 257 pp. $12.95.
A speech pathologist uses a question-and-answer format to inform readers about the causes, treatment, and social implications of hearing loss. Although only two sections deal specifically with hearing loss and aging, the work is valuable for its handling of such concerns as surgery, hearing aids, lipreading, auditory training, hearing maintenance, emotional problems, employment,

resources, and family support. Bibliography appended. Within the limitations of its format, the book is thorough and readable.

Arthritis

Berson, Dvera, with Roy, Sander. *Pain-Free Arthritis.* New York: Simon & Schuster, 1978. 96 pp. $6.95.
Herself a victim of rheumatoid arthritis, osteoarthritis, and two other bone disorders, the author presents her own program of exercise and water therapy that helped transform her from a virtual cripple to an active, productive individual. After describing her medical history, Berson explains how the exercises work and provides step-by-step instructions for other arthritics. She includes numerous illustrations, information on exercise aids, and a brief discussion of diet therapies and quack cures that she considers ineffective. The program is praised by a physician with the New York Arthritis Foundation and the Arthritis Clinic at Maimonides Hospital, but should be carried out under doctor's supervision. Recommended.

Dong, Collin H., and Banks, Jane. *New Hope for the Arthritic.* New York: Crowell, 1975. 269 pp. $6.95; New York: Ballantine, 1976. $1.95 (paper); St. Albans, Herts: Hart-Davis, 1976. £2.50.
Asserting that arthritis can successfully be treated with dietary measures, a physician describes the types of arthritis, causal theories, and common therapies; explains his own hypothesis that chemicals and allergic reactions are causal factors; and proposes a diet that eliminates milk, fruit, red meat, alcohol, and additives. Although he approves of vegetables, he claims that after a single serving of asparagus, his arthritic symptoms returned. The book also contains advice on exercise, menu planning and cooking, a lengthy recipe section, and a scientific bibliography. Criticizing both the Arthritis Foundation and traditional rheumatologists, Dr. Dong has written a sensational but unconvincing work.

Engleman, Ephraim, and Silverman, Milton. *The Arthritis Book: A Guide for Patients and Their Families.* New York: Dutton, 1979. 225 pp. $9.95.
Dr. Engleman, an expert on arthritic diseases, and Milton Silverman, nationally known science writer, discuss in simple language the many forms of arthritis that affect thirty-one million victims, the newly discovered immunogenetic factors, recent advances in treatment (some still unknown by most patients and even many physicians), and some of the crushing personal and social problems arthritis patients and their families face. They conclude that proper care can provide relief and a normal life for arthritis sufferers.

Freeman, Julian. *Arthritis: The New Treatments.* Chicago: Contemporary, 1979. 158 pp. $8.95.
A good overview of arthritis and its manifestations. Freeman writes in a

sensible, direct, and honest manner. The chapters on rheumatoid arthritis, gout, and the use of medication are particularly good. A comprehensive, informative book recommended for the more sophisticated reader.

Fries, James F. *Arthritis: A Comprehensive Guide.* Reading, MA: Addison-Wesley, 1979. 258 pp. $11.95, $6.95 (paper).
The author is director of the Stanford University Arthritis Clinic and is coauthor with Donald Vickery, M.D., of *Take Care of Yourself.* In this work, Fries has produced the best book to date on arthritis for the education of the general reader. In an informative, lucid manner, the author describes the major types of treatment, medications to help arthritis victims, tests, quackery, saving money, how to cope with pain and the side effects of medications, problems in getting around, difficulties in enjoyment and sexual activity. Certainly a landmark book. Highly recommended.

Kitay, William. *Understanding Arthritis.* New York: Monarch, 1977. 152 pp. $2.95 (paper).
In this concise and uncomplicated handbook on arthritis, the author begins with historical and demographic information and follows with descriptions of 12 little-known forms of arthritis, as well as osteoarthritis, rheumatoid arthritis, gout, and infectious arthritis. Diagnostic procedures and various treatment modalities are explained thoroughly. In a chapter on the patient's role in therapy, Kitay emphasizes cooperation and emotional balance, exercise and proper nutrition, and other helpful measures. He includes warnings about ineffective diet therapy, and information about functional therapy, self-help devices, and sexual relations. Appended are a directory of Arthritis Foundation chapters and a glossary. A current, practical guide.

Malone, Fred. *Bees Don't Get Arthritis.* New York: Dutton, 1979. 178 pp. $8.95.
Alleging that bee products can alleviate a myriad of disorders, from acne to cancer, the author concentrates his private research on bee venom as an arthritis treatment. Though not a medical professional, Malone takes great care to warn his readers about allergenic hazards and documents his work with a respectable four-page bibliography. His claims demand skepticism and further study, but his book is both novel and thought provoking.

Rosenberg, Alan L., ed. *Living with Your Arthritis: A Home Program for Arthritis Management.* New York: Arco, 1979. 226 pp. $8.95; $3.95 (paper).
This work is the composite product of several contributors, including rheumatologists, orthopedic surgeons, physical therapists, occupational therapists, and social service personnel. Equipping the average arthritic with self-help skills, this program covers posture and exercise for increasing joint mobility, suggestions for facilitating everyday activities, helpful devices, appraisals of common medications, alternative forms of therapy such as biofeedback and nerve stimulation, surgical options, nutritional factors,

communication tips for interacting with health workers, psychosocial and sexual insights, and therapeutic recreation. Also discussed are several common forms of quackery. Exercises, glossary, and a resource directory are appended. A simple, sensible aid to coping. Recommended.

Nursing Homes

Burger, Sarah Greene, and D'Erasmo, Martha. *Living in a Nursing Home: A Complete Guide for Residents, Their Families and Friends.* New York: Seabury, 1976. 178 pp. $8.95; New York: Ballantine, 1979. $2.50 (paper).

Beginning with a vignette about one woman's deterioration in a reasonably adequate home, two registered nurses with expertise in the area provide a thorough introduction to the nursing-home experience. They explore the physiology of aging and the socioeconomic factors leading to displacement, advise readers on shopping for a nursing home, and itemize the necessary preparations a family should make. Patient and family reactions to placement, the patient's legal status, nursing-home personnel, and death of a resident are covered thoroughly. In every chapter, the author warns against common mistakes and provides specific advice on making the most of a particular situation. Notes and glossary are appended, along with directories of federal and state agencies, nursing-home ombudsmen, licensing offices, and concerned organizations. Practical and compassionate: Indispensable.

Glasscote, Raymond M., and others. *Old Folks at Homes: A Field Study of Nursing and Board-and-Care Homes.* Washington, D.C.: Joint Information Service of the American Psychiatric Assn. and the Natl. Assn. for Mental Health, 1976. 148 pp. $6.50.

A group of 13 psychiatrists, social workers, nurses, and health administrators conducted a study into nursing-home conditions, two years after the Senate investigation that exposed numerous gross deficiencies. Covered in the study are state hospitals, community mental health centers, and nursing homes in particular. Within this last category are skilled nursing facilities, intermediate care facilities, and board-and-care homes. Federal and state regulations are explained in detail, including scopes of Medicare and Medicaid. Following a section of vignettes, the authors share their findings that specially trained physicians and support staff are scarce, pay is low, locales remote or unsafe, volunteers and relatives poorly mobilized, and psychosocial needs neglected. Despite these observations, the authors note improvement over previous years and are puzzled by continuing horror stories in the press. Extremely balanced and constructive.

Horn, Linda, and Griesel, Elma. *Nursing Homes: A Citizen's Action Guide.* Boston: Beacon, 1977. 190 pp. $3.95 (paper).

Horn and Griesel provide advice on how to organize citizen's action groups, how to use the Freedom of Information Act to obtain Medicare Inspection

Reports, how to remedy complaints, and how to plan, publicize, and lobby for reform. A summary of the activities of major citizens' action groups in the United States is supplied together with sources of government information. An excellent insight into the Gray Panthers movement. Recommended.

Mendelson, Mary Adelaide. *Tender Loving Greed: How the Incredibly Lucrative Nursing Home "Industry" is exploiting America's Old People and Defrauding Us All.* New York: Random, 1975. $2.45 (paper).
The classic expose of the nursing-home "industry" that talks about loving care while mistreating the old and helpless. Mendelson describes how the munificence of federal aid, together with the lack of effective control, has made the nursing-home industry into a giant profit machine. Based on case histories and extensive research, this is a very pessimistic view of nursing homes. However, it is a magnificent statement of the problem and has contributed greatly to the achievement of nursing-home reform. Highly recommended.

Moss, Frank E., and Halamandaris, Val J. *Too Old, Too Sick, Too Bad.* Germantown, MD: Aspen Systems, 1977. 326 pp. $15.95; Corte Madera, CA: Anthelion, 1979. $4.95 (paper).
An outgrowth of hearings by the Senate's Special Committee on Aging, this work is an indictment of the nursing-home system in America. The authors examine the problems and their causes, as well as the positive aspects and reforms of long-term care. Especially informative are the chapters on nursing-home drugs, fires, profiteering, inadequate staffing and medical concern, the types of programs that succeed, and guidelines for selecting a facility. Included in the appendixes is a thorough directory of resources. Balanced and well-documented.

Hospices

Cohen, Kenneth P. *Hospice: Prescription for Terminal Care.* Germantown, MD: Aspen Systems, 1979. 303 pp. $17.50.
A hospital administrator and participant in two hospice committees traces the history of hospices and contrasts the care given to that found in hospitals and nursing homes. Also covered are the different attitudes toward death and bereavement, ethical questions regarding the right to die, and elements of a hospice program. The second half of the book is directed more to administrators than to general readers but does contain interesting material on the right-to-die issue. Appended hospice and organizational addresses are especially useful. Recommended.

DuBois, Paul M. *The Hospice Way of Death.* New York: Human Sciences Pr., 1980. 223 pp. $16.95.
Providing comparative case studies of two hospices and an aborted attempt at

establishing another, the author evaluates not only hospices in general but also specific programs within the movement. Terminal care in traditional health facilities is clearly inadequate, but the hospices themselves have flaws. DuBois includes chapters on the components of hospice care, federal response to the movement, leading causes of death, the quality of dying, and personal responses. Bibliography appended. A most provocative work that highlights policy and planning failures. Recommended.

Hamilton, Michael P., and Reid, Helen F., eds. *A Hospice Handbook: A New Way to Care for the Dying.* Grand Rapids, MI: Eerdmans Publishing, 1980. 196 pp. $3.95 (paper).
One of the newest hospice books, this work brings together 13 experts who reflect on the process of dying and the advantages of the hospice approach. Three sections cover the needs of the dying, the response of the hospice, and elements of organization. Especially valuable are the personal testimonies of patients and relatives, the observations of a medical anthropologist who pretended to be dying to gather data for a study, and a series of report forms on a terminal patient in a palliative care service. Other contributions include the perspectives of a doctor and a chaplain, a comparison of the hospice approach to those found in nursing homes and hospitals, and a description of a hospice volunteer program. Bibliography and list of slides and films are appended. A most revealing work that presents several unusual perspectives on the hospice movement.

Rossman, Parker. *Hospice: Creating New Models of Care for the Ill.* New York: Association Pr., 1977. 240 pp. $8.95; New York: Fawcett, 1979. $4.95 (paper).
A clergyman analyzes the experience of American hospices. Chapters include "The Dilemma of the Family"; "Healthcare Professionals and the Dying"; "The New Haven Hospice: An American Adaptation"; "The Hospice Concept as Program"; "Advice to Other Communities"; and "Home Care for the Dying." Chapter notes are appended, as are materials for orienting volunteers and an "official" definition of hospice. The work has a more clinical tone than other works on the same subject.

Warburg, Sandol Stoddard. *The Hospice Movement: A Better Way of Caring for the Dying.* Briarcliff Manor, NY: Stein & Day, 1977. 266 pp. $8.95; London: Cape, 1979. £5.95.
A former volunteer at St. Christopher's Hospice in London explains the aims and functions of the hospice movement, which helps terminally ill persons face death without pain, fear, or abandonment. Using case histories and her personal experience, the author presents specific information about patient care, medication techniques, funding, staffing, home care programs. Three technical appendixes describe the drugs used for pain control. A combination journal and report, the work is compassionately written and filled with enlightening details. A poetic and inspiring book. Highly recommended.

Death and Dying

Barton, David, ed. *Dying and Death: A Clinical Guide for Caregivers*. Baltimore:
    Williams & Wilkins, 1977. 238 pp. $14.95.
Although this work is aimed at professionals, some chapters will be undeniably
helpful to certain terminal patients and their families. Divided into two parts,
the book begins with general discussions of the subject. Despite its nontechnical terminology, this section will have limited value for the layperson. The
second part, consisting of nine articles by various contributors, includes several notable chapters, including two by terminal cancer victims, and one on
caring for the dying child.

Caughill, Rita E., ed. *The Dying Patient: A Supportive Approach*. Boston: Little,
    1976. 228 pp. $7.95 (paper).
A series of essays by several contributors, which cover such topics as dying and
society, grieving, dying with dignity, coping with death in acute-care units, the
dying child, supportive care, and the age of the patient. It is aimed at an
educated audience, both professional and lay.

Feifel, Herman, ed. *New Meanings of Death*. New York: McGraw-Hill, 1977.
    367 pp. $11.95; $4.95 (paper). Maidenhead: McGraw-Hill. £8.95; £3.70
    (paper).
An excellent anthology of essays by 21 distinguished contributors, this work
includes such titles as "Meanings of Death to Children"; "Dying They Live: St.
Christopher's Hospice"; "Make Today Count"; "Dying and Preparing for
Death: A View of Families." Providing comprehensive coverage of the subject,
this book can give the terminal cancer patient and his family a framework that
is both philosophical and practical. Included are personal accounts of cancer
victims.

Grof, Stanislav, and Halifax, Joan. *The Human Encounter with Death*. 1st ed.
    Foreword by Elisabeth Kubler-Ross. New York: Dutton, 1977. 240 pp. $3.95
    (paper); London: Souvenir, 1978. £4.95, £2.95 (paper).
Written by a psychiatrist and an anthropologist, this book describes a program
in psychedelic therapy with terminal cancer patients. Using passages of
monologue and constructing what they term "psychedelic biographies," the
authors attempt to depict the emergence of peaceful attitudes in several
persons. Although the work centers on the use of lysergic acid diethylamide
(LSD) and its psychological effects on the dying, it is valuable chiefly for the
philosophical insights it may provide to other terminal cancer victims. The
therapy itself is decidedly controversial.

Hanlan, Archie J. *Autobiography of Dying*, ed. by Muriel E. Nelson. Garden City,
    NY: Doubleday, 1979. 193 pp. $8.95.
In this posthumously published journal, a professor of social work tells of his

three years with amytropic lateral sclerosis or Lou Gehrig's disease. Dying is perceived as a complex process: dehumanizing in some respects and dynamic in others. Included is a postscript entitled "Living with a Dying Husband" by Hanlan's wife and colleague. Both introspective and remarkably objective.

Kubler-Ross, Elisabeth, ed. *Death: The Final Stage of Growth*. Human Development Series. Englewood Cliffs, NJ: Prentice-Hall, 1975. 175 pp. $10.95; $2.95 (paper); Hemel Hempstead, Herts: Prentice-Hall, £8; £2.15 (paper).
Contents are essays by various contributors, and styles range from diary to report form. The tone of the book is established through a combination of philosophic, religious, and sociological approaches. In general, it has a very personal flavor, but in parts it appears almost saccharine. Recommended nevertheless.

Kubler-Ross, Elisabeth. *To Live Until We Say Goodbye*. Englewood Cliffs, NJ: Prentice-Hall, 1978. 160 pp. $8.95.
A beautiful and moving book produced by Dr. Kubler-Ross and Mal Warshaw, a photographer. Dr. Kubler-Ross portrays what can and will happen to human beings, young and old, child and adult alike, when they are in the process of being destroyed by a malignant growth. Through relationships with Beth, Jamie, Louise, and Jack, the author shows how courage and love can make the person "emerge as a butterfly emerges from a cocoon with a sense of peace and freedom, not only in themselves, but in those who are willing to share their final moments and who have the courage to say goodbye, knowing that every goodbye also includes a hello." Finally, Dr. Kubler-Ross describes hospices and other alternatives to hospital care. The splendid photography serves to enhance the impact of the very moving text. Truly outstanding. Highly recommended.

Lamerton, Richard. *Care of the Dying*. Westport, CT: Technomic Co. 160 pp. $11.50.
Written by a professional at two British hospices, this work is focused on all levels of readership. As a guide for anyone caring for the terminally ill, it deals with such topics as dying at home, hospices, dying children, and counseling the dying. Laced with case histories, many of which relate to cancer, the text is presented in a straightforward and compassionate manner. Includes references, bibliography, and index.

Lifton, Robert Jay. *The Broken Connection: On Death and the Continuity of Life*. New York: Simon & Schuster, 1979. 495 pp. $11.95.
This heavily philosophical work by a renowned, post-Freudian psychiatrist examines the blending of continuity and mortality in the human mind. According to Lifton the individual's sense of being necessarily includes an awareness of death, but when the notion of continuity is lost, so also is the person's ability to function fully. Topics include the various emotions involved

in death anxiety, the image of death in neurosis and schizophrenia, the effects of the Nazi holocaust and Hiroshima. Documentation is provided through extensive notes and four appendixes. A most impressive and intriguing book that philosophically oriented readers will welcome.

Miller, Marv. *Suicide after Sixty: The Final Alternative.* Springer Series on Death and Suicide, Vol. 2. New York: Springer, 1979. 118 pp. $6.95 (paper).
An expert on geriatric suicide identifies such common predicaments as early retirement, fixed incomes, social isolation, poor health, and dependency as the roots of suicide after sixty. The various losses the elderly must endure can trigger a suicidal reaction that is unmistakably genuine. Rarely does an elder's suicide attempt fail. Also discussed are suggestions for research in suicidology and the relation between geriatric suicide and euthanasia. Bibliography included. A most intriguing, chilling work appropriate for all levels of readership.

Pattison, E. Mansell, ed. *The Experience of Dying.* Englewood Cliffs, NJ: Prentice-Hall, 1977. 335 pp. $12.95; $4.95 (paper).
Twenty-four contributors specializing primarily in psychiatry examine the dying process in its many forms. Among the titles applying specifically to cancer are "Childhood Leukemia"; "Cancer in the School Age Child"; "The Adolescent with Cancer"; "A Father with Leukemia"; "Living in a Cancer Unit"; and "Acute Leukemia: A Personal Encounter." Several of the remaining articles are also relevant to the emotional aspects of terminal cancer.

Prichard, Elizabeth R., and others, eds. *Home Care: Living with the Dying.* New York: Columbia Univ. Pr., 1979. 290 pp. $18.50.
Forty-five professionals reflect on the history, goals, and modalities of home-care services. Although the scope of this work is general, there are several sections that apply to the geriatric patient. Relevant topics include the family's perspective, hospice-based services, senior companion programs, dying and the aged person, homemaker aides as thanatologists, and others. A clear and readable exploration of community response to illness and dying; not as clinical as similar efforts, attuned to the whole patient.

Shepard, Martin. *Someone You Love Is Dying: A Guide for Helping and Coping.* New York: Harmony, 1976. 223 pp. $7.95.
In this sensible guidebook, a psychiatrist addresses the everyday problems that accompany the dying process. Using interviews with patients and their families and friends, the author asserts that open communication is essential to control the fear of death. Shepard discusses the major terminal illnesses and provides information on telling the dying person, retaining a sense of humor, pain and pain relievers, the family's suffering, religious attitudes, economic and funeral matters. Included is a section of short meditations, some secular in tone. Both practical and uplifting. Highly recommended.

Weir, Robert F., ed. *Ethical Issues in Death and Dying.* New York: Columbia
   Univ. Pr., 1977. 405 pp. $20; $8 (paper).
A collection of 26 articles written by persons in the life sciences, medicine, law,
philosophy, and religion. Aimed at terminal patients and their families in
addition to professionals, it focuses on the interface of the various concerns
involved in death and dying. Chapters include "Do Cancer Patients Want to Be
Told?"; "What to Tell Cancer Patients: A Study of Medical Attitudes"; "Medical Diagnosis: Our Right to Know the Truth," by a layperson; "A Patient's
Decision to Decline Life-saving Medical Treatment."

Wright, H. T. *The Matthew Tree.* New York: Pantheon, 1975. 115 pp. OP;
   London: Hale, 1976. £3.95.
This is the journal of a family's seven-year vigil, waiting for the death of the
father. Despite multiple strokes and months of confinement in bed, it appeared he would survive indefinitely. With a clipped style and acute insight,
his middle-aged daughter describes the vigil and her own efforts at
euthanasia. Recommended.

PAMPHLETS

American Association of Retired Persons/National Retired Teachers Association, 1099 K St. N.W., Washington, DC 20049.
Membership includes such literature as:

   Modern Maturity, bimonthly magazine.
   National Community Service Programs, booklet.
   News Bulletin, monthly periodical.
   Pharmacy Products List.
   Your Retirement Health Guide.

American Dental Association, 211 E. Chicago Ave., Chicago, IL 60611.
Available booklets include:

   Dentures: What You Don't Know Can Hurt You.
   Don't Do It Yourself (denture repair).
   Keep Your Teeth All Your Life.
   They're Your Teeth . . . You Can Keep Them.
   Your New Dentures.

American Foundation for the Blind, Inc., 15 W. 16 St., New York, NY 10011.

   Aging and Blindness: A Public Symposium, 19 pp., AFB Offprint Series.
   Cataracts and Their Treatment, by Arthur S. Freese, 24 pp., 1977, FIL053.
   Facts about Aging and Blindness, 1976, FAL030.

Outreach to the Aging Blind: Some Strategies for Community Action, by Irving R. Dickman, 168 pp., 1977, PAP078. $3.50.

American Health Care Association, 1200 15 St. N.W., Washington, DC 20005. Publications include the monthly periodical *Modern Nursing Home, Weekly Notes* newsletter, and such consumer literature as *Thinking about a Nursing Home?* 29 pp.

American Heart Association, 7320 Greenville Ave., Dallas, TX 75231. Materials on stroke such as:

Aphasia and the Family, No. 50-002-A.
Body Language, No. 51-003-A.
Do It Yourself Again, on self-help devices, No. 50-005-A.
Facts about Strokes, No. 51-008-A.
Seven Hopeful Facts about Stroke, No. 51-016-A.
Stand Up to Stroke, No. 50-033-A.
Strike Back at Stroke, care of patients, No. 50-024-A.
Stroke: Why Do They Behave That Way? No. 50-035-A.
Strokes, A Guide for the Family, No. 50-024-A.
Up and Around, for newly ambulatory patients, No. 50-026-A.

American Medical Association, 535 N. Dearborn St., Chicago, IL 60610. Material on aging includes:

How the Older Person Can Get the Most Out of Living.
What to Look for in a Nursing Home.
Your Age and Diet.

American National Red Cross, 17 and D Sts. N.W., Washington, DC 20006. Literature such as the free publications *Caring* and *Telephone Reassurance.*

American Podiatry Association, 20 Chevy Chase Circle N.W., Washington, DC 20015. Among the free pamphlets are:

Foot Health and Aging: You're as Young as Your Feet.
Podiatrists' Services under Medicare.

Arthritis Foundation, 3400 Peachtree Rd. N.E.. Atlanta, GA 30326: and local chapters.. Annual reports, fact sheets, booklets, and reprints are available, including:

The Arthritis Foundation: What It Is and What It Does, 4-page leaflet, 1977.
Arthritis: The Basic Facts, booklet, 27 pp., 1976.

Clinic List.
Living with Arthritis, and Where to Turn for Help, booklet, 31 pp., 1976.
Osteoarthritis: A Handbook for Patients.
Physician Referral List.
Rheumatoid Arthritis: A Handbook for Patients, 20 pp., 1977.
The Truth about Aspirin for Arthritis, 1978.

Better Vision Institute, 230 Park Ave., New York, NY 10017.

Vision Problems of the Aging.

Blue Cross and Blue Shield of Central New York, 433 S. Warren St., Box 4809, Syracuse, NY 13221.

Health Insurance After 65: A Consumer's Guide, 1978.

Channing L. Bete Co., Inc., 45 Federal St., Greenfield, MA 01301.

Arthritis, 16 pp., C210-1133.

Citizens for Better Care, 960 E. Jefferson Ave., Detroit, MI 48207.

How to Choose a Nursing Home: A Shopping and Rating Guide.

Concerned Relatives of Nursing Home Patients, 3137 Fairmount Blvd., Cleveland Heights, OH 44118.

Insight, monthly newsletter.
Nursing Home Check List, 40-question leaflet.

Consumer Information Center, Pueblo, CO 81009.
Pamphlets on concerns of the aging include the following:

A Brief Explanation of Medicare, 13 pp., 1979, 571H.
Fitness Challenge . . . in the Later Years, 28 pp., 1979, 202H.
How to Cope with Arthritis, 26 pp., 1978, 139H.
What You Should Know about Stroke and Stroke Prevention, 10 pp., 1979, 178H.
A Woman's Guide to Social Security, 12 pp., 1979, 539H.
Your Right to Question the Decision on Your Hospital Insurance Claim, 8 pp., 1979, 583H.
Your Social Security, 31 pp., 1978, 540H.

Hospice Inc., 765 Prospect St., New Haven, CT 06511.
Sample print materials are:

Frequently Asked Questions about Hospice, $3.00.
Hospice Quarterly Newsletter.

Merck Sharp & Dohme, Public Relations Dept., West Point, PA 19486.

Understanding Arthritis: Information and Advice for Patients, booklet, 16 pp., 1976.

National Alliance of Senior Citizens, Inc., Box 40031, Washington, DC 20016.

Senior Services Manual.

National Clearinghouse on Aging, Administration on Aging, 330 Independence Ave. S.W., Washington, DC 20201.
Among the numerous materials available are:

Basic Concepts of Aging.
Consumer Guide for Older People, compact checklists.
Facts about Older Americans, DHEW Pubn. No. (OHD) 75-20006.
The Fitness Challenge in the Later Years, AOA Pubn. No. (OHD) 75-20802.
Home Delivered Meals.
Increasing Mobility among Isolated Elderly.
Information and Referral Services.
Publications of the Administration on Aging.
To Find a Way, brochure on services.
Traffic Accidents and Older Drivers.

National Council for Homemaker–Home Health Aide Services, Inc., 65 Irving Pl., New York, NY 10003.
Directory of Homemaker-Home Health Aide Services, $3, in addition to a quarterly newsletter and brochure literature.

The National Council on the Aging, 1828 L St. N.W., Washington, DC 20036.
Extensive literature includes:

Facts and Myths about Aging, 1976 booklet.
Memo, monthly newsletter.
Perspective on Aging, a bimonthly periodical for members.

National Institute of Arthritis, Metabolism, and Digestive Diseases, National Institutes of Health, 9000 Rockville Pike, Bethesda, MD 20014.

How to Cope with Arthritis, booklet, 27 pp., 1978, DHEW Pubn. No. (NIH) 78-1092.

National Institute on Drug Abuse, 5600 Fishers La., Parklawn Bldg., Rockville, MD 20857.
Using Medicines Wisely, 4-pamphlet kit, 1979, DHEW Pubn. No. (ADM) 78-705, consisting of:

Do's and Don'ts of Wise Drug Use.
Keeping Track of Your Medicines.
Saving Money with Generic Drugs. Can You? Should You?
Using Your Medicines Wisely: A Guide for the Elderly.

Office of Nursing Home Affairs, Public Health Service, 5600 Fishers La., Rockville, MD 20857.

How to Select a Nursing Home, booklet, 52 pp., DHEW Pubn. No. (OS) 76-50045.

Public Affairs Committee, Inc., 381 Park Ave. S., New York, NY 10016. Among the pamphlets available are:

After 65: Resources for Self-reliance, No. 501.
Better Health in Later Years, No. 446.
Cataracts and Their Treatment, No. 545.
The Dying Person and the Family, No. 485.
Getting Ready to Retire, No. 182A.
How to Keep Your Teeth after 30, No. 443.
Light on Your Feet, No. 345A.
Sex after Sixty-five, No. 519.
Vitamins, Food, and Your Health, No. 465.
What Can We Do about Limited Vision? No. 491.

Sight Center, Cleveland Society for the Blind, 1909 E. 101 St., Cleveland, OH 44106.

Don't Fear Cataract . . . Now There is Help!
Don't Gamble with Glaucoma: You May Lose Your Sight.

Social Security Administration, Altmeyer Bldg., 6401 Security Blvd., Baltimore, MD 21235; and local offices.
Available materials include:

A Brief Explanation of Medicare, 1979, DHEW Pubn. No. (SSA) 79-10043.
A Guide to Supplemental Security Income, 1979, DHEW Pubn. No. (SSA) 79-11015, 15 pp.
How Medicare Helps during a Hospital Stay, 1979, DHEW Pubn. No. (SSA) 79-10039.
How SSI Can Help, 1979, DHEW Pubn. No. (SSA) 79-11051, 7 pp.
How to Complete the Request for Medicare Payment, 1976, DHEW Pubn. No. (SSA) 76-10083.
Medicare Coverage in a Skilled Nursing Facility, 1976, DHEW Pubn. No. (SSA) 76-10041.
Social Security Information Items, monthly newsletter.
SSI for the Aged, Blind, and Disabled, 1979, DHEW Pubn. No. (SSA) 79-11000.
What You Have to Know about SSI, 1977, DHEW Pubn. No. (SSA) 77-11011.

A Woman's Guide to Social Security, 1979, DHEW Pubn. No. (SSA) 79-10127, 12 pp.
Your Medicare Handbook, 1979, DHEW Pubn. No. (SSA) 79-10050, 62 pp.
Your Social Security, 1979, DHEW Pubn. No. (SSA) 79-10035, 31 pp.
Your Social Security Rights and Responsibilities: Retirement and Survivors Benefits, 1979, DHEW Pubn. No. (SSA) 79-10077, 19 pp.

AUDIOVISUAL PRODUCERS AND DISTRIBUTORS

Abbott Laboratories
Abbott Park, D-383
North Chicago, IL 60064
Degenerative arthritis is among the topics covered in 3/4" video, available for free loan.

Arthritis Foundation Film Library
3400 Peachtree Road, N.E.
Atlanta, GA 30326
The library offers 16mm films on arthritis, quackery, manual rehabilitation, demographics, for sale or rental.

Benchmark Films
145 Scarborough Rd.
Briarcliff Manor, NY 10510
Motion picture or videocassette on death and dying.

Robert J. Brady Company
A Prentice-Hall Company
Bowie, MD 20715
Hearing aids, rheumatoid arthritis, cosmetic surgery, aging, death, and bereavement are among the programs available in filmstrip-audiocassette format. Audiocassettes on dying, flipchart package on stroke. Sale and leasing.

Department of Human Resources
Bureau of Health Services
275 E. Main St.
Frankfort, KY 40601
Among the relevant topics covered in

16mm filmstrips are the concerns of the aged, death.

Hear Center
301 E. Del Mar Blvd.
Pasadena, CA 91101
Hearing disorders relevant to the aging are among the topics covered in 16mm films for purchase or rental.

International Films Bureau, Inc.
332 S. Michigan Ave.
Chicago, IL 60604
Among the topics covered are aging, glaucoma, in 16mm or 35mm film for rental or purchase.

McGraw-Hill Films
110 15 St.
Del Mar, CA 92014
Videocassettes and 16mm films for purchase or rent cover aging, including emotional adjustments.

Milner-Fenwick, Inc.
2125 Green Spring Dr.
Timonium, MD 21093

National Association for Human Development
1750 Pennsylvania Ave. N.W.
Washington, DC 20006
Slide/script presentations and 16mm film are available on the subject of physical fitness for the elderly.

National Audiovisual Center
General Services Administration
National Archives and Records Service
Washington, DC 20409
Topics available on the concerns of the
elderly include day hospital care.

**National Council for
 Homemaker—Home Health Aide
 Services, Inc.**
67 Irving Pl.
New York, NY 10003
Films are available on the benefits of
in-home services.

National Council on the Aging
1828 L St. N.W.
Washington, DC 20036
Films and tapes on various aspects of
aging are available for purchase.

National Pharmaceutical Council
1030 15 St. N.W.
Washington, DC 20005
Proper use of prescriptions and
over-the-counter medications is
covered in 16mm film.

**National Society for the Prevention of
 Blindness, Inc.**
79 Madison Ave.
New York, NY 10016
Materials include posters, 16mm films,
and super 8mm on blindness.

Pfizer Laboratories
Div. of Pfizer, Inc.
Film Library
267 W. 25 St.
New York, NY 10001
Arthritis is among the relevant topics
covered in 16mm films; free loan.

Phoenix Films
470 Park Ave. S.
New York, NY 10016
Communicating with the elderly,

family relationships, death with
dignity, are among the topics
covered in 16mm film, for rent or
purchase.

Professional Research, Inc.
12960 Coral Tree Pl.
Los Angeles, CA 90066
Several formats are available on such
pertinent topics as glaucoma,
cataracts, menopause, rheumatoid
arthritis, dentures, living with dying.

Schering Corporation
Professional Services
Galloping Hill Rd.
Kenilworth, NJ 07033
Aging and nutrition are topics covered
in 16mm films available for free
loan and for sale.

Sister Kenny Institute
27 St. at Chicago Ave.
Minneapolis, MN 55407
Slide-sound series of stroke
programs covering causes, effects,
and rehabilitation. Sales and
rentals.

Society for Nutrition Education
2140 Shattuck Ave.
Berkeley, CA 94704
Nutrition in later years is covered in
16mm film.

Soundwords, Inc.
56-11 217 St.
Bayside, NY 11364
Audiocassettes are offered on
such relevant topics as strokes,
baldness, vitamins and minerals,
understanding menopause,
hearing problems, arthritis,
osteoarthritis, gout, sex in later
years, glaucoma and cataracts,
grief, death and dying.

Spenco Medical Corporation
Box 8113
Waco, TX 76710
Slides and audiocassettes are
available on musculoskeletal
diseases like arthritis, neurological
disorders like stroke, dental care,
hearing loss, living with senior
citizens. Other media include
folding displays and posters.

Teach'em, Inc.
Department 3-C
625 N. Michigan Ave.
Chicago, IL 60611
Films, videotapes, and audiocassettes
for sale cover such topics as death,
osteoarthritis, cataracts.

Time-Life Films
Multimedia Div.
100 Eisenhower Dr.
Box 644
Paramus, NJ 07652
Old age and death in various
societies are among the largely

sociological topics covered in
16mm film and videocassettes with
discussion guides. Sales and rental.

Trainex Corporation
Box 116
Garden Grove, CA 92642
Audiovisual materials cover
biological changes of aging both in
functions and in physical
appearance, loss in aging,
psychological crises, rheumatoid
arthritis, sexuality in aging, death
and dying, grief, stroke,
menopause. Formats include
cartridge programs, slides, and
filmstrip programs for purchase
or rental.

TV Film Library
Rm. 860
475 Riverside Dr.
New York, NY 10027
Audiovisual material is available on
hospice care.

RESOURCE ORGANIZATIONS

Aging Research Institute
342 Madison Ave.
New York, NY 10017

**American Academy of
Ophthalmology**
15 Second St. S.W.
Rochester, MN 55901

American Aging Association
Univ. of Nebraska
College of Medicine
Omaha, NE 68105

**American Association of Homes for
the Aging**
1050 17 St. N.W.
Washington, DC 20036

**American Association of Retired
Persons/National Retired Teachers
Association**
1909 K St. N.W.
Washington, DC 20049

American Dietetic Association
430 N. Michigan Ave.
Chicago, IL 60611

American Geriatrics Society
10 Columbus Circle
New York, NY 10019

American Health Care Association
1200 15 St. N.W.
Washington, DC 20005

American Medical Association
Committee on Aging
535 N. Dearborn St.
Chicago, IL 60610

American Psychological Association
Div. of Adult Development and Aging
1200 17 St. N.W.
Washington, DC 20036

**American Society for Geriatric
    Dentistry**
431 Oakdale Ave.
Chicago, IL 60657

**American Speech and Hearing
    Association**
10801 Rockville Pike
Rockville, MD 20852

**Ethel Percy Andrus Gerontology
    Center**
Univ. of Southern California
Los Angeles, CA 90007

Arthritis Foundation
3400 Peachtree Rd. N.E.
Atlanta, GA 30326

Arthritis Information Clearinghouse
Box 34427
Bethesda, MD 20014

Better Hearing Institute
1430 K Street N.W.
Suite 600
Washington, DC 20005

**The Center for Death Education and
    Research**
1167 Social Science Bldg.
Univ. of Minnesota
Minneapolis, MN 55455

**Center for Studies of the Mental
    Health of the Aging**
Division of Special Mental Health

Programs
National Institute of Mental Health
5600 Fishers La.
Rockville, MD 20857

**Center for the Study of Aging and
    Human Development**
Duke University
Durham, NC 27710

Central Bureau for the Jewish Aged
31 Union Sq. W.
New York, NY 10003

**Citizens for Better Care in Nursing
    Homes, Homes for the Aged and
    Other After-Care Facilities**
960 E. Jefferson Ave.
Detroit, MI 48207

Council on Stroke
American Heart Association
7320 Greenville Ave.
Dallas, TX 75231

**The Dwight D. Eisenhower Institute
    for Stroke Research, Inc.**
785 Mamaroneck Ave.
White Plains, NY 10605

Federal Council on the Aging
U.S. Dept. of Health and Human
    Services
330 Independence Ave. S.W.
Washington, DC 20201

**The Forum for Death Education and
    Counseling, Inc.**
Box 1226
Arlington, VA 22210

**Friends and Relatives of
    Institutionalized Aged**
129 E. 79 St.
New York, NY 10021

The Gerontological Society
One Dupont Circle N.W.
Suite 520
Washington, DC 20036

Gerontology Research Center
National Institute on Aging
Baltimore City Hospitals
Baltimore, MD 21224

Gray Panthers
3700 Chestnut St.
Philadelphia, PA 19104

Homemakers Home and Health Care Services
3651 Van Rick Dr.
Kalamazoo, MI 49001

Institute of Gerontology
The University of Michigan/
Wayne State University
Ann Arbor, MI 48106

International Federation on Aging
1909 K St. N.W.
Washington, DC 20006

International Senior Citizen Association
11753 Wilshire Blvd.
Los Angeles, CA 90025

Jewish Association for Services for the Aged
222 Park Ave. S.
New York, NY 10003

National Alliance of Senior Citizens, Inc.
Box 40031
Washington, DC 20016

National Association for Human Development
1750 Pennsylvania Ave. N.W.
Washington, DC 20006

National Association for Mental Health
1800 N. Kent St.
Arlington, VA 22209

National Association for Visually Handicapped
305 E. 24 St.
New York, NY 10010

National Association of Area Agencies on Aging
1828 L St. N.W.
Washington, DC 20036

National Association of Jewish Homes for the Aged
2525 Centerville Rd.
Dallas, TX 75228

National Association of State Units on Aging
1828 L St. N.W.
Washington, DC 20036

National Association of the Deaf
814 Thayer Ave.
Silver Spring, MD 20910

National Caucus/Center on the Black Aged
1730 M St. N.W.
Washington, DC 20036

National Citizens Coalition for Nursing Home Reform
National Paralegal Institute
2000 P St. N.W.
Washington, DC 20036

National Clearinghouse on Aging
Administration on Aging
Office of Human Services
300 Independence Ave. S.W.
Washington, DC 20201

**National Council for Homemaker
–Home Health Aide Services**
67 Irving Pl.
New York, NY 10003

National Council of Senior Citizens
1511 K St. N.W.
Washington, DC 20005

National Council on Black Aging
Box 8522
Durham, NC 27707

National Council on the Aging, Inc.
1828 L St. N.W.
Washington, DC 20036

National Geriatrics Society
212 W. Wisconsin Ave.
Milwaukee, WI 53203

National Hospice Organization
1750 Old Meadow Rd.
McLean, VA 22101

**National Institute of Arthritis,
Metabolism, and Digestive
Diseases**
National Institutes of Health
Bethesda, MD 20014

National Institute on Aging
National Institutes of Health
Bethesda, MD 20014

**National Society for the Prevention
of Blindness**
79 Madison Ave.
New York, NY 10016

Office of Nursing Home Affairs
Public Health Service
U.S. Department of Health and
Human Services
5600 Fishers La.
Rockville, MD 20857

**Scripps Foundation Gerontology
Center**
Miami University
Oxford, OH 45056

**Senior Actualization and Growth
Exploration (SAGE)**
National Association for Humanistic
Gerontology
Claremont Office Pk.
41 Tunnel Rd.
Berkeley, CA 95705

Senior Advocates International
1825 K St. N.W.
Washington, DC 20006

Social Security Administration
U.S. Department of Health and
Human Services
6401 Security Blvd.
Baltimore, MD 21235

Stroke Foundation
898 Park Ave.
New York, NY 10021

U.S. House of Representatives
Select Committee on Aging
House Office Bldg.
Annex 1
300 New Jersey Ave. S.E.
Washington, DC 20515

U.S. Senate
Special Committee on Aging
New Senate Office Bldg.
Washington, DC 20510

Visiting Nurses
National League for Nursing
10 Columbus Circle
New York, NY 10019

Western Gerontological Association
785 Market St.
San Francisco, CA 94103

Chapter 12

Heart Disease and Stroke

BOOKS

General

American Heart Association. *Heartbook: A Guide to Prevention and Treatment of Cardiovascular Diseases.* New York: Dutton, 1980. 370 pp. $25.
An authoritative and comprehensive compendium of the latest information on heart attack, stroke, hypertension, and cardiac emergencies. In clear, nontechnical language, 32 cardiac specialists provide answers to questions: What is a heart attack? what should one do? how does salt affect the heart? is cholesterol a killer? is hypertension inherited? Excellent illustrations. Highly recommended.

DeBakey, Michael, and Gotto, Antonio. *The Living Heart: Two Famous Heart Specialists Tell How Your Cardiovascular System Works, Why It Fails and What Can Be Done about It.* New York: McKay, 1977. 256 pp. $14.95.
Two cardiovascular specialists collaborate to provide a detailed guide to the circulatory system, its diseases, and their prevention and correction. In the first six chapters, DeBakey and Gotto describe the nature of the system together with the history of cardiovascular knowledge and surgery. The next ten chapters cover specific conditions and corrective measures involving pacemakers and other devices. The final chapter emphasizes prevention and control of the primary and secondary risk factors. With technical jargon and anatomical drawings, the work resembles a textbook, although the authors are careful to tailor their discussions for the educated nonprofessional, explaining terminology and processes and appending a glossary. Despite the absence of such topics as rehabilitation and the role of the emotions, the work is clearly excellent.

Haft, Jacob I., with Berlin, Saretta. *Consultation with a Cardiologist: Coronary Heart Disease and Heart Attacks: Prevention.* Chicago: Nelson-Hall, 1979. 317 pp. $13.95.
An authoritative discussion of heart disease, this work covers heart anatomy and function as well as the effects of hypertension, cholesterol, stress, weight, exercise, vitamins, and drugs. Also examined are methods of diagnosis, treatment, management, and control. Emphasis is on the impact of personal behavior.

Kezdi, Paul. *You and Your Heart.* New York: Atheneum, 1977. 245 pp. $9.95; $4.95 (paper); London Proteus. £5.50.
The director of the Cox Heart Institute discusses heart function and disease, as well as 13 risk factors and specific preventive behavior. Particularly helpful are chapters on true symptoms vs. false, eating sensibly without drastic change, quitting smoking, initiating an exercise program, and living well after a heart attack. There are appendixes with low-fat, low-cholesterol menus and weight, calorie, and exercise tables. Also included are charts and line drawings, glossary, and bibliography. Simply written for the layperson, this book has a dispassionate approach and a depth of coverage that render it far superior to most similar works.

Lamb, Lawrence E. *Your Heart and How to Live with It,* rev. and updated ed. New York: NAL, 1975. 302 pp. $1.95 (paper).
A cardiologist at Baylor University provides a detailed explanation of heart and circulatory function, including the effects of altitude and environmental factors on the cardiovascular system. The book also contains chapters on nutrition and fat, exercise, stress, and prevention or management of specific conditions. Includes comparative tables by which the reader can calculate the probability of developing cardiovascular disease and the American Heart Association Meal Plan. Recommended in the *Journal of the American Medical Association.*

Levitas, Irving M., with Machal, Libby. *You Can Beat the Odds on Heart Attack.* Indianapolis: Bobbs-Merrill, 1975. $7.95; $3.95 (paper).
A heart specialist describes the experience of one man's heart attack and continues by examining its nature and causes, the major risk factors, and basic corrective behavior. Of special interest is a chapter urging preliminary stress tests for moderate-to-high-risk individuals contemplating exercise programs. In the last chapter, a questionnaire is provided by which the reader can calculate his or her own risk. Readable, but not unique. No index.

Lynch, James J. *The Broken Heart: The Medical Consequences of Loneliness.* New York: Basic, 1979. 271 pp. $11.95 (paper); London: Basic, £6.95.
A specialist in psychosomatic medicine claims that loneliness has a negative influence on health, and especially on the heart. Companionship, on the other

hand, may have a positive effect. Lynch's arguments are well presented, with references to numerous studies and statistics. Interesting.

Nash, David T. *Coronary! Prediction and Prevention.* New York: Scribner's, 1979. 256 pp. $12.50.
A cardiologist discusses various factors affecting cardiovascular health, including diet, exercise, and smoking. He discusses the role of stress and Type-A behavior, as well as the development and symptoms of atherosclerosis. Describing a few simple methods of perceiving imminent trouble, he recommends specific tests to confirm suspicions. Nash also discusses the actual experience of a coronary, possible complications, diagnostic tools and techniques, surgery and drug treatment. Prevention and patient cooperation are given major attention. Included in appendixes are a cereal-based diet for reducing weight and cholesterol and charts indicating a person's probability of developing cardiovascular disease, given certain factors. Glossary and bibliography.

Phibbs, Brendan. *The Human Heart: A Guide to Heart Disease,* 3rd ed. St. Louis: Mosby, 1979. 280 pp. $12.95 (paper); London: Mosby. £7.25.
Believing that heart patients should be involved in the management of their own conditions, a cardiologist provides simple but comprehensive explanations of cardiovascular function and disease. With five other contributors, Phibbs covers a variety of ailments and topics such as electrocardiograms, surgery, pregnancy and heart disease, the heart patient and work, what to do about a heart attack, and catheterization of the heart. Illustrations not only clarify explanations but demonstrate how to administer emergency care when medical help is not available. An excellent book; recommended.

Ross, John, Jr., and O'Rourke, Robert A. *Understanding the Heart and Its Diseases.* New York: McGraw-Hill, 1975. 182 pp. $9.95; $6.95 (paper); London: McGraw-Hill. £6.70; £4.45 (paper).
Directed toward both general readers and students of the health sciences, this work by two doctors covers broad topics such as blood circulation; heart structure and circulatory regulation; factors affecting the cause, prevention, and treatment of heart disease; diseases of the valves, electrical system, coronary arteries, and the heart muscle itself; high blood pressure; congenital defects; and surgery. Although medical terminology is used throughout, an effort is made to assist the general reader, and a glossary is appended. After each chapter, both general and scientific works are suggested. Recommended for the more educated layperson.

Roth, Oscar, with Galton, Lawrence. *Heart Attack! A Question and Answer Book.* Philadelphia: Lippincott, 1978. 262 pp. $8.95.
A Yale cardiologist replies to questions on angina and other chest pains, the occurrence and effects of a coronary, healing and rehabilitation, decreasing

the risks, diagnostic tests, medications, and surgical procedures. Other topics covered include psychosocial concerns; emergency care, such as cardiopulmonary resuscitation; Social Security and compensation; choosing a physician or surgeon; and heart failure vs. heart attack. In seven appendixes Roth and Galton provide weight, calorie, and cholesterol tables; the American Heart Association Meal Plan: a sodium-restricted diet; and suggestions for quitting cigarette smoking. Glossary included. Although the format discourages in-depth response to specific questions, this book is recommended for its breadth of coverage and for the straightforward, reassuring style.

Silverstein, Alvin, and Silverstein, Virginia B. *Heart Disease.* Chicago: Follett, 1976. 122 pp. (Grades 5 and up.) OP.
An introduction to the heart and to diseases that affect it, this work covers causes and risks, symptoms, treatments, and ways to prevent illness.

Springarn, Natalie Davis. *Heartbeat: The Politics of Health Research.* Bethesda, MD: Luce, 1976. 202 pp. OP.
A journalist examines the politics and workings of the National Institutes of Health, focusing especially on the National Heart, Lung and Blood Institute. According to Springarn, the role of the government in directing policy has inhibited scientists and blurred some very basic priorities of heart research. Exceptionally well written; controversial.

Vineberg, Arthur. *How to Live with Your Heart: The Family Guide to Heart Health.* New York: Times Bks., 1977. 219 pp. $8.95; $2.95 (paper); London: Canada Bks. £5.85.
A renowned cardiac surgeon examines heart function and coronary-artery disease, risk factors, and preventive measure. Included are two chapters comparing other surgical methods with the "Vineberg Procedure" for implanting arteries. Appendixes give cholesterol, calorie, and exercise charts, plus step-by-step resuscitation instructions. Glossary and bibliography.

Hypertension

Brams, William A. *Living with Your High Blood Pressure.* New York: Arco, 1977. 160 pp. $1.75 (paper).
A physician discusses the complications that can result from hypertension, what patients can do to help themselves, and the value of specific medications. Especially noteworthy is Brams's explanation of the two different types of hypertension and their particular symptoms. Includes "rules" for living with high blood pressure.

Feinman, Max L., and Wilson, Josleen. *Live Longer: Control Your Blood Pressure.* New York: Coward, McCann, 1977. 225 pp. $7.95.
Focusing on a major cardiovascular risk factor, a physician and a medical

writer thoroughly examine the demographics, characteristics, and consequences of hypertension. Special attention is given to its effect on the heart, brain, kidneys, and eyes; and to those diseases that actually produce high blood pressure. After relating hypertension to other factors, Feinman and Wilson detail corresponding corrective behavior and other means of prevention or control. Among these are medications, checkups, and screenings. Numerous miscellaneous data enhance this valuable work.

Freis, Edward D., and Kolara, Gina Bari. *The High Blood Pressure Book: A Guide for Patients and Their Families.* New York: Dutton, 1979. 140 pp. $9.95.
Dr. Freis, an authority on drugs used to reduce blood pressure, and Gina Bari Kolata, writer for *Science* and winner of the American Heart Association's Blakeslee Award, discuss in lay terms a major killing disease. Discussion includes the effect of salt (harmfully high in the American diet), altered life-style, diet, exercise, and biofeedback. The authors conclude that with proper diagnosis and treatment, the twenty to thirty million Americans affected by high blood pressure can be successfully treated either by drugs or by other means.

Nutrition

Ferguson, James M., Taylor, C. Barr, and Ullman, Phyllis. *A Change for Heart: Your Family and the Food You Eat.* Palo Alto, CA: Bull Publg. Co., 1978. 183 pp. $4.95 (paper).
Two physicians and a dietician map a program to help families reduce their risk of heart disease by altering their eating habits. The program as outlined in this workbook is introduced gradually over a six-week period. The book contains explanations of the risks of the program, checklists for measuring progress, refrigerator analysis sheets, shopping lists, and suggestions for further improvement after completing the program. Appended are "tips for a healthy diet," menus and recipes, glossary, and recommended readings. Rather bleakly presented, but valuable when dietary change requires strong reinforcement.

Passwater, Richard. *Supernutrition for Healthy Hearts.* New York: B.J. Publg. Group, 1978. 386 pp. $2.50 (paper).
A biochemist contends that elevated cholesterol is caused by heart disease, instead of the reverse. Discussing and then dismissing the "cholesterol myth," Passwater recites a litany of studies to support his claim. He issues warnings about polyunsaturates, sugar, and soft and chlorinated water, and recommends specific nutrients and eating habits. Also covered are blood pressure and drugless ways to control it, quitting smoking, exercise and relaxation, and chelation therapy. Passwater offers a rather involved "total protection plan," with quizzes and charts by which reader's can rate themselves. There are 11 appendixes, a glossary, and suggested readings. This polemical work will fatigue the skeptic.

Shute, Wilfrid E. *Dr. Wilfrid E. Shute's Complete Updated Vitamin E Book*. New
    Canaan, CT: Keats, 1975. 228 pp. $8.95; $2.25 (paper); London: Keats. £6.
Written by a Canadian cardiologist, this work claims that large doses of Vitamin E, alpha tocopherol, are highly instrumental in preventing and treating
cardiovascular diseases. Chapters include discussions of the causes, survival,
and avoidance of heart attacks, and the effect of Vitamin E on several specific
conditions. Written for both professionals and general readers; the work
contains an index; end-of-chapter references; and three appendixes discussing the cholesterol problem, Vitamin E in dermatology, and the findings of
an Australian doctor on its role in managing heart disease. Although one
chapter covers the professional controversy, opponents to Shute's opinionated position are given short shrift.

Shute, Wilfrid E. *Health Preserver: Defining the Versatility of Vitamin E*. Emmaus,
    PA: Rodale, 1977. 167 pp. $7.95; London: Rodale. £4.75.
Shute discusses at length the role of Vitamin E in preventing or alleviating
cardiovascular problems such as varicose veins, intermittent claudication,
thrombophlebitis, rheumatic heart disease, heart attacks, and angina. Several
case histories and letters support the author's arguments, but Shute admits
that the medical establishment has been slow to endorse this "miracle"
nutrient.

Cookbooks

Brown, W. Jann, Liebowitz, Daniel, and Olness, Marlene. *Cook To Your Heart's
    Content on a Low-Fat, Low-Salt Diet,* rev. ed. New York: Van Nostrand
    Reinhold, 1976. 150 pp. $6.95 (paper); London: Van Nostrand. £5.30
    (paper).
Two doctors and a dietician explain how fat, salt, and other factors affect the
body; suggest ways for altering habits; and provide menus for controlled-fat
and low-sodium diets. In the recipe section, all items include calorie and
sodium contents together with recommendations for making low-sodium
modifications. Appendix presents tables of calories, fat, sodium, potassium;
includes comparisons of oils and margarines; lists companies offering special
diet foods. Bibliography.

Eshelman, Ruthe, and Winston, Mary. *The American Heart Association Cookbook,*
    new, rev. and expanded ed. New York: Ballantine, 1977. $6.95 (paper).
In addition to the main recipe section, this book contains a minisection on
low-calorie, quickly made dishes. There are also suggestions for interpreting
labels and advice on adapting existing recipes to low-fat cookery. Charts on
herb and spice substitutes for salt, and on fat-cholesterol-calorie contents of
foods.

Jones, Jeanne. *Diet for a Happy Heart*. San Francisco: 101 Prodns., 1975. 192
    pp. $5.95 (paper).

Introduces "rules" for reducing saturated fats; lists foods in groups, marking those rich in specific nutrients and those very low or high in saturated fats. Menus; bibliography.

Leviton, Roberta. *The Jewish Low-Cholesterol Cookbook.* Middlebury, VT: Eriksson, 1978. 370 pp. $14.95; New Amer. Lib. $2.50 (paper).
Preliminary materials cover heart disease. There are sections on cholesterol and saturated fats giving their content in foods and a guide on preparing and shopping and how to identify acceptable and unacceptable foods. Also gives advice on adapting recipes, eating out, feeding children, Jewish dietary customs, weight reduction. Appendix includes table of fatty acid composition in selected foods.

Margie, Joyce Daly, and Hunt, James C. *Living with High Blood Pressure: The Hypertension Diet Cookbook.* Radnor, PA: Chilton, 1979. 309 pp. $13.95.
This readable and practical cookbook, produced by two experts from the Mayo Clinic for the dietary management of persons with high blood pressure, assists in the daily regulation of sodium and energy intake, which are essential adjuncts to total patient management. The authors define the rationale for drug and dietary management of hypertension and provide a wide range of menus and recipes to achieve nutritional objectives. Highly recommended by reviews in *American Family Physician.*

Norman, Cecilia. *The Heart-Watcher's Cook Book: Low Cholesterol Cookery.* New York: Hippocrene, 1975. 224 pp. OP.
Contains introductory material on cholesterol, dietary recommendations by nutritional group, and table of cholesterol content of common foods. Especially noteworthy is the author's advice on replacing vitamins formerly obtained from restricted foods. Includes bibliography. Helpful, but not recommended for those on strict diets.

Page, Helen Cassidy, and Schroeder, John Speer. *The Whole Family Low Cholesterol Cookbook.* New York: Grosset & Dunlap, 1976. 334 pp. OP.
A cooking instructor and a cardiologist mark each recipe with a "signpost" for calories, saturated fat, and cholesterol levels, and append a chart for rapid comparisons. Introductory material covers the reasons for—and means to achieve—dietary change, including various helpful tables and a six-month plan to ease the transition. Excellent.

Payne, Alma, and Callahan, Dorothy. *The Fat and Sodium Control Cookbook,* 4th ed. Boston: Little, 1975. 539 pp. $8.95.
In addition to providing menus and recipes, this book discusses the reasons for controlling fats, carbohydrates, and sodium; suggests appropriate food substitutes and cooking techniques; and provides comparative tables. Comprehensive.

Rosenthal, Sylvia. *Live High on Low Fat,* new enl. ed. Philadelphia, PA: Lippincott, 1975. 439 pp. $9.95.
Introductory sections cover general dietary safeguards, the cholesterol problem, analysis of certain foods with recommendations, suggestions for weight
control. There are menus; cholesterol chart of foods to have often, occasion-
ally, or never; tables of cholesterol, fat, and calorie contents.

Thorburn, Anna Houston, and Turner, Phyllis. *Living Salt Free and Easy.* Los
Angeles: Douglas-West, 1975. 152 pp. $5.95; New York: NAL. $1.50
(paper).
Recommended by Salem Hospital in Massachusetts, this book is both a cookbook and a manual for adapting existing recipes to low-sodium diets. Provides
useful information on identifying foods by sodium content; on shopping,
preparation, and storage; on observing restrictions while dining out. Appendix compares sodium, potassium, fat, protein, carbohydrate, and calorie content of specific recipes.

Exercise

Cantwell, John Davis. *Stay Young at Heart.* Chicago: Nelson-Hall, 1975. 199 pp.
$8.95.
A physician discusses the usual risk factors associated with heart disease,
placing major emphasis on sedentary living. To correct this, Cantwell outlines
exercise routines tailored to each person's metabolism and pulse rate. He also
urges that cardiacs receive exercise therapy and that children be taught preventive behavior. Glossary included. Despite a rather juvenile style of writing,
the author presents worthwhile material.

Kavanagh, Terence. *Heart Attack? Counterattack!* Toronto: Van Nostrand
Reinhold; 1976. 232 pp. $9.95; London: Van Nostrand Reinhold. £7.55.
By way of introduction, the medical director of the Toronto Rehabilitation
Centre recalls the 1973 Boston Marathon, which seven of his cardiac patients
completed. He then examines the nature of heart disease, with its risks, and
discusses the beneficial effects of exercise. In the second part of the book, the
author describes the rehabilitation program in Toronto and offers suggestions and warnings for would-be runners, including people whose degree of
illness precludes such activity. In detail, and with scrupulous attention to pulse
rate and other indicators, Kavanagh presents an exercise program that can be
tailored to individual conditions. Also discussed are "fads, facts, and fallacies"
about heart disease. Included at the end is an appendix with training tables,
windchill factors, and other relevant information. A serious, highly detailed
guide for sophisticated readers.

Kiell, Paul J., and Frelinghuysen, Joseph S. *Keep Your Heart Running: A
Graduated Total Health and Fitness Program for People of All Ages.* New York:
Winchester, 1976. 264 pp. $8.95.

A psychiatrist and a writer collaborate to produce this systematic guide to healthful running. Stressing the importance of exercise to the cardiovascular system and advocating other beneficial activities, the authors illustrate calisthenics for beginners, as well as advice on walking and running, biking and swimming. Also discussed are nutrition, weight, and harmful agents such as cigarettes. An entire chapter is devoted to fluid and electrolyte management. Included are an appendix of calories expended for various activities, a glossary, and selected references.

Sheehan, George A. *Dr. Sheehan on Running.* Mountain View, CA: World Pubns., 1975. 205 pp. $5.95; $3.95 (paper); New York: Bantam, $2.50 (paper); London: Bantam. £0.85 (paper).
A heart specialist discusses running and dispenses advice from personal experience on both minor and critical questions. Although the author devotes little direct attention to the effect of running on the heart, his chapters on sports and medicine are excellent. In a chapter on the cardiovascular system, Sheehan addresses the physiological benefits of athletic activity and also the problems it can create. Provocative.

Treatment and Rehabilitation

Armellino, Donna. *CPR: It Could Save Your Life.* Chicago, IL: Contemporary, 1979. 91 pp. $4.95.
A nurse discusses cardiopulmonary resuscitation (CPR), a lifesaving technique that can be administered to heart-attack victims and also to victims of drowning, electric shock, automobile accidents, drug reactions, choking, smoke inhalation, and carbon monoxide poisoning. The basic technique is described and demonstrated with high-quality photographs. The Heimlich Maneuver is also well illustrated. Enhancing the value of the book is the material on anatomy, normal cardiac activity, and factors that influence heart function. An excellent book, with great visual appeal from the viewpoint of print and illustrations. Highly recommended.

Cohn, Keith, Duke, Darby, and Madrid, Joseph A. *Coming Back: A Guide to Recovering from Heart Attack and Living Confidently with Coronary Disease.* Reading, MA: Addison-Wesley, 1979. 240 pp. $10.95; $5.95 (paper).
A cardiologist, a coronary-care unit nurse, and a health communications specialist combine to provide a simple step-by-step guide to what a heart attack is, the kinds of care available, hospital stay, posthospital convalescence, and rehabilitation. Technical terms such as atherosclerosis, angina pectoris, myocardial infarction, electrocardiogram, coronary bypass surgery, and coronary angiography are explained in lay terms. Information on cardiovascular drugs, diet, menu planning, and physical activity is presented. The emphasis is on how to cope intelligently and effectively with a heart attack and how to minimize the risk of suffering one. Informative explanation at a very elementary level.

Haft, Jacob I., with Berlin, Saretta. *Consultation with a Cardiologist: Coronary Heart Disease and Heart Attacks: Management.* Chicago, IL: Nelson-Hall, 1979. 215 pp. $11.95.
Written for and about people with heart disease, this work provides advice on living after an angina or heart attack. Besides offering strategies for rehabilitation and postcoronary life, Haft describes coronary arteriography, surgery, and drugs. A special chapter is devoted to women. Succinct; encyclopedic.

Karpman, Harold L., and Locke, Sam. *Your Second Life.* New York: B. J. Publishing Group, 1977. 266 pp. $1.75 (paper).
Using a series of personal narratives, a physician and a professional writer explain the problems encountered by people with various cardiovascular conditions and provide advice and encouragement. Excellent passages of dialogue illustrate the concerns of heart patients when confronting and adjusting to their illness. In addition, there are four question-and-answer appendixes on sexual activity, diet, exercise, and cigarette smoking. Also included are a four-page glossary and a bibliography. Highly recommended.

Schindler, Paul E., Jr. *Aspirin Therapy.* New York: Walker, 1978. 134 pp. $8.95.
In addition to its general coverage of the subject, this work provides substantial information about the role of aspirin in preventing cardiovascular crises. The drug's "bright promise" derives from its effect on blood clotting. According to several studies, aspirin may help prevent thromboembolism, stroke, and heart attack. Although Schindler recommends cautious use, he also disarms many myths regarding this substance. A fair appraisal, presented rather flatly.

Stroke and Aphasia

Ancowitz, Arthur. *Strokes and Their Prevention: How to Avoid High Blood Pressure and Hardening of the Arteries.* New York: Van Nostrand, 1975. 255 pp. OP; London: Van Nostrand Reinhold. £7.25.
Written by a physician, this work is a handbook on stroke, its causes, effects, and prevention. In Part One, Ancowitz discusses the nature of the illness, its victims, atherosclerosis ("hardening of the arteries") and hypertension, emotions and exercise, environment, food faddism—including the supposed benefit of Vitamin E, smoking and drinking; "the anatomy of a stroke," and rehabilitation. Part Two emphasizes prevention, with chapters on diet, including recipes; advice on quitting cigarette smoking; controlling high blood pressure; and research. Especially valuable are ten suggestions for reducing the risk of suffering a stroke. Appendixes include a glossary, lists of calorie and cholesterol content of common foods, references by subject. Highly recommended.

Brown, Arnold. *Physiological and Psychological Considerations in the Management of Stroke.* St. Louis, MO: Green, 1976. 83 pp. $10.
A physical therapist gives an overview of stroke that covers causes, onset, incidence, physical effects, and treatment. In detail Brown examines various perceptual and sensory dysfunctions plus many stroke-related emotional problems. In a section on the patient at home, he discusses family involvement, ambulation, the hemiplegic hand. sexual problems, acceptance of disability, driving, agency help, exercise, the elderly patient, and death. Includes references and glossary. Aimed at therapists, the work is presented clearly enough for the average general reader.

Crickmay, Marie C. *Help the Stroke Patient to Talk.* Springfield, IL: Charles C. Thomas, 1977. 121 pp. $8.75 (paper).
A speech pathologist describes a wide range of communication problems that may affect stroke victims. Attention is also given to the influence of emotional disturbance on prognosis. Using numerous examples, the author explains in detail the therapeutic processes by which specific disorders are alleviated. Aiming her book at relatives of stroke victims, Crickmay argues extensively for their active involvement in patient rehabilitation. Sophisticated yet highly readable.

Feldenkrais, Moshe. *The Case of Nora: Body Awareness as Healing Therapy.* New York: Harper, 1977. 91 pp. $6.95.
A case history of a stroke victim in therapy, this highly intellectual work is also an exposition of the author's theory of body awareness in rehabilitation. With sensitivity and determination, Feldenkrais reacquaints a physically and emotionally disoriented woman with her own body, its functions and patterns of movement.

Gardner, Howard. *The Shattered Mind: The Person after Brain Damage.* New York: Knopf, 1975. 488 pp. $12.95; London: Routledge. £9.75.
Despite its concern with brain damage in general, this work has several sections on aphasia (impairment or loss of ability to speak) as a result of stroke. Included are the case histories of four patients, whose different degrees of impairment are subsequently contrasted. Informative for educated individuals who are personally involved with stroke victims.

Hodgeman, Karen, and Warpeha, Eleanor. *Adaptions and Techniques for the Disabled Homemaker.* Minneapolis, MN: Sister Kenny Inst., 1976. 30 pp. $3.50.
Though general in application, this aid is especially valuable to the hemiplegic stroke victim. It suggests tools and techniques by which the disabled can accomplish everyday tasks in the kitchen and elsewhere around the house. Practical, step-by-step instructions are accompanied by ample photographs

and line drawings. When special equipment is recommended, addresses of suppliers are given. Highly recommended.

Sarno, John E., and Sarno, Martha Taylor. *Stroke: A Guide for Patients and Their Families*. New York: McGraw-Hill 1979. 215 pp. $9.95; $4.95 (paper).
A professor of rehabilitation medicine and a speech pathologist describe causes of stroke; physical consequences, including speech disorders: intellectual and emotional aspects; rehabilitation; and prognosis. Advice is given concerning practical measures that can be taken to lessen the risk factors. More than 100 basic questions of interest to victims and their families are answered lucidly and precisely. This is a most practical book that will doubtless be a source of great assistance to those confronted with the problem of stroke. Highly recommended.

Sister Kenny Institute. *About Stroke*. Minneapolis, MN: The Institute, 1975. 38 pp.
Providing an overview of stroke, this illustrated book includes anatomical descriptions of the brain and the cerebral vascular system and basic facts about stroke's underlying conditions, diagnosis, and treatment, and spontaneous recovery. Substantial coverage is given to the various effects of stroke: motor, sensory, hemiplegic, perceptual, intellectual, emotional, and communication disorders. The factors affecting prognosis are also discussed. Glossary. An elegantly simple, attractive aid.

Sister Kenny Institute. *Self-Care for the Hemiplegic*, rev. ed. Rehabilitation Publication No. 704. Minneapolis, MN: The Institute, 1977. 26 pp. $2.10.
Useful to lay people and professionals alike, this excellent guide is designed to help stroke victims manage everyday activities. For those with partial paralysis or other muscular impairment, instructions cover eating, personal hygiene, and dressing. Suggestions are also given for improving posture when one side of the body is affected by stroke. Step-by-step photographs clearly show how to perform the actions discussed. Address provided for obtaining additional materials.

Smith, Genevieve Waples, *Care of the Patient with a Stroke*, 2nd ed. New York: Springer, 1976. 166 pp. $11.50; $6.95 (paper).
A registered nurse whose husband is a stroke victim provides a superb guide for the layperson. Smith begins by discussing the physiological effects of a stroke and then advises on developing a workable home routine. With a straightforward, compassionate style she covers such problems as gradually expanding physical activity, handling personality and mental changes, overcoming speech difficulties. The book's second part has instructions for meal management, nursing care and hygiene, massage, exercises, basic activities and movements. Includes suggested readings. Practical and reassuring.

Stryker, Stephanie. *Speech after Stroke: A Manual for the Speech Pathologist and the Family Member.* Springfield, IL: Charles C. Thomas, 1978. 422 pp. $17.25 (paper).
Written by a certified speech pathologist, this aid is designed to help rehabilitate victims of aphasia. Composed of numerous exercises, the workbook uses large bold-faced type and simple pictures to test and promote comprehension, articulation, muscular coordination, vocabulary and grammar, reading and time-telling, and writing skills. In addition, Stryker touches on the emotional aspects of therapy and stresses the need for patience. Includes a list of references and further readings and an index. Especially valuable to relatives who want to supplement the work of the professional therapist.

Personal Narratives

Armstrong, April Oursler. *Cry Babel.* New York: Doubleday, 1979. 252 pp. $8.95.
In an unusual, introspective work, a middle-aged stroke victim describes the onset of her condition and her subsequent effort to recover from severe aphasia. The author succeeds well in communicating the verbal effect of aphasia, with disjointed phrases and highly repetitive expressions. This aspect of Armstrong's personal narrative is exceptional. In its heavy emphasis on religion, however, the work may be too much for some readers. Numerous passages represent personal dialogues with Christ that, though skillfully composed, are almost painfully private. But the author has written a unique and inspirational book, re-creating the chaos of aphasia and striving to make sense of it.

Colman, Hila. *Hanging On.* New York: Atheneum, 1977. 216 pp. $8.95.
In an intensely personal journal of her husband's final year, the author describes the gradual development of stroke-related symptoms until a massive stroke completely cripples his body while leaving his mind intact. Anger, frustration, and awareness of life's absurdities are present, but, also candor, perseverance, and love. In addition, this book acquaints the reader with many of the practical difficulties associated with devastating illness. An exceptionally well-written narrative.

Cook, Fred J. *Julia's Story: The Tragedy of an Unnecessary Death.* New York: Pocket Bks., 1977. 180 pp. $1.75 (paper).
An account of the experiences of a woman who underwent heart surgery, the work is something of a muckraker. The author, a journalist, emphasizes the numerous blunders that occurred during years of treatment and especially after his wife's operation had been pronounced successful. Despite hallucinations and "bubbles in the head," her complaints were continually dismissed, and she ultimately died because the thinning of her blood had not been adequately monitored. In addition to relating his wife's story, Cook describes

how the errors altered the careers of the doctors involved and prompted several reports of similar blunders. Although the author plays down the effect of his wife's depression, his criticism of the medical system is lucid.

Dahlberg, Charles Clay, and Jaffe, Joseph. *Stroke: A Doctor's Personal Story of His Recovery.* New York: Norton, 1977. 200 pp. $8.95.
Collaborating with a colleague, a psychiatrist describes his own experiences as a stroke victim, attempting to overcome aphasia and muscular impairment on his right side. Not only is the account filled with hope and the steady progress toward recovery, it is also unique for the victim's dual perspective as a patient and as a doctor observing the stroke's effects. Before Dahlberg's illness, the two authors had conducted linguistic research together, and the book reflects this interest with its emphasis on aphasia. Although much space is given to examining scientific theories, the work is not overly technical but is aimed at educated lay people. Especially helpful to concerned readers is the last chapter, which offers advice to stroke victims and their families. Highly recommended.

Dossick, Philip. *Transplant: A Family Chronicle.* New York: Viking, 1978. 274 pp. $10.95.
This is the story of John Hurley's heart transplant, as told to the author by both John and his wife. They take turns describing their experiences and feelings from the time of his massive coronary through the first anniversary of the transplant. With candor and spontaneity they tell of emotional strain, financial worries, and their personal growth. Absorbing.

Halberstam, Michael, and Lesher, Stephan. *A Coronary Event.* Philadelphia: Lippincott, 1978. 208 pp. $1.95 (paper).
Dr. Michael Halberstam and journalist Stephan Lesher collaborate on this personal narrative about the latter's heart attack. Largely concerned with the emotional interaction between physician and patient, the book also highlights the diagnostic problems Halberstam faced and the fears that beset Lesher as he attempted to reconcile his life-style to his condition. Well written in the style of a novel, the chapters alternate between the perspective of the patient and that of the doctor.

Keiser, Bea, with Booker, Janice. *All Our Hearts Are Trump.* Durham, NC: Moore, 1976. 103 pp. $8.95.
The wife of a heart-attack victim describes her family's teamwork during her husband's coronaries and rehabilitation. More than a personal narrative, the book focuses on the health hazards in their life-style as well as the modifications they made to avert further trouble. Included are practical suggestions and literature for wives of cardiacs, low-fat recipes, and "do's and don'ts." Well done.

Levine, Louis S. *Heart Attack!* New York: Harper, 1976. 121 pp. $6.95.
An attorney describes his struggle against cardiovascular disease, beginning
with intermittent chest pains and culminating with both a stroke and a heart
attack, within days of each other. This introspective work highlights Levine's
panic and helplessness during the crisis, the support of the medical team, and
his emerging hope of recovery. During his convalescence, Levine consulted
"many books written about heart attacks for lay consumption," and here he
attempts to alert others to the warnings he himself ignored.

Nolen, William A. *Surgeon under the Knife.* New York: Coward, McCann, 1976.
  223 pp. $8.95.
A surgeon and popular medical writer describes his own experience with a
coronary-artery bypass operation. Seeing hospital procedures from a patient's
viewpoint, Nolen discusses the mistakes that were made during his treatment,
his reactions to both the illness and its resolution, and the risk factors of heart
disease. At the end of this fascinating narrative, he not only examines the
causes and effects of his own problem but also offers advice on prevention.
Also included are five short case histories of other bypass patients. Highly
readable narrative.

PAMPHLETS

American Heart Association, National Center, 7320 Greenville Ave., Dallas,
  TX 75231, or local affiliate.
A complete listing of publications is given in the *Master Catalog of Materials,*
June 1978. Typical titles available are:

  After a Coronary, 7 pp.
  Anticoagulants: Your Physician and You, leaflet.
  "The Attack," by William A. Nolen, MD. *Esquire* reprint.
  CPR: A Death Defying Act, leaflet.
  Children with Heart Disease: A Guide for Teachers, 15 pp.
  Dr. . . . We Have a Question, 7 pp.
  "E" is for Exercise, 3 pp.
  Eat Well but Eat Wisely to Reduce Your Risk of Heart Attack, leaflet.
  A Guide for Weight Reduction, 14 pp.
  The Heart and Blood Vessels, 18 pp.
  Heart Attack: How to Reduce Your Risk, 15 pp.
  High Blood Pressure and How to Control It, 12 pp.
  How the Doctor Examines Your Heart, 31 pp.
  "How to Recognize—and Survive—A Heart Attack." *Reader's Digest* reprint.
  How to Stop Smoking, leaflet.
  How You Can Help Your Doctor Treat Your High Blood Pressure, 12 pp.
  "I Am Joe's Heart." *Reader's Digest* reprint.
  If You Have Angina, 7 pp.

If Your Child Has a Congenital Heart Defect, 44 pp.
Inside the Coronary Care Unit: A Guide for the Patient and His Family, 7 pp.
Nutrition Labelling: Food Selection Hints for Fat Controlled Meals, 8 pp.
Plan to Reduce the Risk of Heart Attack, 5 pp.
Reduce Your Risk of Heart Attack, 15 pp.
Save Food $$ and Help Your Heart, 14 pp.
Smoking and Your Heart, 15 pp.
Stroke: Why Do They Behave That Way? 31 pp.
Strokes: A Guide for the Family, 18 pp.
Varicose Veins, 10 pp.
The Way to a Man's Heart: A Fat-Controlled, Low Cholesterol Meal.
What Everyone Should Know about Smoking and Heart Disease, leaflet.

Merck, Sharp and Dohme, Public Relations Dept., West Point, PA 19486.

The Dentist's Role in High Blood Pressure Detection, 1977, 7 pp.
High Blood Pressure: Health Enemy No. 1, 1978, 8 pp.
High Blood Pressure: Your Doctor's Advice Could Save Your Life If You Follow It, leaflet.
Hypertension Is High Blood Pressure, 1978, 12 pp.
Life with High Blood Pressure, 1977, 12 pp.
Measuring Blood Pressure, 1978, 9 pp.

National Dairy Council, 6300 W. River Rd., Rosemont, IL 60018.

Coronary Heart Disease: Risk Factors and the Diet Debate, by Dr. Lawrence Hursh, 1976, 16 pp.

National Heart, Lung and Blood Institute, Bldg. 31, Rm. 5A-03, 9000 Rockville Pike, Bethesda, MD 20014.

Aspirin Myocardial Infarction Study Questions and Answers, 1975, 2 pp. DHEW Pubn. No. (NIH) 76-972.
Cardiovascular Surgery, 1968, 58 pp. DHEW Pubn. No. (NIH) 1701.
Don't Take Chances with High Blood Pressure, leaflet.
Fact Sheet: Congestive Heart Failure, 1976, reprinted 1977, 6 pp. DHEW Pubn. No. (NIH) 77-923.
Fact Sheet: Diabetes and Cardiovascular Disease, 1977, 11 pp. DHEW Pubn. No. (NIH) 77-1212.
Fact Sheet: Extrasystoles, 1975, reprinted, 1977, DHEW Pubn. No. (NIH) 77-733.
Fact Sheet: Heart-Lung Machines, 1975, reprinted 1977, 3 pp. DHEW Pubn. No. (NIH) 77-734.
Fact Sheet: Hyperlipoproteinemia, 1975, rev. 1977, 10 pp. DHEW Pubn. No. (NIH) 77-734.

Fact Sheet: Venous Thrombosis and Pulmonary Embolism, 1975, reprinted 1977, 3 pp. DHEW Pubn. No. (NIH) 77-737.

A Handbook of Heart Terms, 1964, rev. 1977, 70 pp. DHEW Pubn. No. (NIH) 78-131.

High Blood Pressure: Facts and Fiction. 4 pp. DHEW Pubn. No. (NIH) 78-1218.

How Doctors Diagnose Heart Disease, 1965, rev. 1978, 20 pp. DHEW Pubn. No. (NIH) 78-753.

The Human Heart—A Living Pump, 1976, reprinted 1978, 6 pp. (Arranged to open as an 11 × 24-inch chart.) DHEW Pubn. No. (NIH) 78-1058.

If You're Black Here Are Some Facts You Should Know about High Blood Pressure, 4 pp. DHEW Pubn. No. (NIH) No. 78-1057.

Inborn (Congenital) Heart Defects, 1964, reprinted 1977, 8 pp. DHEW Pubn. No. (NIH) 77-1085.

Pacing the Heart Electrically, 1974, 7 pp. DHEW Pubn. No. (FDA) 74-4002.

References Relating to Diet and Heart Disease, 1967, rev. 1976, reprinted 1977, 4 pp.

So, I Have the Sickle Cell Trait (English and Spanish). DHEW Pubn. No. (NIH) 78-421.

Special Report: Chronic Respiratory Disease, 1978, 7 pp.

Special Report: Hemophilia, 1978, 8 pp.

Special Report: Hypertension (High Blood Pressure), 1978, 7 pp.

Varicose Veins, 1959, reprinted 1975, 9 pp. DHEW Pubn. No. (NIH) 76-752.

Your Employee with Sickle Cell. DHEW Pubn. No. 78-1523.

What Every Woman Should Know about High Blood Pressure.

National Hemophilia Foundation, 25 W. 39 St., New York, NY 10018.

State and Federal Resources for Hemophiliacs.
What You Should Know about Hemophilia.
Your Child and Hemophilia: A Manual for Parents.

Prudential Insurance Company, Public Relations Department, Box 36, Newark, NJ 07101.

How to Extend Your Life Span, by Paul Dudley White, 1970, 10 pp.
It's Your Heart, 1973, 6 pp.

Public Affairs Committee, Inc., 381 Park Ave. S., New York, NY 10016.

Living with a Heart Ailment, by Theodore Irwin, 1975, 28 pp. No. 521.
Watch Your Blood Pressure, by Theodore Irwin, 28 pp. No. 483B.

Smith, Kline and French, 1500 Spring Garden St., Philadelphia, PA 19101.

High Blood Pressure: What It Is. What It Can Do. What You Can Do About It., 9 pp.

AUDIOVISUAL PRODUCERS AND DISTRIBUTORS

A T & T — Long Lines
Medical Department
Rm. 2B 200
Bedminster, NJ 07921

Abbott Laboratories
Abbott Park, D-383
North Chicago, IL 60064

American Heart Association Film Library
8615 Directors' Row
Dallas, TX 75247

American Learning Systems
1106 Jeanette Ave.
Columbus, GA 31906

Robert J. Brady Co.
A Prentice-Hall Company
Bowie, MD 20715

CRM Educational Films
110 15 St.
Del Mar, CA 92014

Churchill Films
662 N. Robertson Blvd.
Los Angeles, CA 90069

Medfact Inc.
1112 Andrew Ave. N.E.
Massillon, OH 44646

Milner-Fenwick, Inc.
2125 Green Spring Dr.
Timonium, MD 21093

Modern Talking Picture Service
2323 Hew Hyde Park Rd.
New Hyde Park, NY 11040

National Audiovisual Center
General Services Administration
National Archives and Records Service
Washington, DC 20409

Pritchett & Hull Associates, Inc.
2122 Faulkner Rd. N.E.
Atlanta, GA 30324

Professional Research, Inc.
12960 Coral Tree Pl.
Los Angeles, CA 90066

Pyramid Films
Box 1048
Santa Monica, CA 90406

Time-Life Films
Multimedia Division
100 Eisenhower Dr.
Box 644
Paramus, NJ 07652

Trainex Corporation
Box 116
Garden Grove, CA 92642

West Glen Communications, Inc.
565 Fifth Ave.
New York, NY 10017

RESOURCE ORGANIZATIONS

American Heart Association
7320 Greenville Ave.
Dallas, TX 75231
(or local affiliate)

Cooley's Anemia Foundation
420 Lexington Ave.
New York, NY 10017

High Blood Pressure Information Center
120/80 National Institutes of Health
Bethesda, MD 20014

The Mended Hearts Inc.
721 Huntington Ave.
Boston, MA 02115

National Heart, Lung and Blood Institute
Office of Information
Bethesda, MD 20014

National Hemophilia Foundation
25 W. 39 St.
New York, NY 10018

Public Affairs Committee
381 Park Ave. S.
New York, NY 10016

Stroke Clubs of America
Box 15186
860 North Highway
Austin, TX 78701

Chapter 13

Cancer

BOOKS

See also the Cancer section of Chapter 9, Children's Health, and the Breast Care and Breast Cancer section of Chapter 10, Women's Health.

General

Braun, Armin C. *The Story of Cancer: On Its Nature, Causes, and Control.* Reading, MA: Addison-Wesley, 1978. 308 pp. $21.50; $9.50 (paper). Emerging from a series of lectures given to exceptional high school students, this work provides an overview of cancer, delving into the biological complexities of the disease and examining various methods of detection and treatment. In spite of its often highly technical jargon, the book is valuable to the sophisticated nonprofessional, especially for its illumination of the intellectual processes of cancer research.

Brody, Jane E., and Holleb, Arthur I. *You Can Fight Cancer and Win.* New York: Times, 1977. 338 pp. $12.50; New York: McGraw-Hill, 1978. $4.95 (paper). A medical journalist and a physician with the American Cancer Society provide a handbook for the layperson seeking an understanding of cancer. Included are sections on prevention and treatment; the emotional and financial upheavals that the illness can trigger; and the nature, causes, and demographics of the disease. Of special interest are the chapters with advice on quitting smoking and avoiding quackery. Several specific types of cancer are covered in detail. Five appendixes list various cancer services throughout North America, with addresses and other useful information. Breast, larynx, and gastrointestinal cancers are emphasized. Index.

Harper, Harold W., and Culbert, Michael L. *How You Can Beat the Killer Diseases*. New Rochelle, NY: Arlington, 1977. 240 pp. $8.95.
Condemning the medical establishment's refusal to use innovative treatment against cardiovascular disease and cancer, the authors argue that economic considerations have influenced this stand. Proposing that these diseases result from improper cell metabolism, they assert that prevention and control must be found in changes of diet and life-style. For cancer, Laetrile is among the authors' prescriptions. In advancing unorthodox treatment, the work nevertheless may fit within a balanced collection.

Israel, Lucien. *Conquering Cancer*, trans. from *Le Cancer Aujourd'hui* by Joan Pinkham. New York: Random, 1978. 218 pp. $10; $2.95 (paper).
Written by an eminent French oncologist, this work explores the nature and types of cancer and brings the reader up-to-date on the diverse methods of detection and treatment. Advocating more applied research, Israel attempts to raise the consciousness of his audience concerning newer forms of treatment. Although many of his views are controversial, his perspective is refreshingly optimistic and balanced. Highly recommended for the educated layperson.

Lehrer, Steven. *Alternative Treatments for Cancer*. Chicago: Nelson-Hall, 1979. 192 pp. $11.95; $6.95 (paper).
Dr. Lehrer is a radiation therapist for the Veterans Administration in New York City. His objective is to provide information to cancer patients and their families to enable them to ask the right questions about treatment. Both traditional and new alternative treatments are discussed in terms of relative effectiveness, and up-to-date information is given about types of cancer, symptoms, and diagnostic techniques. Many laypersons, and doctors, are unaware that new diagnostic and treatment tools are available that can effect cures without the disfigurement caused by traditional surgical procedures.

Levitt, Paul, and others. *The Cancer Reference Book: Direct and Clear Answers to Everyone's Questions*. New York: Paddington, 1979. 188 pp. $10.
Several hundred questions most people would like to ask are answered in a concise, lucid style. What is cancer? Where does a cancer begin? Which cancers respond poorly to surgery? How does radiotherapy work in cancer treatment? When is chemotherapy used? What are the side effects of chemotherapy? Also, twenty-one most common types of cancer are briefly described with information presented on the description of the organ (e.g., colon-rectum); symptoms, diagnosis; treatment; possible side effects of treatment; prognosis; geographic, ethnic, occupational, and age patterns; and specific causes. Of particular interest are questions related to the psychological state of the cancer patient. Why do some doctors abandon the dying patient? What is a modern hospice? Do the religious die more easily than the nonreligious? Who should be with the dying patient at the end? The authors are two professors of English and two physicians, who have produced a book

that is informative and supportive. The literary sophistication of the authors is evidenced by the effective use of quotations from Dylan Thomas, George Elliot, John Milton, and Plato, among others. Recommended.

Nierenberg, Judith, and Janovic, Florence. *The Hospital Experience: A Complete Guide to Understanding and Participating in Your Own Care.* Indianapolis, IN: Bobbs-Merrill, 1978. 273 pp. $12.50; $7.95 (paper).
Supplies extensive information on both overall treatment and specific procedures. In addition to such general concerns as patients' rights and the needs of hospitalized children, this work also discusses the 38 most frequently performed diagnostic tests, 22 types of surgery, and the treatment of certain diseases. Detailed explanations are given for radiotherapy, chemotherapy, and immunotherapy. The rights of the dying are also considered. Selected bibliography; index.

Rapaport, Stephen A. *Strike Back at Cancer: What to Do and Where to Go for the Best Medical Care.* Englewood Cliffs, NJ: Prentice-Hall, 1978. 478 pp. $12.95. London: Prentice-Hall. £9.45.
An absolutely essential book for any consumer health collection, this is billed as "the world's leading reference guide for cancer treatment." Written for both lay and professional people, the work is an encyclopedia of cancer treatment centers, organizations, and qualified oncologists. Although most of the book is composed of directories, there is also substantial material on cancers and their effects, specific sites, and the organizations fighting cancer. Of special note are the illustrated instructions for self-examination for oral and breast cancer. Symptoms are provided for major sites covered: breast, lung, colon and rectum, prostate, leukemia, and mouth.

Renneker, Mark, and Leib, Steven. *Understanding Cancer: A Text for Self-Education for University Courses in Cancer Such as "The Biology of Cancer,"* 2nd ed. Palo Alto, CA: Bull Publg., 1979. 463 pp. $19.95; $12.95 (paper).
Although this book is a compilation prepared for an academic course at the University of California, Santa Cruz, it has much to offer the layperson. Essentially, it is a collection of readings drawn from authoritative books, journal articles, American Cancer Society publications, and so on. The coverage is broad: cancer statistics, biology of cancer, etiology, pathology, major sites of cancer, therapies, rights of the cancer patient, psychological aspects of cancer, death and dying, smoking, cancer self-examination, breast cancer, and quackery. A bibliography and glossary are supplied. Highly recommended as an encyclopedic reference work that presents in one volume a clearly written text suitable for both professional and lay use.

Rettig, Richard. *Cancer Crusade: The Story of the National Cancer Act of 1971.* Princeton, NJ: Princeton Univ. Pr., 1977. 382 pp. $16.50.
A social scientist assesses the National Cancer Act, focusing on the controversy that surrounded its origins, enactment, and implementation. Providing an

account of the legislative debate, the work highlights the practical problems that affected the final outcome. Readable and of value as a history of the national effort against cancer.

Richards, Victor. *Cancer: The Wayward Cell: Its Origins, Nature and Treatment,* 2nd ed. Perspectives in Medicine. Berkeley, CA: Univ. of California Pr., 1978. 407 pp. $12.50; London: I.B.E.G. £8.75.
Written by a surgeon, the book is divided into four parts: the biology of the cell; history, ecology, and environmental origins of the cell; current methods of treatment; and psychological and social aspects. Emphasizing prevention and control, the author analyzes the research being done on the problem. According to Richards, his work is "directed to laymen willing to make a modest effort to understand the biology of cells," as well as to professionals in other specialties.

Richardson, John, and Griffin, Patricia. *Laetrile Case Histories: The Richardson Cancer Clinic Experience.* New York: Am Media, 1977. 265 pp. $5.95 (paper); London: Thorsons. £4.00 (paper).
Written by a doctor and a registered nurse, this work records over 60 case histories that support the benefits of the controversial drug Laetrile (trade name for the drug amygdalin, believed by its promoters to be a cure for cancer). In addition, the authors discuss the history of Laetrile, arguments against its value, legal and political considerations, conventional treatments, and "the Cancer Establishment." An unorthodox but useful source of information for those desiring information on Laetrile.

Rosenbaum, Ernest H., and Rosenbaum, Isadora. *A Comprehensive Guide for Cancer Patients and Their Families.* Palo Alto, CA: Bull Publg., 1980. $11.95 (paper).
A patient's guide to cancer and rehabilitation. The authors provide well-written and comprehensive coverage on major topics of concern: what cancer is; the will to live; stress and cancer; treatment; nutrition; rehabilitation exercises; sexuality; hospital, home, and office support teams; social services; and resource organizations. The Rosenbaums present a total rehabilitation approach involving the patient's mind, exercise, nutrition, sexuality, and supportive care. Their book is informative, positive, and practical. Particularly helpful are the lists of recommended books, pamphlets, national organizations, and regional and local supportive services. Highly recommended.

Silverstein, Alvin, and Silverstein, Virginia. *Cancer,* rev. ed. New York: John Day, 1976. 102 pp. $6.79. (Grades 3 and up).
Two science writers who have coauthored several children's books explain the nature of the cancer cell and disease, possible treatments, the body's immune defenses, cancer research, and environmental dangers. The last chapter, "What You Can Do about Cancer," includes the seven warning signals and the

address of the American Cancer Society. Although billed as a children's book with "easy to understand language," the book contains many complex names and terms that the authors do not explain. Filled with more details than many adult books, it seems more appropriate for older children and young adults.

Sontag, Susan. *Illness as Metaphor.* New York: Farrar, 1978. 87 pp. $5.95; New York: Random, 1979. $1.95 (paper); London: Lane. £3.95.
In elegant prose, the author examines the misconceptions and fantasies that have developed around cancer and tuberculosis over the centuries. Considering the unreal and often punitive uses that these illnesses have within our culture, Sontag believes that the words have become synonymous with death. She finds an analogy between the idea of the cancer-prone personality and the belief in the last century that there were certain tuberculosis "types." With this discussion Sontag hopes to demythologize the diseases and promote healthier attitudes in those confronting them. Recommended.

Whelan, Elizabeth M. *Preventing Cancer: What You Can Do to Cut Your Risks up to 50 Percent.* New York: Norton, 1978. 284 pp. $9.95.
Written by an epidemiologist, this work provides a series of specific recommendations that may help to reduce a person's chances of developing cancer. Part I covers "Factors Known to Increase Your Odds"; Part II discusses "Some Much Talked-about Factors Which Have Never Been Shown to Increase Your Odds" (including chemicals in food, stress, and air pollution). There are three appendixes: tips for quitting smoking, prudent-eating advice, and the warning signals of cancer. Recommended.

Environmental Influences

Agran, Larry. *The Cancer Connection: And What We Can Do about It.* Boston: Houghton, 1977. 220 pp. $9.95; $3.95 (paper).
Written by an attorney, this work examines the national policies that either permit carcinogens to affect Americans or ineffectively combat their presence. Divided into six parts, the book covers "job-caused cancer," "human test animals," occupational cancer, cigarettes and other marketed carcinogens, "childhood cancer," and the need for a new national "ethic." In addition, there are six personal accounts, each accompanying one of the above topics.

Brodeur, Paul. *The Zapping of America: Microwaves, Their Deadly Risk, and the Coverup.* New York: Norton, 1977. 343 pp. $11.95; $4.95 (paper).
In a piece of investigative reporting, a journalist addresses the possible dangers of microwave exposure. Although its scope is broad, the book includes a chapter on "the cancer connection." The author, something of a muckraker, emphasizes the period in which microwaves were directed at the U.S. embassy in Moscow. Brodeur voices concern over changes in white blood counts and other health effects.

Corbett, Thomas H. *Cancer and Chemicals*. Chicago: Nelson-Hall, 1977. 210 pp. $8.95; $5.95 (paper).
A clinical investigator discusses chemical causes of cancer, including food substances, industrial chemicals, drugs, and cigarettes. Corbett attempts to show which chemicals are dangerous, where they are, how they got there, and their health effects. In the final chapter he provides information on decreasing the risk. He stresses the need for prevention through the cooperation of government, industry, and individuals. In the style of an exposé, the work's message is harsher than most.

Eckholm, Erik P. *The Picture of Health: Environmental Sources of Disease*. New York: Norton, 1977. 256 pp. $9.95; $3.95 (paper).
Although this work is concerned with the broad spectrum of environmentally caused diseases, cancer is a prominent topic. Possible causative factors, according to Eckholm, include food additives and industrial chemicals. In the final chapter, he stresses the need for change—from government priorities to personal behavior patterns. Written in the form of a documentary with numerous notes and suggested readings, the work has a sense of urgency.

Epstein, Samuel S. *The Politics of Cancer*. San Francisco, CA: Sierra Club, 1978. 583 pp. $12.50; New York: Doubleday. $5.95 (paper).
An expert in environmental medicine supplies documentation in support of the growing consensus that most cancers are environmentally induced or related. The book is divided into three parts: cancer research and test results; various carcinogens found in industry, consumer products, and the general environment; and the policies that poorly regulate them or fail to enforce laws that presently exist. Seven appendixes include information on known carcinogenic chemicals, regulated substances, concerned public interest groups, human cancers following drug treatment, specialized treatment centers. Highly critical of both government and industry for allowing these hazards to persist, this authoritative work alerts lay people to their own public and private role in cancer prevention.

Gardner, Archibald Ward, and Taylor, Peter. *Health at Work*. New York: Halsted, 1975. 170 pp. $18.95.
Two occupational health physicians discuss the broad area of industrial hygiene and occupational health services. Among the topics covered are examinations and screenings, causes of absenteeism, and occupational hazards and how to deal with them. Cancer is discussed primarily with respect to chemical causes. The authors use language that lay people can easily understand, explaining technical terms and distinctions when necessary. Appendixes include a draft for investigating and reporting incidents.

Glasser, Ronald J. *The Greatest Battle*, 1st ed. New York: Random, 1976. 180 pp. $6.95.
A doctor concentrates on the environmental causes of cancer and the possibil-

ity of eliminating more than 75 percent of its incidence by preventative measures. Contents include discussions of the nature of cancer; the detrimental effects of cigarettes, certain drugs and chemicals, and food substances; and radiation hazards. Also described is a test to determine if a chemical is carcinogenic. The author calls for vigilance not only in identifying carcinogens, but also in dealing with industrial and governmental resistance or apathy.

Randall, Willard S., and Solomon, Stephen D. *Building 6: The Tragedy at Bridesburg*. Boston: Little, 1977. 317 pp. $9.95.
An investigative report on the hazards of the chemical BCME for workers exposed to it, this book by two journalists presents the story of the problem and the resultant fight about occupational lung cancer at one chemical company. The authors also provide historical background to occupational disease and level an indictment against the government for not enacting protective legislation. The style is narrative, with some dialogue.

Nutritional Influences

Berkeley, George. *Cancer: How to Prevent It and How to Help Your Physician Fight It*. Englewood-Cliffs, NJ: Prentice-Hall, 1978. 242 pp. $9.95; $4.95 (paper); London: Prentice-Hall. £6.25; £2.75 (paper).
Written by a social scientist, this work concentrates on nutritional measures for preventing cancer. Contents include a strong argument for the role of Vitamin C in the anticancer diet; discussion of the value of other nutrients; mention of such topics as the psychological element, exercise, breast-feeding, and Laetrile; and a review of factors increasing risk. The author's presentation is balanced; he considers opposing views and documents his statements well.

Cheraskin, E., and others. *Diet and Disease*. New Canaan, CT: Keats, 1977. 369 pp. $5.95; Berkhamsted: Rodale, £4.95.
In this heavily documented work, Dr. Cheraskin argues that diet plays a significant role in the occurrence of cancer, heart disease, birth defects, mental retardation, and several other chronic conditions. Devoting a chapter to each disease, the author includes animal and human correlative observations, therapeutic findings, a summary, and references. In the final section, he proposes an optimal diet for diminishing risks.

Flath, Carl I. *The Miracle Nutrient: How Dietary Fiber Can Save Your Life*. New York: Evans, 1975. 169 pp. $6.95; London: Bantam. £0.60 (paper).
Written by a health-care administrator and consultant in community health services, this work addresses several health problems associated with the gastrointestinal system, including cancer of the colon. Flath advocates a diet of "high-residue, high-fiber, low-fat foods" as a means of preventing these ailments. Includes an appendix of recipes using bran.

Fredericks, Carlton. *Breast Cancer: A Nutritional Approach.* New York: Grosset & Dunlap, 1979. 196 pp. $4.95 (paper).
A nutrition expert advances the theory that estrogen is responsible for much breast cancer and that the indiscriminant prescription of this hormone is dangerous. Fredericks argues that the medical community as well as the public needs to recognize the role that proper diet can play in preventing cancer. He presses for diets low in refined sugar and processed carbohydrates, supplemented by specific vitamins and minerals. With these nutritional measures, he argues, estrogen can be broken down into a harmless substance. Includes a list of "multiple vitamin-mineral supplements" and a 3-page chart on the "distribution of sugar in common foods." Contains many highly controversial claims.

Germann, Donald R. *The Anti-Cancer Diet.* New York: Wideview Bks., 1979. 305 pp. $4.95 (paper).
In 52 chapters a doctor discusses nutritional measures to prevent cancer. The work is divided into three parts: "Eating the Anti-Cancer Way"; "How to Follow the Anti-Cancer Diet"; "Meal Plans and Recipes." Covered are food additives, fiber, harmful and beneficial foods. Pleasantly written and well researched, the book contains many useful lists, including an "anti-cancer diet at a glance."

Timms, Moira, and Zar, Zachariah. *Natural Sources: Vitamins B-17/Laetrile.* Millbrae, CA: Celestial Arts, 1978. 150 pp. $4.95 (paper); Wellingborough, Northants: Thorsons, £3.40 (paper).
Timms and Zar restate the importance of dietary measures in prevention and control of the disease. Recommended are unprocessed raw food, certain recipes, and avoidance of dangerous substances. Includes references to both standard and esoteric sources of information.

Psychological Aspects

Abrams, Ruth D. *Not Alone with Cancer: A Guide for Those Who Care; What to Expect; What To Do.* Springfield, IL: Charles C. Thomas, 1976. 98 pp. $5.75.
The work is divided into four sections, each on a specific degree of the disease (localized stage, regional involvement, advanced stage, and late advanced stage). Using numerous case histories, Abrams addresses the emotional and psychological aspects from a family orientation. Includes discussions of very practical considerations that worry a patient's family.

Cantor, Robert C. *And a Time to Live: Toward Emotional Well-Being during the Crisis of Cancer.* New York: Harper, 1978. 280 pp. $10.95; $3.95 (paper).
The author, a former coordinator of a cancer rehabilitation clinic and a psychologist, states: "I write for those who choose to understand: for those, be they patient, friend, nurse, family member or physician, who want to examine

the cancer experience and come to know it better; for those who see themselves as active participants in the process of treatment and recovery." Emphasis is placed on understanding and coping with the threatening experience of cancer treatment. Cantor analyzes the fear, anxiety, stress, and lack of personal control faced by the cancer patient. He discusses the impact of cancer on different kinds of marriages and suggests ways for dealing with stress. Finally, he points out the ability to grow beyond the crisis of cancer by finding a personal meaning in it. A tender, sensitive, and powerful insight into the dark cloud of unknowing, valuable for those who confront cancer in themselves, friends, or families. Highly recommended.

Kelly, Orville, and Becker, Randall. *Make Today Count.* New York: Delacorte, 1975. 203 pp. $7.95; $3.95 (paper).
The story of Orville Kelly, founder of the Make Today Count organization for terminally ill persons and their families, which attempts to provide emotional support for those dying of cancer, helping them to learn to *live,* despite their situation. Biographical to a large extent, the book also helps to explain the rationale and goals of the self-help organization. Includes a foreword by Elisabeth Kubler-Ross.

LeShan, Lawrence. *You Can Fight for Your Life: Emotional Factors in the Causation of Cancer.* New York: Evans, 1977. 192 pp. $7.95.
An experimental psychologist outlines the psychological factors that may determine the development and course of cancer in an individual. Contents include sections on psychological patterns, the emotional life history of the disease, stress and susceptibility, patient psychotherapy, and the will to live. LeShan urges self-acceptance and assertiveness as the keys to a healthy personality.

Rosenbaum, Ernest H. *Living with Cancer: Guide for the Patient, the Family and Friends.* New York: Praeger, 1975. 214 pp. OP.
A timely and practical aid to dealing with cancer in one's own life or in that of relatives or friends, its style is intimate and compassionate. The author views the psychological consequences of the disease from every angle: informing the patient, the doctor-patient relationship, the patient's self-image, the family. Also covered is quackery and patient dignity in life and death. Appendixes include a patient's bill of rights and actual forms for informed consent and the living will.

Simonton, O. Carl, and others. *Getting Well Again: A Step-by-Step Self-Help Guide to Overcoming Cancer for Patients and Their Families.* Los Angeles, CA: Tarcher, 1978. 268 pp. $8.95.
Written by a radiologist, this work strongly emphasizes the emotional factors affecting cancer development and recovery. Contents include an analysis of mental attitudes and stress and a program for dealing with the disease. The

authors provide advice on learning to relax, developing positive mental images, overcoming resentment, and managing pain. Also discussed are the psychological "benefits" of being ill. The supportive, psychological approach supplements conventional methods of treatment. Recommended.

Sveinson, Kelly M. *Learning to Live with Cancer.* New York: St. Martin's, 1978. 112 pp. $7.95.
A victim of Hodgkin's disease details his technique for maintaining a positive attitude and overcoming the problems of physical weakness, treatments, hospitalization. Contents include suggested readings and advice for both hospital personnel and families of cancer victims. Rather than being a personal narrative, the work is a psychological handbook for the patient. Indispensable despite the absence of an index.

Rehabilitation

Hardy, Richard E., and Cull, John G., eds. *Counseling and Rehabilitating the Cancer Patient.* American Lectures in Social and Rehabilitation Psychology Series. Springfield, IL: Charles C. Thomas, 1975. 147 pp. $13.25.
Primarily for professional rehabilitation workers, this book also has value for the layperson, enabling him to read about the medical, psychological, and vocational problems of cancer victims. Among the sections defined in the work are those on psychotherapeutic work with patients, psychosexual effects of some cancer surgery, and vocational rehabilitation case studies.

Nelson, Charles R. *You Can Speak Again: A Guide to Speech after a Laryngectomy,* 2nd ed., rev. and updated by Joan Steen Wilentz. New York: Funk & Wagnalls, 1977. 105 pp. OP.
A revision of a 1949 learning aid by a laryngectomy patient, this work contains step-by-step instructions on learning to speak again by using muscles other than the larynx. The revision includes new medical data on the operation, the problems that necessitate it, and medical devices and learning techniques. There are 11 lessons provided for self-instruction in speaking, plus appendixes on sources of information, assistance, books, and supplies. An extremely valuable tool.

Winkler, Win Ann. *Post-Mastectomy: A Personal Guide to Physical and Emotional Recovery.* New York: Hawthorn, 1976. 197 pp. $7.95.
A mastectomy patient provides several practical aids for postsurgical recovery. Among the topics covered are rehabilitation; anxiety and depression; active recovery measures such as diet, beauty care, and exercise; prosthesis; sexual relations; and physical activity. Appendixes include approved cancer-detection centers; comprehensive cancer centers; shopping for clothing, prostheses, and other items (with brand names, illustrations, and prices supplied). Suggested readings, tapes and records; index. A thorough handbook, essential for any consumer health collection.

Personal Narratives

Beatty, Robert O., with his family. *Still a Lot of Living: Coping with Cancer*, ed. by Melissa Lloyd Dodworth. New York: Macmillan, 1979. 196 pp. $8.95.
Written by a former assistant secretary of the Department of Health, Education, and Welfare, this personal narrative describes Beatty's last five years after he was diagnosed as having prostate cancer. It provides compassionate advice on dealing with cancer—physically, psychologically, socially, medically, and sexually. In addition, the author discusses his experiences with both conventional treatments and those involving acupuncture and Laetrile. In lay terms, he reviews questions concerning the nature of cancer, its demographics and mortality patterns. The "afterward" by his wife lists the seven signals of cancer and advises early diagnosis and treatment. A handbook for coping, the work is clearly written and emphasizes the family perspective. Further readings; index.

Brady, Mari. *Please Remember Me*. New York: Doubleday, 1977. 104 pp. $5.95.
A personal narrative by a recreation aide at Memorial Sloan-Kettering Cancer Center tells of the author's friendship with a 15-year-old boy with terminal cancer. It is simply written and sensitive but not excessively maudlin.

Buchanan, William J. *A Shining Season*. New York: Coward, McCann, 1978. 240 pp. $8.95; New York: Bantam. $2.25 (paper).
A cancer biography of a distance runner named John Baker, this books tells of the last 18 months of his life, his thoughts of suicide, and his determination to suppress his pain. Also described are his efforts in training troubled children to compete athletically.

Lee, Laurel, *Walking through the Fire: A Hospital Journal*. New York: Dutton, 1977. 113 pp. $6.95; New York: Bantam. $1.95 (paper); London: Macmillan. £3.95.
This journal is a personal narrative by a victim of Hodgkin's disease, discovered when the author was six-months pregnant. As her story progresses, the reader witnesses such emotionally charged experiences as the birth of her daughter, her treatment, and the disintegration of her marriage. Woven into her diary are drawings and poetic passages by the author, which accent the unique sensitivity and humor of the work. This is a narrative unusual not only in its style and layout but also in the complexity of its case history and philosophy.

Lerner, Gerda. *A Death of One's Own*. New York: Simon & Schuster, 1978. 269 pp. $10.
A historian writes a personal account of the death of her husband from a malignant, incurable brain tumor. The attitude of the author is that her husband shaped his own dying, just as a person shapes his own life. Philosophical in flavor, the work presents the positive emotions of courage and trust as the victim faces death openly. The author also provides three

possible endings, in an attempt to show how complex death really is and how impossible it is to adequately project this complexity.

McGrail, Joie Harrison. *Fighting Back: One Woman's Struggle against Cancer.* New York: Harper, 1978. 196 pp. $10.95.
A personal narrative by a victim of inoperable lung cancer, this book traces the author's search for successful treatment during her remaining three years. In addition to conventional treatments, McGrail attempted to arrest her disease through various kinds of therapies here and overseas. These included nutritional strategies and use of the chemical Trophosphamide, available in Germany but outlawed by the Food and Drug Administration. Written in a precise but flowing style, the book radiates the hope that fueled her battles. Includes an "after-note" written by McGrail's son after her death.

Oden, Clifford E. *Thank God I Have Cancer!* New Rochelle, NY: Arlington, 1976. 174 pp. $7.95.
Written by a Baptist minister and victim of cancer of the colon, this book promotes the use of Vitamin B-17 and other natural substances in preventing or controlling cancer. Oden espouses the trophoblast theory that sees the cancer cell as a normal part of the body. The book provides practical advice and appends information on an early detection test, doctors and others who favor B-17 and metabolic therapy, and recommended readings. Highly religious in flavor, the work may be of value to those patients needing spiritual encouragement. Some may find its approach unacceptable in the light of current medical practice.

Parker, Joan H., and Parker, Robert B. *Three Weeks in Spring.* Boston: Houghton, 1978. 183 pp. $7.95; $2.25 (paper); London: Deutsch. £3.95.
A personal narrative by a victim of breast cancer written in a flowing conversational style. Laced with introspective passages, it tells of the fears of one woman as she faces mastectomy, and of the emotional support she receives from family and friends. It is a positive work, emphasizing love, hope, and recovery.

Pradeau, Jean *I Had This Little Cancer* . . . , trans. by June P. Wilson from *Un Petit Truc de Rein de Tout.* New York: Abelard-Schuman, 1976. 147 pp. OP.
Written by a French journalist, this work describes the author's struggle with cancer of the salivary gland. The book is filled with introspection, where fear and hope are constant adversaries. And in a market overflowing with personal narratives, most written by women, this book is valuable in offering a male perspective.

Rollin, Betty. *First, You Cry.* Philadelphia: Lippincott, 1976. 206 pp. $7.95; New York: NAL, $1.95 (paper).
Probably the best-known personal narrative about cancer, Rollin's work de-

scribes the discovery of a lump in her breast and follows through a period of emotional adjustment and the accompanying changes in her interpersonal relationships. Analytical rather than moving.

Rosenfeld, Stephen S. *The Time of Their Dying.* New York: Norton, 1977. 189 pp. $7.95.
An editorial writer and columnist for the *Washington Post* presents a personal narrative about the death of his parents, within months of each other, from cancer. Written in an intimate style, the work blends the subjective feelings of a bereaved son with the professional reserve and perspective of a journalist.

Sanes, Samuel. *A Physician Faces Cancer in Himself.* Albany, NY: State Univ. of New York Pr., 1979. 201 pp. $12.95.
A frank and honest narrative of a physician-educator who discovers that he has disseminated reticulum cell sarcoma. Dr. Sanes describes his discovery of the disease, definitive diagnosis, his treatment with chemotherapy, radiation, and immunotherapy. Of particular interest is the description of the heavy psychological and emotional burden placed on both patients and their physicians. The author feels that patients are deprived of much support because physicians see their therapeutic function almost solely in terms of control, recovery, and cure. They cannot accept defeat. Dr. Sanes discusses with great sensitivity the responses of professional colleagues, relationships with other cancer patients, effects of cancer on the patient's family, and the problem of communication. Shortly after completion of the book, the author died. Highly recommended.

Smith, JoAnn Kelley. *Free Fall.* Foreword by Elisabeth Kubler-Ross. Valley Forge, PA: Judson, 1975. 138 pp. $5.95.
Written by a victim of breast cancer, this personal narrative is primarily a philosophical discussion of the art of dying and of patients' rights. Religious in tone, much of it is introspective and interwoven with aphorisms. The book is intended as an aid for families and friends seeking spiritual answers.

Snow, Lois Wheeler. *A Death with Dignity: When the Chinese Came.* New York: Random, 1975. 149 pp. OP.
Another personal narrative, this one contrasts Western techniques of caring for terminal cancer patients with those used in the People's Republic of China. The author's husband, Edgar Snow, benefited from the Chinese concept of "total care" when a team of doctors and nurses from that country responded to the news that he had inoperable cancer of the pancreas. During an extended visit, living with the family, these professionals demonstrated a unique "attitude toward the illness, the patient, and all engaged in the struggle."

Wallin, Bernice, with Wallin, Fred. *I Beat Cancer.* Chicago: Contemporary, 1978. 193 pp. $8.95.

A personal narrative by a cancer victim, this work is also an account of the experimental immunotherapy for which the patient opted. It is a story of her struggle with the medical establishment at the University of California at Los Angeles Hospital over her rights to this form of treatment and of her apparent recovery from widespread cancer. Also included are passages relating her disenchantment with Laetrile. A well-written, intimate book.

Weingarten, Violet. *Intimations of Mortality.* New York: Knopf, 1978. 243 pp. $8.95.
This posthumously published work by a cancer victim is a diary of her emotions and experiences during the treatment and spread of her disease. Confronting death as something no one really expects, the author juxtaposes fear and humor in a narrative almost stream-of-consciousness in style.

Research

Berger, Melvin. *Cancer Lab.* New York: John Day, 1975. 127 pp. $8.79. (Ages 8–11).
Providing a behind-the-scenes view of the cancer research laboratory, this book is composed largely of photographs. Accompanying text explains the work done at such major facilities as the National Cancer Institute and the Sloan-Kettering Institute for Cancer Research, in language that is somewhat technical but within the reach of the layperson. Children may have to struggle to comprehend it at times.

Dunn, Thelma Brumfield. *The Unseen Fight against Cancer: Experimental Cancer Research—Its Importance to Human Cancer.* Charlottesville, VA: Batt Bates, 1975. 204 pp. OP.
Highly recommended for the educated layperson, this clearly written work provides an overview of cancer research, discussing its various kinds and implications. Among the topics covered are: cancer definitions, transplantation of neoplasms, genetic and geographic strains, carcinogenesis, viruses, and the branches of medicine concerned with the disease. Includes bibliography, although the works cited tend to be older and/or technical.

Goodfield, June. *The Siege of Cancer.* New York: Dell, 1976. 240 pp. $1.95 (paper).
The author presents a kind of diary of her observations and study of several cancer research institutions and key personalities associated with them. Although concentrating on the United States, the work also includes material on foreign research, particularly among the Turkomans of Iran. Intelligently written for the general reader, it contains adequately explained, technical information.

Hixson, Joseph R. *The Patchwork Mouse*. New York: Anchor, 1976. 228 pp. OP.
A medical science reporter reviews an incident in which a Sloan-Kettering researcher was guilty of faking test results. Of concern to the author is the possibility that such occurrences emerge from the overwhelming pressure for results exerted by government and institutions. The work has value for the reader interested in the history and problems of cancer research.

Maugh, Thomas H., II, and Marx, Jean L. *Seeds of Destruction: The Science Report on Cancer Research*. New York: Plenum, 1975. 251 pp. $22.50.
An assessment of cancer research and progress, this work emphasizes the area of molecular biology. It includes sections on cancer etiology, therapy, and specific forms of cancer. Illustrated. Recommended for the educated lay reader as well as the professional.

National Cancer Institute. *U.S. International Cancer Research Data Bank: Directory of Cancer Research Information Resources*. Bethesda, MD: Natl. Cancer Inst., Off. of Cancer Communications, 1977. 226 pp.
Valuable as a reference tool, this work is organized into 12 sections: primary and secondary publications, classification schemes, libraries and special collections, automated services, audiovisuals, dial-access, research projects, information sources, registries, organizations, National Institutes of Health programs and services. Although some of the material is inappropriate for consumer health purposes, the book is indispensable. Includes four indexes: title, organizations, geographic, and subject.

PAMPHLETS

American Cancer Society, 777 Third Ave., New York, NY 10017.
Answering Your Questions about Cancer, No. 2025-LE (ACS), 1971, 9 pp.
Answers to the Most Often Asked Questions about Cigarette Smoking and Lung Cancer, No. 2023 LE (ACS), 1975, 6 pp.
The Beleaguered Lung—Cancer Invades, (ACS), 1965, 3 pp.
Cancer Facts & Figures—1979, (ACS), 31 pp.
Cancer of the Breast, No. 2003-LE (ACS), 1972, 4 pp.
Cancer of the Colon and Rectum, No. 2004-LE (ACS), 1967, 3pp.
Cancer of the Mouth, No. 2630 LE (ACS), 1968, 4 pp.
Cancer of the Prostate, No. 2654 LE (ACS), 1968, 4 pp.
Cancer of the Skin, No. 2049-LE (ACS), 1967, 3 pp.
Cancer of the Stomach, No. 2655 LE (ACS), 1974, 4 pp.
Cancer Word Book, No. 2097-LE (ACS), 1976, 8 pp.
Facts on Hodgkins's Disease, No. 2093-LE (ACS), 1978, 4 pp.
Facts on Lung Cancer, (ACS), 1978, 3 pp.
Facts on Oral Cancer, No. 2630 LE (ACS), 1978, 4 pp.

Facts on Uterine Cancer, No. 2006 LE (ACS), 1978, 5 pp.

The Hopeful Side of Cancer, No. 2012-LE (ACS), 1977, 9 pp.

Laetrile-Cancer Quackery, No. 2063-LE (ACS), 1977, 6 pp.

Leukemia, No. 2629-LE (ACS), 1977, 4 pp.

Take Joy! (A Teacher's Guide to Six Systems of the Body), 2056 LE (ACS), 1973, 10 pp.

Teacher's Guide—*Decision for Mike,* 2010 LE (ACS), 1975, 8 pp.

Teaching about Cancer, No. 2040-LE (ACS), 1975, 37 pp.

Understanding Chemotherapy (Franklin County Unit—Ohio Division, ACS), 4 pp.

Understanding Immunotherapy (Franklin County Unit—Ohio Division, ACS), 3 pp.

Understanding Radiation Therapy (Franklin County Unit—Ohio Division, ACS), 4 pp.

Youth Looks at Cancer (ACS/Lib. of Cong. Cat. Card No. 60-7733, 1975, 68 pp.

Cancer Information Clearinghouse, Office of Cancer Communications, National Cancer Institute, 7910 Woodmont Ave., Suite 1320, Bethesda, MD 20014.

Asbestos Exposure—A Desk Reference for Communicators, DHEW Pubn. No. (NIH) 78-1622, 8 pp.

Asbestos Exposure—What it Means, What to Do, DHEW Pubn. No. 78-1594, 6 pp.

Breast Self Examination, DHEW Pubn. No. (NIH) 76-649, 6 pp.

Chemotherapy and You, DHEW Pubn. No. (NIH) 78-1136, 8 pp.

Childhood Leukemia—A Pamphlet for Parents, DHEW Pubn. No. (NIH) 78-212, 15 pp.

Cigarette Smoking among Teen-Agers and Young Women, DHEW Pubn. No. (NIH) 77-1203, 15 pp.

Clearing the Air—A Guide to Quitting Smoking, DHEW Pubn. No. (NIH) 78-1647, 18 pp.

Did You as A Child or a Young Adult Have X-ray Treatments Involving Your Head or Neck? DHEW Pubn. No. 77-1206, 3 pp.

Drugs vs. Cancer,. DHEW Pubn. No. (NIH) 78-786, 8 pp.

Feeding the Sick Child, DHEW Pubn. No. (NIH), 78-795, 68 pp.

The Leukemia Child, DHEW Pubn. No. (NIH) 78-863, 80 pp.

Progress against Cancer of the Bladder, DHEW Pubn. No. (NIH) 78-722, 4 pp.

Progress against Cancer of the Bone, DHEW Pubn. No. (NIH) 78-721, 4 pp.

Progress against Cancer of the Breast, DHEW Pubn. No. (NIH) 78-328, 4 pp.

Progress against Cancer of the Colon and Rectum, DHEW Pubn. No. (NIH) 79-95, 4 pp.

Progress against Cancer of the Lung, DHEW Pubn. No. (NIH) 78-526, 7 pp.

Progress against Cancer of the Larynx, DHEW Pubn. No. (NIH) 78-448, 4 pp.

Progress against Cancer of the Mouth, DHEW Pubn. No. (NIH) 79-118, 4 pp.

Progress against Cancer of the Prostate, DHEW Pubn. No. (NIH) 77-528, 4 pp.

Progress against Cancer of the Stomach, DHEW Pubn. No. (NIH) 77-527, 4 pp.

Progress against Cancer of the Testis, DHEW Pubn. No. (NIH) 78-1492, 2 pp.

Progress against Cancer of the Uterus, DHEW Pubn. No. (NIH) 78-171, 3 pp.

Progress against Hodgkin's Disease, DHEW Pubn. No. (NIH) 78-172, 4 pp.

Progress against Leukemias, Lymphomas, Multiple Myeloma, DHEW Pubn. No. (NIH) 79-329. 5 pp.

Were You or Your Daughter Born after 1949? DHEW Pubn. No. (NIH) 77-1226, 4 pp.

What Black Americans Should Know about Cancer, DHEW Pubn. No. (NIH) 78-1635, 16 pp.

What You Need to Know about Adult Leukemia, DHEW Pubn. No. (NIH) 79-1572, 10 pp.

What You Need to Know about Cancer, DHEW Pubn. No. (NIH) 79-1566, 10 pp.

What You Need to Know about Cancer of the Bladder, DHEW Pubn. No. (NIH) 79-1559, 8 pp.

What You Need to Know about Cancer of the Bone, DHEW Pubn. No. (NIH) 79-1571, 8 pp.

What You Need to Know about Cancer of the Brain and Spinal Cord, DHEW Pubn. No. (NIH) 79-1558, 8 pp.

What You Need to Know about Cancer of the Breast, DHEW Pubn. No. (NIH) 79-1556, 8 pp.

What You Need to Know about Cancer of the Colon and Rectum, DHEW Pubn. No. (NIH) 78-1552, 8 pp.

What You Need to Know about Cancer of the Esophagus, DHEW Pubn. No. (NIH) 79-1557, 7 pp.

What You Need to Know about Cancer of the Kidney, DHEW Pubn. No. (NIH) 79-1569, 8 pp.

What You Need to Know about Cancer of the Larynx, DHEW Pubn. No. (NIH) 79-1568, 8 pp.

What You Need to Know about Cancer of the Lung, DHEW Pubn. No. (NIH) 79-1553, 7 pp.

What You Need to Know about Cancer of the Mouth, DHEW Pubn. No. (NIH) 79-1574, 8 pp.

What You Need to Know about Cancer of the Ovary, DHEW Pubn. No. (NIH) 79-1561, 8 pp.

What You Need to Know about Cancer of the Pancreas, DHEW Pubn. No. (NIH) 79-1560, 8 pp.

What You Need to Know about Cancer of the Prostate, DHEW Pubn. No. (NIH) 79-1576, 10 pp.

What You Need to Know about Cancer of the Skin, DHEW Pubn. No. (NIH) 79-1564, 7 pp.

What You Need to Know about Cancer of the Stomach, DHEW Pubn. No. (NIH) 79-1554, 8 pp.

What You Need to Know about Cancer of the Testis, DHEW Pubn. No. (NIH) 79-1565, 8 pp.

What You Need to Know about Cancer of the Uterus, DHEW Pubn. No. (NIH) 79-1562, 8 pp.

What You Need to Know about Childhood Leukemia, DHEW Pubn. No. (NIH) 79-1573, 8 pp.

What You Need to Know about Hodgkin's Disease, DHEW Pubn. No. (NIH) 79-1555, 8 pp.

What You Need to Know about Melanoma, DHEW Pubn. No. (NIH) 79-1563, 8 pp.

What You Need to Know about Multiple Myeloma, DHEW Pubn. No. (NIH) 79-1575, 7 pp.

What You Need to Know about Non-Hodgkin's Lymphoma, DHEW Pubn. No. (NIH) 79-1567, 8 pp.

What You Need to Know about Wilms' Tumor, DHEW Pubn. No. (NIH) 78-1570, 8 pp.

Public Affairs Committee, Inc., 381 Park Ave. S., New York, NY 10016.

Can We Conquer Cancer? No. 496, 1974, 28 pp.
Cigarettes—America's No. 1 Health Problem, No. 439A, 1975, 10 pp.
When a Family Faces Cancer, No. 286, 1978, 28 pp.
Women and Smoking, No. 475, 1978, 12 pp.

AUDIOVISUAL PRODUCERS AND DISTRIBUTORS

Abbott Laboratories
Abbott Park, D-383
North Chicago, IL 60064

American Cancer Society
777 Third Ave.
New York, NY 10017

M. D. Anderson Hospital and Tumor Institute
Department of Medical Communication
Houston, TX 77030

Robert J. Brady Co.
A Prentice-Hall Company
Bowie, MD 20715

Cancer Care
One Park Ave.
New York NY 10016

Cancer Center of University Hospitals At-Home Rehabilitation Center
2074 Abington Rd.
Cleveland, OH 44106

Concept Media
Box 19542
Irvine, CA 92714

Core Communications in Health, Inc.
919 Third Ave.
New York, NY 10022

Health Film Library
Box 309
Madison, WI 53701

Hollister, Inc.
211 E. Chicago Ave.
Chicago, IL 60611

International Association of Cancer
  Victims and Friends
434 S. San Vincente Blvd.
Los Angeles, CA 90048

International Union Against Cancer
3 Rue de Conseil General
CH-1205 Geneva, Switzerland

Jeppersen Sanderson
8025 E. 40 Ave.
Denver, CO 80207

Leukemia Society of America
211 E. 43 St.
New York, NY 10017

Medfact, Inc.
1112 Andrew Ave. N.E.
Massillon, OH 44646

Milner-Fenwick, Inc.
2125 Green Spring Dr.
Timonium, MD 21093

St. Louis Park Medical Research
  Foundation
5000 W. 39 St.
St. Louis Park, MN 55416

Train-Aide Educational Systems
1015 Grandview
Glendale, CA 91201

Trainex Corporation
Box 116
Garden Grove, CA 92642

United Ostomy Association
1111 Wilshire Blvd.
Los Angeles, CA 90017

Wexler Film Productions
801 N. Seward St.
Los Angeles, CA 90028

RESOURCE ORGANIZATIONS

American Cancer Society
777 Third Ave.
New York, NY 10017

Breast Cancer Advisory Center
Box 422
Kensington, MD 20795

The Candlelighters
123 C St. S.E.
Washington, DC 20003

CanSurMount
c/o American Cancer Society
777 Third Ave.
New York, NY 10017
or local affiliate

CURE Childhood Cancer Association
Box 9627
Rochester, NY 14604

Encore
National Board YWCA
600 Lexington Ave.
New York, NY 10022

International Association of
  Larynegectomees
c/o American Cancer Society
777 Third Ave.
New York, NY 10017
or local affiliate

International Union Against Cancer
3 Rue de Conseil General
CH-1205 Geneva, Switzerland

Leukemia Society of America
211 E. 43 St.
New York, NY 10017
or local affiliate

Make Today Count
Box 303
Burlington, IA 52611
or local affiliate

National Cancer Institute
Cancer Information Service
7910 Woodmont Ave.
Bethesda, MD 20014
Tel: 800-638-6694; or local Regional
  Cancer Center

National Hospice Organization
765 Prospect St.
New Haven, CT 06511

Reach to Recovery Program
c/o American Cancer Society
777 Third Ave.
New York, NY 10017
or local affiliate

United Cancer Council
1803 N. Meridian St.
Indianapolis, IN 46202

United Ostomy Association
1111 Wilshire Blvd.
Los Angeles, CA 90017

Chapter 14

Diabetes

BOOKS

See also Juvenile Diabetes in Chapter 9, Children's Health.

General

Blevins, Dorothy R., ed. *The Diabetic and Nursing Care.* New York: McGraw-Hill, 1979. 366 pp. $13.95.
With contributions by 14 health-care professionals, this guide for nurses approaches several diabetic concerns in a manner and terminology largely comprehensible by educated lay people. Chapters include cultural and social dimensions of caring for the diabetic; personal adjustment of the patient; patient education; and care of diabetic children, elderly, and pregnant women. Seven chapters are too technical for lay use, but the above-mentioned topics include psychological insights from which patients and their families can benefit. Recommended as a reference tool.

Bloom, Arnold. *Diabetes Explained,* 2nd ed. Lancaster: Medical and Technical Publishing Company, 1978. 159 pp. £5.25.
A physician on the executive council of the British Diabetic Association explains the nature, diagnosis, treatment, and complications of the disease. Included are chapters on oral medication; the treatment of mild diabetes; hypoglycemia and diabetic coma; the special situations of children, pregnant women, and the elderly; and research covering insulin, the retina, and other problems. Several dietary options are also detailed. Although this work is intended for lay readers, the terminology and explanations tend to be overly technical. Regarding the oral therapies, moreover, there is little indication of the current controversies.

Brothers, Milton J. *Diabetes: The New Approach.* New York: Grosset & Dunlap, 1978. 229 pp. $5.95 (paper).
In four major sections, a diabetes specialist at New York's Mt. Sinai Hospital discusses the nature of the disorder, therapeutic approaches, diabetic pregnancy, the uses and limitations of oral antidiabetic medication, psychological factors, employability and insurability, the benefits of exercise, and various research leads. Especially informative are the detailed and well-illustrated chapters on blood vessel complications. Glossary is appended, fortunately, because Dr. Brothers is generous in his use of highly technical jargon. Though intended for general readership, this work is recommended only for better-educated laypersons.

Jorgenson, Carol Dow, and Lewis, John E. *The ABC's of Diabetes.* New York: Crown, 1978. 305 pp. $10.95.
The authors have produced a reference compendium, arranged alphabetically in a dictionary format. Some topics are defined in several sentences, while others, such as Food Exchanges (tables indicating the calorie counts of measured portions of food), merit more than 20 pages. The subject matter includes types, treatment, and control of diabetes; diet plans and diets for special situations such as illness, exercise, and travel; insulin injections and sites; blood and urine tests; oral hypoglycemic agents; pregnancy and childbirth; traveling with diabetes; exercise and sports; and research in diabetes. Appendixes include suggested cookbooks, recommended reading, emergency treatment, a directory of organizations, and a bibliography. This is an excellent source book of current information that will be highly useful to the more than six million people in the United States who are known to have diabetes. Highly recommended for the reference shelf and popular usage.

Laufer, Ira J., and Kadison, Herbert. *Diabetes Explained: A Layman's Guide.* New York: Dutton, 1976. 179 pp. $7.95.
Written by a diabetes specialist and one of his patients, this manual explains the disease in straightforward, precise language. The authors carefully profile the high-risk individual, weighing the risk factors and symptoms and identifying the shortcomings of urine tests. Among the topics covered are diet, insulin, oral agents, acute and chronic complications, psychological considerations, and research developments. A concise glossary is appended. A sensible and explicit presentation. Exceptional.

Lowenstein, Bertrand E., and Preger, Paul D., Jr. *Diabetes: New Look at an Old Problem.* New York: Harper, 1976. 274 pp. $11.95.
A physician specializing in metabolic disease and a medical writer with diabetes collaborate on this reappraisal of the disease. Considerable space is given to such key topics as the different types of diabetes, the hazards of too much insulin, the need for carbohydrates, daily self-care, emotional problems, and handling emergencies. There are also chapters exploring the connection

between obesity and diabetes, functional hypoglycemia, juvenile diabetes, the question of diabetes in the elderly, the disease as a major killer. In question-and-answer format, the final chapter addresses some common concerns regarding the disease. Resource addresses are appended. Clearly written, with the average layperson in mind. Recommended.

Silvian, Leonore. *Understanding Diabetes.* New York: Monarch Pr., 1977. 117 pp. $2.95 (paper).
Providing a current view, the author begins with an explanation of the nature, symptoms, and prevalence of diabetes. Two chapters present problems and guidelines for both adult-onset and juvenile-onset diabetes. There are tips for living with diabetics, whether they are infants, older children, teens, or adults; terse advice on diet management; material on insulin and oral medications; detection and follow-ups, especially with self-testing at home. Also included are sections on pregnancy and birth control, complications and therapies, research developments. Appended are a resource directory and a glossary. Adequate but not very detailed.

Living with Diabetes

Biermann, June, and Toohey, Barbara. *The Diabetic's Sports and Exercise Book: How to Play Your Way to Better Health.* New York: B.J. Publg. Group, 1978. 256 pp. $2.25 (paper).
Offended by the condescending attitude that diabetics can lead *nearly* normal lives, the authors recall the three elements of diabetic control: diet, medication, and exercise. Irritated by the scarcity of supportive literature, Biermann and Toohey present several convincing arguments in favor of diabetic exercise. There are tips on avoiding or handling insulin shock; preparations and precautions like Medic Alert bracelets, emergency snacks, and foot care; conscientious diet control; creative forms of fitness; correcting the misconceptions of parents, doctors, and coaches; prejudice, legal sanctions, psychological snags, and other disadvantages; determination, discipline, and health potentials that are seen as advantages. Appended are profiles of active diabetics, blood pressure charts, cholesterol and triglyceride ranges, maximum heartbeat, calorie-expenditure charts, sugar-raising snack list, and a diabetes manual for school personnel. Detailed, sensible advice, enthusiastically proclaimed. Highly recommended.

Boylan, Brian, and Weller, Charles. *The New Way to Live with Diabetes,* rev. and updated. New York: Dolphin, 1976. 140 pp. $2.50 (paper).
Aimed at the newly diagnosed diabetic, this book is the second edition of a 1966 guide, which the authors consider outdated. Since then several developments have occurred, including the theory that diabetes is spread by virus, advances toward transplantation of the pancreas, and growing suspicion of oral drugs. Strongly favoring dietary control, Boylan and Weller are

most vehement in their condemnation of oral therapy. Other topics of interest are diagnostic tests, self-testing in therapy, injections, reactions such as coma, exercise, "stress diabetes," complications, hypoglycemia. There are also chapters on everyday concerns and an interesting piece on traveling with the disease. Four appendixes provide height and weight tables, a calorie/activity chart, lists of forbidden foods, oral hypoglycemic agents. Rather dreary, but informative.

Browning, Norma Lee, and Ogg, Russell. *He Saw a Hummingbird.* New York: Dutton, 1978. 154 pp. $8.95.
The victim of diabetic retinopathy, photographer Russell Ogg faced the prospect of losing his profession as well as his eyesight when the blood vessels in his eyes started hemorrhaging. His wife, a journalist, first describes Ogg's life with "brittle" diabetes, a type that defies control and involves frequent complications. She writes of his bouts with despair and of his eventual triumph over encroaching blindness when he devised a method of photographing hummingbirds without seeing them. Also included in the book are passages on the everyday management of diabetes, a routine much more complex than commonly thought, and on the pain of laser surgery to stop the hemorrhaging. A study in courage, which closes with eight color photographs of his hummingbird subjects.

Colwell, Arthur R., Jr. *Understanding Your Diabetes.* Springfield, IL: Charles C. Thomas, 1978. 171 pp. $12.50; $8 (paper).
Emphasizing the need for balanced and thoughtful daily management, a physician and professor at Northwestern University presents the technical side of diabetes in lay terms. Dr. Colwell begins by explaining the nature, genesis, diagnosis, and physiological effects of diabetes. Illustrating his discussions with case reports, charts, and diagrams, he examines the factors of diet and insulin, the hazards and benefits of oral antidiabetic agents, urine testing and the problems it screens, the unstable nature of "brittle" diabetes and emergencies caused by insufficient or excessive insulin, the cause and treatment of hypoglycemia, chronic complications, pregnancy, travel recommendations. Five appendixes provide more detailed information on diet, insulin, testing techniques, drugs, identification cards. Selected readings and glossary are included. Excellent.

Danowski, T. S. *Diabetes as a Way of Life,* 4th rev. ed. New York: Coward, McCann, 1978. 208 pp. $8.95.
Originally published in 1957, this handbook by a distinguished specialist again provides comprehensive information on the nature, treatment, and complications of diabetes. Dr. Danowski includes material on diagnosis and its emotional impact; the need for a doctor-patient team; stages, types of diabetes; symptoms; diet philosophy, variations, exchange lists; the nature, types, and function of insulin; alternate therapies like oral antidiabetic agents; quackery;

aggravation of the disease by physical inactivity; infections; menstruation and menopause; emotions; irregularities in diet or insulin therapy; insulin shock; disorders of other glands; conditions lessening the disease's severity, occasional remissions; acidosis and coma, insulin shock; problems with the nervous system, eyes, kidneys, blood vessels; injection sites, infections, surgery; travel and socializing; alcohol; diabetes in children; pregnancy; and diabetic attitudes. A question-and-answer checklist for patients, a glossary, and appendixes including a roster of diabetes associations are supplied. Well reviewed in medical journals; highly recommended.

Dolger, Henry, and Seeman, Bernard. *How to Live with Diabetes*, 4th ed. New York: Norton, 1977. 224 pp. $8.95; New York: Schocken, 1978. $4.95 (paper).
The nature, management, and complications of the disease are presented by a physician with Mount Sinai Medical School in New York and a medical writer. Among the areas covered are the demographics of diabetes; insulin and oral drugs; and the special problems of children, adolescents, and women. The cardiovascular risks created by oral medications are briefly reviewed; but in the chapter on general complications, only insulin shock and diabetic coma are adequately explained. The book closes with a section on research prospects, including studies of viral connections, insulin resistance, hemoglobin testing, transplants, and the artificial pancreas. Informative but uneven. Recommended as a supplementary source.

Goodman, Joseph I., with Biggers, W. Watts. *Diabetes without Fear*. New York: Arbor, 1978. 198 pp. $8.95; New York: Avon, 1979. $2.25 (paper).
Aimed at the mass of misinformation that surrounds diabetes, this work is the collaborative effort of an eminent diabetes specialist and a free-lance writer who is married to a diabetic. After reviewing and discounting several "scare stories," the authors present their "rational approach" to diabetes. They discuss basic questions and answers about insulin and its problems, hypoglycemia, oral drugs, self-testing, glucose levels, blood and urine tests, so-called forbidden foods and other dietary misinformation, guilt about cheating, weight control, emotional problems, the myth and truth about heredity, safe pregnancy, wound healing, atherosclerosis, diabetic neuropathy, eyesight, kidney damage, foot lesions and other complications, adolescent diabetics, insulin and children, overprotection, the Juvenile Diabetes Association, the American Diabetes Association, new diagnostic techniques, insulin improvements, pancreas transplants, and other research developments. Personal testimonials are included with notes and references. A comprehensive and entirely realistic guide. Essential.

Joslin Clinic, physicians at. *Joslin Diabetes Manual*. 11th ed. edited by Leo P. Krall. Philadelphia: Lea & Febiger, 1978. 324 pp. $8.50 (paper).
Providing comprehensive health care to a large diabetic population, the

Boston-based Joslin Clinic (a division of the Joslin Diabetes Foundation) has been issuing this manual since 1918. Directed specifically at patients, it covers such broad topics as diet, insulin, oral hypoglycemic agents, and other factors in treatment; testing; acute and long-term complications; diabetes in the young; research issues; and appropriate action in minor and severe emergencies. In the chapter on living with diabetes, the doctors address the problems of emotional acceptance, life expectancy, education, choosing a physician, frequency of visits, economic considerations, identification badges, vehicular operation, exercise and sports, alcohol, smoking, drugs and medication, camps, contact lenses, childbearing, traveling, the older diabetic. Ten appendixes include a wealth of additional material, including useful addresses, advice on dining out, insulins available abroad, and sick-day rules. A conscientious, rather scientific presentation that should be the foundation of the lay diabetic library.

Stephens, John W. *Understanding Diabetes.* Beaverton, OR: Touchstone, 1979. 192 pp. $5.95 (paper).
Designed as a reference book for diabetics and other interested persons, this manual by a professor of medicine at the University of Oregon presents the nature, management, and special problems of the disease in direct, uncluttered terms. In five chapters the author explains the peculiarities of adult-onset and juvenile-onset diabetes; dietary and exchange information; treatment concerns such as oral agents and their risks, insulin treatment and precautions, hypoglycemic reactions, urine testing, treatment during illness, and foot care; special problems of diabetic living like obesity and high blood fats, menstruation and pregnancy, employability and insurance, and travel. Also included are recipes and appended resource lists and glossary. A remarkable book that is concise yet detailed, highly readable yet technically precise. Recommended.

Warner, Rebecca, Wolfe, Sidney, and Rich, Rebecca. *Off Diabetes Pills.* Washington, DC: Public Citizen Health Research Group, 1978. 121 pp. $3.50.
This book is published by the Public Citizen's Health Research Group to convey a warning: "Antidiabetic pills are dangerous to your health." If you are taking Orinase, Tolinase, Diabinase, or Dymelar, "these pills could cost you your life." The advice given is to stop taking antidiabetic pills, go on a diet and lose weight, and stop seeing your present doctor unless he or she genuinely tries to help you lose weight or agrees to switch you to insulin. These recommendations are based on the results of the University Group Diabetes Program (UGDP), a large-scale study commissioned by the National Institutes of Health. The findings of UGDP have been backed by the American Diabetes Association, the American Medical Association Council on Drugs, and the Food and Drug Administration, all of which indicate that oral hypoglycemic agents should be used only when the disease cannot be controlled by diet

alone. The book outlines community resources available to assist diabetics, particularly with respect to diet counseling. A crusading, provocative book that should permit patients and their families to discuss diabetes more intelligently with their physicians. Recommended.

Nutrition and Cookbooks

Majors, Judith S. *Sugar Free That's Me.* Milwaukee, OR: Apple, 1978. 200 pp. $6.95 (paper).
Admitting that she lives to eat, this diabetic author shows her "legal" substitutes for many familiar and delectable dishes. After an introductory section on the diabetic food exchanges, Majors provides recipes in seven categories: appetizers and beverages; eggs, breads and muffins; soups and sandwiches; sauces, toppings, and gravy; main dishes; salads, dressings, and vegetables; and sweets. Appending some "words of wisdom," the author advises on measuring artificial sweeteners and on preparation and creativity. Very bright and in most cases clearly gourmet. Recommended as a supplementary cookbook.

Middleton, Katharine, and Hess, Mary Abbott. *The Art of Cooking for the Diabetic.* New York: NAL, 1979. 387 pp. $2.75 (paper); Chicago: Contemporary, 1978. $12.95; 1979, $5.95 (paper).
A diet counselor and a nutrition educator collaborate on this extremely detailed guide to diabetic food management. Beginning with a glossary of diabetic terminology, the work discusses the "weighed," sugar-free, and "free" diets; explains and inventories the updated Food Exchange system of the American Diabetes Association; identifies 12 dangerous foods; and includes an extraordinary section called "Living with Diabetes." The authors provide superb advice on such concerns as eating out, alcohol and diabetes, food exchanges for fast foods like McDonald's, traveling, grocery shopping, label reading, brown-bagging, recognizing the various types of sugar, and sugar in recipes. The list section provides choice recipes in 13 categories. A guide to further sources of information is appended. Indispensable.

Rhodes, Winnie B. *Cooking for Diabetics at Home and Away.* Springfield, IL: Charles C. Thomas, 1976. 237 pp. $14.50 (paper).
A mother of a diabetic shares the recipes she devised over 20 years. Beginning with an explanation of the food exchanges, the author precedes her recipes with advice on marketing, label reading, and storing; cooking and household tips; and a chapter on artificial sweeteners. The recipes themselves cover beverages, snacks, desserts, bread, meat and meat substitutes, poultry and seafood, favorite family meals, soups and sandwiches, salads and dressing, vegetables, fats. The final section provides a variety of menus for use at home, away from home, and on special occasions. Not only imaginative, but filled with the wisdom of an experienced and sympathetic parent.

West, Betty M. *Diabetic Menus, Meals, and Recipes,* 3rd ed., rev. and expanded
    by Nancy Greene Eash. New York: Doubleday, 1978. 194 pp. $7.95.
This up-to-date version of a 1949 "classic" cookbook was written originally by
a diabetic homemaker and has since been revised by a dietician working with
metabolic disorders. A chapter on the diabetic mechanism is followed by
information on vitamins, nutrition, the saccharine problem. After the recipes
themselves, there are also valuable chapters on home canning; artificial
sweeteners in general; and dietary information for the insulin-dependent, for
the overweight, and for those needing low-sodium or low-fat diets. There are
extensive food lists, including material on alcohol ingestion and diabetic
foods. Instructive. but relatively light on recipes.

Hypoglycemia

Airola, Paavo O. *Hypoglycemia, A Better Approach.* Phoenix, AZ: Health Plus,
    1977. 192 pp. $4.95; Provo, UT: Bi World. $4.95.
A nutritionist and naturopathic physician proposes a holistic approach to
hypoglycemia. His book surveys the nature of the disorder; its myriad of
symptoms; causes and aggravating agents such as sugar, caffeine, tobacco,
nutritional deficiencies; diagnosis via a glucose tolerance test. Advocating
unorthodox diet therapy, Airola condemns the high-protein diet and recommends one that emphasizes vegetables, moderately sweet fruits, and grains,
seeds, and nuts. Contrary to popular belief, he argues, these protein foods are
indeed "complete" and superior to meats. Also included are suggested menus,
supplements, herbs, and recipes; favorable reports from four medical doctors
and from hypoglycemic patients. Holistic therapy involving exercise, relaxation, and pure air is Airola's closing advice. A most persuasive, albeit unconventional, work.

Barnes, Broda O., and Barnes, Charlotte W. *Hope for Hypoglycemia.* Fort
    Collins, CO: Robinson, 1978. 57 pp. OP.
A general practitioner with a special interest in the glands describes hypoglycemia as "a blood sugar low enough to cause symptoms," many of which
involve the central nervous system. Caused in diabetes by insulin overdose,
"hypoglycemic syndrome" can appear in nondiabetics also. According to
Barnes it derives from any of several kinds of liver malfunction and can
accompany other conditions, notably thyroid deficiency. In addition to explaining the importance of glucose to the system and the intricate mechanism
involved in controlling blood sugar, the author discusses the incidence, diagnosis, and treatment of hypoglycemia. Despite some very reasonable arguments, many of Dr. Barnes's views are clearly maverick and require further
study.

Brennan, Richard O., with Milligan, William C. *Nutrigenetics: New Concepts for
    Relieving Hypoglycemia.* New York: Evans, 1976. 258 pp. $8.95.
The founder of the International Academy of Preventive Medicine contends

that hypoglycemia is a metabolic imbalance caused by genetic weakness and malnutrition, working together as a single "nutrigenetic" factor. Hypoglycemia not only mimics several other disorders; it is the forerunner of serious diseases. Criticizing the American diet and calling for preventive education in nutrition, he advocates a high-protein, low-carbohydrate diet, with few calories and generous nutritional supplements. He also criticizes the medical establishment for minimizing hypoglycemia and warns readers in detail about diagnostic problems. Included are several case histories and four appendixes that emphasize "nutrition-wise" menus and recipies. An aggressive and poorly organized work, but one that is basically sound and instructive.

Cleave, T. L. *The Saccharine Disease.* New Canaan, CT: Keats, 1975. 200 pp. $7.95; $4.95 (paper); Bristol, England: John Wright. £3.
A member of the Royal College of Physicians presents his arguments against the "saccharine disease," his umbrella term for any condition adversely affected by sugar. Belonging to the epidemic are constipation, diverticular disease, colon cancer and other gastrointestinal disorders; varicose veins, hemorrhoids, and other venous problems; periodontal disease; obesity; diabetes; coronary disease; peptic ulcers; and others. Regarding diabetes, Dr. Cleave claims that overconsumption of refined carbohydrates, especially sugar, is the "essential cause of diabetes." Appended is a "Guide for the Prevention and Arrest of all the Manifestations of Saccharine Disease." Extensive references. The author's style is florid and tediously academic, but his thesis is thought provoking.

Dufty, William. *Sugar Blues.* Radnor, PA: Chilton, 1975. 194 pp. $7.95; New York: Warner, 1976. $2.50.
A popular version of Dr. Cleave's "saccharine disease" thesis, this work by a journalist is heavy on anecdotes and surprisingly well documented. The material on diabetes is concentrated in a chapter entitled "Blame It on the Bees." Unlike Cleaves, Dufty devotes some space to the other side of the case: Kicking the sugar habit and the rewards of sugarless living are the themes of the closing chapters. Notes and bibliography are appended.

PAMPHLETS

Alcohol, Drug Abuse, and Mental Health Administration, Public Health Service, 5600 Fishers La., Rockville, MD 20857.

Psychosomatic Diabetic Children and Their Families, 1977, DHEW Pubn. No. (ADM) 77-477.

American Diabetes Association, Inc., 600 Fifth Ave., New York, NY 10020; or local affiliate.
Among the materials available from this nonprofit voluntary health organization are the following:

Diabetes Forecast, bimonthly magazine.
Exchange Lists for Meal Planning, 1976, 24 pp.
Helping Your Child Live with Diabetes.
Identification Cards.
School Children with Diabetes.
School Record: What School Personnel Should Know about the Student with Dia-
betes, 8 1/2 x 11'' sheet.
Warning Signal Leaflet.
What Everyone Should Know about Diabetes, 16 pp.
What Is Diabetes?
What Is the American Diabetes Association?
What You Need to Know about Diabetes, 1976, 28 pp.
A Word to Police and Fire Personnel.

American Foundation for the Blind, Inc., 15 W. 16 St., New York, NY 10011.

Blindness and Diabetes, 1979, 16 pp.
Devices for the Visually Impaired Diabetic.

American Medical Association, 535 N. Dearborn St., Chicago, IL 60610.

Diabetes, 1977, 8 pp.

American Podiatry Association, 20 Chevy Chase Circle N.W., Washington, DC
20015.

Diabetics Take Care of Your Feet, by A.E. Helfand, reprinted from *Alive and Well 1,*
No. 6 (Feb. 1975): 63–64.

Ames Company, Division of Miles Laboratories, Inc., 1127 Myrtle St., Elkhart,
IN 46514.

Care of the Child with Diabetes: Guidebook for Parents and Teachers of Diabetics,
1977, 20 pp.
Diabetes in the News, quarterly.
Mr. Hypo is My Friend: A Handbook for the Young Diabetic, 1975, 38 pp.
Straight Talk about Diabetes: Guidebook for the Teenager and Young Adult Dia-
betic, 18 pp.
Toward Good Control: Guidebook for Diabetics, 1977, 45 pp.

Becton, Dickinson & Company, Consumer Product Division, Rutherford, NJ
07070.

Some Questions and Answers on Insulin Injection Equipment.

Canadian Diabetic Association, 1491 Yonge St., Toronto, ON M4T 1Z5,
Canada.

Alcohol and Diabetes: Do They Mix?
Basics of the Diabetic Way of Eating.

Channing L. Bete Co., Inc., 45 Federal St., Greenfield, MA 01301.

Diabetics, scriptographic booklet (C210-1136).

Consumer Information Center, Pueblo, CO 81009

Diabetes, (135H), 1978, 16 pp.

Diabetes and Arthritis Program, Division of Chronic Diseases, Department of Health and Human Services, 200 Independence Ave. S.W., Washington, DC 20201.

Foot Care for the Diabetic Patient, 1979.

Diabetes Association of Greater Cleveland, 2022 Lee Rd., Cleveland Heights, OH 44118.

Better Meals for You, 1978 rev. ed.
Better Meals for You with Low Calorie Gourmet Recipes, 1977, $3.
Diabetes and Foot Care: A Step in the Right Direction, 4 pp.
Diabetes Is the Third Most Prevalent Cause of Death in the United States, 3 pp.
The Diabetic's Duty during Illness, 29 pp.
The Diabetic's Insight about the Eye, 4 pp.
Diet Treatment for the Diabetic, 8 pp.
Easy Weight Control with Diet and Exercise, by Joanne Lane and Mary Ellen Rosenlund, 2nd ed., 1980, $3.50.
Insulin Injections for Diabetics, 21 pp.
Pertinent Information for the Teacher of a Diabetic Student, 8 1/2 x 11" card, printed both sides.
Some Children Have Diabetes.
Urine Testing for the Diabetic, 29 pp.

Diabetes Education Center, 4959 Excelsior Blvd., Minneapolis, MN 55416. Sample materials include:

Calculation of a Diabetic Diet Prescription, 1977.
Convenience Food Lists (Based on 1979 Products), ed. by M. Franz, 31 pp.
Exchanges for Special Occasions, by M. Fruin, M. Hargrave, and M. Lavelle.
Labeling Activities for Diabetics, 9 pp.
Menu Magic with Exchanges, by A. Larson, M. Hargrave, and M. Lavelle.
Steps for Calculating Diabetic Diet Exchanges in Recipes, 1976, 2 pp.
Your Meal Plan in Exchanges, 12 pp.

Joslin Clinic, Joslin Diabetes Foundation, Inc., One Joslin Pl., Boston, MA 02215.

The Bulletin, periodical reporting research progress and treatment news.
Diabetes Teaching Guide, comp. by G. P. Kozak, 1977, 61 pp., $4.
Diet and Exercise, 1976, 12 pp.

Juvenile Diabetes Association, 23 E. 26 St., New York NY 10010; and local affiliates.

This nonprofit association focuses on insulin-dependent diabetes, with a quarterly newsletter called *Dimensions in Diabetes* and instructional print material such as the following:

Are You DIABETIC, symptom card.
Children Believe in Miracles, JDF Is Working to Make Them Happen, 8 pp.
Diabetes: There Is Hardly a Family It Doesn't Touch, 1978.
Fact Sheets, 8 1/2 x 11" sheets.
Facts about Diabetes, 9 1/2 x 6" card with personalized section on insulin reaction.
Having Children . . . A Guide for the Diabetic Woman, by Richard Hausknecht, M.D., 12 pp.
Helping Research Find a Cure: A Summary of Research Support, July 1, 1979–June 30, 1980, 48 pp.
In Her Own Words, interview reprinted from July 11, 1977, *People Weekly* magazine, 3 pp.
Juvenile Diabetes Isn't Just for Kids, leaflet.
Just Delicious and Sugar Free: Favorite Sweets, by Ida Ellinson, recipe booklet, 1977, 22 pp.
Parent to Parent, 6-page foldout.
Parent to Parent: Babies with Diabetes, 8-panel foldout.
What You Should Know about Insulin, by Charles Nechemias, M.D., and Norman Lewis Smith, 12 pp.
What You Should Know about Juvenile Diabetes, 10 pp.
What You Should Know about the Student with Diabetes, leaflet with personal records section.

Eli Lilly and Company, Box 618, Indianapolis, IN 46206.

Basic Facts about Diabetes, 1975, 6 pp.
Diet Planner, 1977, 44 pp.
A Guide for the Diabetic, 1976, 79 pp.
Menu Sheets for 6 Different Caloric Allowances, 1977.
Tony and Mark Score a Winning Run Over Diabetes, 1975, 18pp.
What Is Diabetes? 1978, 31 pp.

Medic Alert Foundation, Box 1009, Turlock, CA 95380.

This Could Save Your Life, rev. 1980.

Metropolitan Medical Center, Diabetes Education, 900 S. Eighth St., Minneapolis, MN 55404.

A Survival Kit for Diabetics, by A. Christy, J. Skaalure, and S. Weinzierl, 1978, $10. 210 pp.
Time Out for Foot Care, 1977, 3pp.

National Association of Patients on Hemodialysis and Transplantation, 505 Northern Blvd., Great Neck, NY 11021.
NAPHT News at $8.50 per year. Pamphlets include:
"Renal Failure and Diabetes."

National Diabetes Information Clearinghouse, 805 15 St., N.W., Suite 500, Washington, DC 20005.
Numerous source materials, including:
Diabetic Aids-Selected Products, booklet, 16 pp.

National Eye Institute, National Institutes of Health, Building 31, Bethesda, MD 20014
Diabetic Retinopathy, 1976, DHEW Pubn. No. (NIH) 75-406.

National Institute of Arthritis, Metabolism, and Digestive Diseases, National Institutes of Health, 9000 Rockville Pike, Bethesda, MD 20014.
Foot Care for the Diabetic Patient, DHEW Fact Sheet, 1978, GPO Pubn. No. 1701-00026, 3 pp.
How to Cope with Diabetes, 1977, DHEW Pubn. No. (NIH) 77-987, 16 pp.

National Institute of Neurological and Communicative Disorders and Stroke, National Institutes of Health, Bethesda, MD 20014.
The Diabetic Neuropathies, 1978, DHEW Pubn. No. (NIH) 79-1651, 13 pp.

National Institute on Aging, National Institutes of Health, 9000 Rockville Pike, Bethesda, MD 20014.
Diabetes and Aging, 1978, DHEW Pubn. No. (NIH) 78-1408, 6 pp.

National Society for the Prevention of Blindness, Inc., 78 Madison Ave., New York, NY 10016.
Some Plain Talk on Diabetic Retinopathy, by Stuart L. Fine, M.D., reprinted from *The Sight-Saving Review* 46, No. 1 (Spring 1976): 3–9.

Nutrition in the Life Cycle, Box 24770, Los Angeles, CA 90024.
Dietary Management of Diabetes Mellitus by J.G. Bringas and T.Y. Chan, 1978, 22 pp.

The Sodium Restricted Diabetic Diet, by J. G. Bringas and T. Y. Chan, 1978, 37 pp.

Squibb & Sons, Box 4000, Princeton, NJ 08540.

Don't Be Afraid of Diabetes: A Handbook for Diabetics, by Stanley Mirsky, M.D., 1978, 27 pp.

Vacationing with Diabetes Not from Diabetes, by Stanley Mirsky, M.D., 1978, 18 pp.

Upjohn Company, 7000 Portage Rd., Kalamazoo, MI 49001.

You and Diabetes, 1977, 26 pp.

Your Guide for Meal Planning, 1979, 12 pp.

AUDIOVISUAL PRODUCERS AND DISTRIBUTORS

Abbott Laboratories
Abbott Park, D-383
North Chicago, IL 60064
Films are available for purchase or rental on the nature and symptoms of diabetes, eye complications, etc. Color, 16mm.

American Hospital Association
840 N. Lake Shore Dr.
Chicago, IL 60611
Comprehensive diabetes patient pamphlets and flip-chart or 35mm slides cover urine testing, insulin injection, oral medications, diet, exercise, long-term complications.

American Podiatry Association
20 Chevy Chase Circle N.W.
Washington, DC 20015
Materials include rentable 16mm films on diabetic foot problems.

Ames Co.
Division of Miles Laboratories, Inc.
1127 Myrtle St.
Elkhart, IN 46514
Free loan of 16mm films on diabetes.

Baptist Medical Center—Montclair
800 Montclair Rd.
Birmingham, AL 35213
Review of exchange tables in a game format.

Becton, Dickinson & Co.
Consumer Products Div.
Rutherford, NJ 07070
An educational audiocassette for the newly diagnosed diabetic, with supplementary print materials and diabetic aids. For purchase.

Robert J. Brady Co.
A Prentice-Hall Company
Bowie, MD 20715
Flip-charts on diabetes and its diet control, including material on symptoms of uncontrolled diabetes and three kinds of insulin injection. Packages include 10″ x 13″ charts and patient pamphlets. An alternative format is slides with a narrative supplement. Also available are filmstrips with audiocassettes on living with diabetes, both insulin-dependent and non-insulin-dependent,

self-injection, foot care, diabetes acidosis, and insulin reaction. Programs include patient pamphlets. Purchase and rental.

The Canadian Diabetic Association, Inc.
1491 Yonge St.
Toronto, ON M4T 1Z5, Canada
Films and slide sets such as a six-program set with tape cassettes. Purchase available.

Communications in Learning, Inc.
2929 Main St.
Buffalo, NY 14214
Purchase or rental of slide-cassette program on dietary exchange lists.

Diabetes Education Center
4959 Excelsior Blvd.
Minneapolis, MN 55416
Available slide sets, free or reasonably priced, cover such topics as insulin administration, urine testing, handling insulin reactions, foot care, diet, meal planning during illness, food labeling, exchange lists, glucagon administration.

Educational Activities, Inc.
1937 Grand Ave.
Baldwin, NY 11510
Diabetes filmstrips are available for purchase.

Juvenile Diabetes Foundation
23 E. 26 St.
New York, NY 10010
Topics include low blood sugar emergencies. Apply for either purchase or rental of 16mm film.

Lilly Film Library
Eli Lilly and Co.
Box 100 B
Indianapolis, IN 46206

Among the materials available for free rental are the 8mm *My Friend EDI* by Robert B. Schultz, M.D., an animated film for children on exercise, diet, and insulin.

Medfact, Inc.
1112 Andrew Ave. N.E.
Massillon, OH 44646
Available in formats such as Labelle and Audiscan cartridges, 3/4″ videocassettes, 35mm filmstrips, and 35mm slides with cassettes are programs covering the nature of diabetes, its biological malfunction, symptoms, treatment modalities, insulin therapy, U-100 insulin, foot care, pregnancy, urine testing, hypoglycemia, diet, and the new American Diabetes Association exchange lists.

Medi-Cine Sales Corporation
8201 Pendleton Pike
Indianapolis, IN 46226
Videocassettes on diabetes cover such topics as hygiene, principally dental and foot care, diet and exchanges, emergencies and chronic complications. Rental and purchase are both available.

Milner-Fenwick, Inc.
2125 Green Spring Dr.
Timonium, MD 21093
Diabetic programs in various formats include insulin self-care, diet, home tests, and avoiding complications such as hypoglycemia, ketoacidosis, insulin shock, and vision problems. Also available is the diabetic children's program *My Friend EDI*. Both purchase and rental available.

Monoject
Division of Sherwood
Medical Department
1831 Clive St.
St. Louis, MO 63103
Diabetic topics include instructions
in taking insulin. Slide-sound or
color filmstrip available for free
loan.

National Health Films
Box 13973
Sta. K
Atlanta, GA 30324
Diabetes diet and meal planning,
alcohol, hypoglycemia,
ketoacidosis, coma, exchange lists,
and food variety. Filmstrips with
audiocassettes, slides.

Pfizer Laboratories
Division of Pfizer, Inc.
Film Library
267 W. 25 St.
New York, NY 10001
Free loan of 16mm films about
diabetes mellitus.

**Pharmaceutical Manufacturers
Association**
1155 15 St. N.W.
Washington, DC 20005
Among the numerous topics covered
in 16mm film is diabetes; available
for rental.

Pritchett & Hull Associates, Inc.
2122 Faulkner Rd.
Atlanta, GA 30324
Topics include diabetes footcare in
slide-audiocassette packages or
videocassettes, for rental or
purchase.

Professional Research, Inc.
12960 Coral Tree Pl.
Los Angeles, CA 90066

Available in Super 8, 3/4'' video, and
16mm are programs on diabetes in
adults and on the exchange diet.
In English and Spanish with
supplementary pamphlet and
quizzes. Both rental and purchase.

St. Mary's Hospital Medical Center
Community Relations Department
707 S. Mills St.
Madison, WI 53715
Puppet show for sale on juvenile
diabetes, including coloring book
and other print materials.

Soundwords, Inc.
56-11 217 St.
Bayside, NY 11364
Audiocassettes available for
purchase include programs on
juvenile diabetes, diet and other
therapies, foot care, chronic
complications, and general
information about the disease.

Spenco Medical Corporation
Box 8113
Waco, TX 76710
Numerous health materials are
represented in a 79-page catalog,
including slide-sound sets on the
nature, treatments, and problems
of diabetes.

Teach'em, Inc.
Department 3-C
625 N. Michigan Ave.
Chicago, IL 60611
Psychological aspects of diabetes,
patient acceptance; for rental or
purchase in various formats.

Train-Aide Educational Systems
1015 Grandview Ave.
Glendale, CA 91201
Filmstrips or slide-audiocassette sets
on living with diabetes and
managing the diet.

Trainex Corporation
Box 116
Garden Grove, CA 92642
Comprehensive coverage in
filmstrip, slide, and cartridge
formats includes the nature and
types of diabetes, diet and
management of both
insulin-dependent and
noninsulin-dependent forms,
preventing problems in both types,
urine testing for sugar and
ketones, insulin treatment, and
helping someone with diabetes.
Teen through adult audience
levels. Both rentals and sales.

University of British Columbia
P. A. Woodward Instructional
   Resource Centre
Rm. 105
Vancouver, British Columbia
   V6T 1W5, Canada
Carbohydrates and other dietary
components, exchange lists,
insulin, dining out, traveling, are
among the topics covered in
slide-tape presentations available
for purchase.

**University of Kansas Medical
   Center**
Education Resource Ctr.

College of Health Sciences
Rainbow Blvd. at 39th
Kansas City, KS 66103
Videocassettes for purchase or
rental include dietary
self-management information on
meal components and exchange
lists. Suitable material for
children.

Upjohn
Professional Film Library
7000 Portage Rd.
Kalamazoo, MI 49001
Films and videocassettes for free
loan or purchase on the nature of
diabetes, detection, insulin
injections.

**Vision Multimedia Communication,
   Inc.**
Box 8527
Orlando, FL 32806
Set of six programs with slides and
audiocassettes on various aspects
of the disease, including diabetic
sugar metabolism, noninsulin
diabetics, diet and exchange lists,
foot care, injecting insulin, site
rotation, urine testing. Purchase
individually or by set.

RESOURCE ORGANIZATIONS

American Diabetes Association, Inc.
600 Fifth Ave.
New York, NY 10020; and local
   affiliates

American Dietetic Association
620 N. Michigan Ave.
Chicago, IL 60611

Canadian Diabetic Association
1491 Yonge St.
Toronto, ON M4T-1Z5, Canada

Diabetes Education Center
4959 Excelsior Blvd.
Minneapolis, MN 55416

Joslin Diabetes Foundation, Inc.
One Joslin Pl.
Boston. MA 02215

Juvenile Diabetes Foundation
23 E. 26 St.
New York, NY 10010; and local
    affiliates.

Medic Alert Foundation
Box 1009
Turlock, CA 95380

**Michigan Diabetes Research and
    Training Center**
University of Michigan Medical School
2715 Medical Science II
Ann Arbor, MI 48109

**National Diabetes Information
    Clearinghouse**
805 15 St. N.W.
Suite 500
Washington, DC 20005

**National Institute of Arthritis,
    Metabolism, and Digestive Diseases**
National Institutes of Health
9000 Rockville Pike
Bethesda, MD 20014

Chapter 15

Mental Health

BOOKS

General

Berne, Eric. *A Layman's Guide to Psychiatry and Psychoanalysis.* New York: Ballantine, 1976. $1.95 (paper); London: Penguin. £1.25.
A clear discussion of normal and abnormal mental development covering neuroses, psychoses and character disorders: methods of treatment; and drugs. Does not discuss the delivery of psychiatric services. Somewhat outdated.

Bry, Adelaide. *Getting Better.* New York: Rawson, Wade, 1979. 239 pp. $8.95.
A clinical psychologist provides a consumer's guide to therapy that includes advice on recognizing warning signals, self-help tactics, and choosing a therapist. Dr. Bry explains the purpose and benefits of several therapies and provides cautions where necessary. Among the methods discussed are behavior, Gestalt, group, and sex therapy; hypnotherapy; transactional analysis; growth techniques; Arica training; Silva Mind Control; transcendental meditation; bioenergetics; biofeedback; rolfing; yoga; and Erhard Seminars Training. A resource guide is appended. Although the presentation tends to be simplistic and overly subjective, the work is an adequate introduction that stresses the mind-body connection and the importance of optimum psychological wellness.

Fabrikant, Benjamin, Krasner, Jack, and Barron, Jules. *To Enjoy Is to Live: Psychotherapy Explained.* Chicago: Nelson-Hall, 1977. 278 pp. $9.95.
Explores the purpose, history, applications, theories, forms, and techniques of psychotherapy. Simple explanations.

Jacobs, Jerome. *Interplay: A Psychiatrist Explains What He Does (And What He Does Not Do) and How and Why.* New York: Reader's Digest, 1979. 229 pp. $10.
In a series of composite case histories, Dr. Jacobs, a psychiatrist, shows what goes on in the minds of patients and how the psychiatrist does his job. Readable, well-written text reveals the imprecise and subjective methodology of modern psychiatry. A good attempt to explain mental illness by the use of anecdotal writing.

Kovel, Joel. *A Complete Guide to Therapy: From Psychoanalysis to Behavior Modification.* New York: Pantheon Bks., 1976. 284 pp. $10; $3.95 (paper); London: Harvester. £8.50; Harmondsworth, Middx: Penguin. £1.50 (paper).
A good explanation of a variety of therapies including Freudian, Jungian, Rogerian, and Gestalt, together with encounter groups, sex therapy, behavior therapy, transactional analysis, primal therapy. Leans very heavily on Freudian psychoanalysis. Omits any discussion of the use of drugs in psychotherapy.

Melville, Jay. *Phobias and Obsessions.* New York: Coward, McCann, 1977. 190 pp. $7.95; Penguin. $2.50 (paper).
An excellent, literate guide to dozens of common and uncommon phobias including fear of flying, spiders, insects, and thunderstorms and animal phobias such as cats, dogs, horses, chickens, feathers, birds, and snakes. Rare phobias are described such as fear of work (ergasiophobia), fear of sacred things (hierophobia), and fear of string (linonophobia). Causes and treatment are discussed with a list of treatment centers in Britain and the United States.

Miller, Milton. *If the Patient Is You (Or Someone You Love): Psychiatry Inside-Out.* New York: Scribner's, 1977. 266 pp. OP.
By means of an existential approach, the author—a psychiatrist—attempts to explain what it is like to be schizophrenic, neurotic, perverse, or normal. A hopeful attitude toward coping with neurotic and psychotic patterns of living.

Mishara, Brian, and Patterson, Robert. *The Consumer's Guide to Mental Health: How to Find, Select, and Use Help.* New York: Times, 1977. 278 pp. $9.95.
Eschewing any rigid definition of "mental health," the authors suggest a variety of symptoms that indicate psychological problems; explore the possible causes; and discuss such major dilemmas as suicide, sexual difficulties, drug and alcohol abuse, and terminal illness. Information is provided on selecting and interacting with a therapist, getting emergency help, types of services, and economic considerations. The authors, who have credentials in psychology and psychiatry, discuss various treatment modalities, including individual psychotherapies, group therapies, self-help organizations and programs, inpatient treatment, and alternatives such as residential programs and nursing homes, medication and electroshock therapy. Also covered are

mental health care for children and adolescents, advice on evaluating patients, and patient's rights information. Suggested readings and resource addresses are appended. Readable and encyclopedic. Highly recommended.

Park, Clara Clairborne, with Shapiro, Leon N. *You Are Not Alone: Understanding and Dealing with Mental Illness. A Guide for Patients, Families, Doctors and Other Professionals.* Boston: Little, 1979. $15; $6.95 (paper).
Provides an overview of the entire mental health field, from diagnosis of illness to treatment, from family support and care to public action. It is a useful compendium of existing knowledge on mental illness. Controversial subjects such as deinstitutionalization, drug therapy, and insurance benefits to the mentally ill are covered, and both laypersons and professionals will find the extensive bibliography and appendixes excellent sources for additional information. The book challenges the mentally ill, their families, and communities to work for self-reliance, mutual help, and concerted citizen action.

Rogers, Julie. *Understanding People or How to Be Your Very Own Shrink.* Chicago: Nelson-Hall, 1979. 232 pp. $10.95; $6.95 (paper).
A guide to talking, listening, and accepting, this book cuts through psychological jargon and comes up as a straightforward training manual for anyone who either takes or gives advice. The author surveys the cause-and-effect dynamics of behavior and interaction, and uses casework examples, exercises, and practice sheets to illustrate effective strategies for overcoming destructive tendencies and strengthening feelings of potency and acceptance.

Therapies

Benziger, Barbara. *Speaking Out: Therapists and Patients; How They Cure and Cope with Mental Illness Today.* New York: Walker, 1976. 298 pp. $15.
Review of the basic types of therapy available in a variety of settings such as hospitals, clinics, halfway houses. Contains a list of addresses of mental health associations, research institutes, clinics.

Binder, Virginia, Binder, Arnold, and Rimland, Bernard, eds. *Modern Therapies.* Englewood Cliffs, NJ: Prentice-Hall, 1976. 230 pp. $9.95; $3.95 (paper); London: Prentice-Hall. £7.25; £2.90 (paper).
Key practitioners describe the new emphasis placed on short-term, group, and nonconventional psychotherapies. Good coverage is given to rational-emotive therapy, transactional analysis, reality therapy, Gestalt therapy, transcendental meditation, sex therapy, behavior modification, and assertion training. A good, clear summary.

Friedberg, John. *Shock Treatment Is Not Good for Your Brain.* San Francisco: Glide Pubns., 1976. 176 pp. $6.95.
Friedberg, a psychiatrist, considers that shock treatment is a betrayal of the

Hippocratic Oath and denies that it is of any use in the treatment of depression and schizophrenia. The author is an admirer of Thomas Szasz (*The Myth of Psychotherapy*) and holds that mental illness is a myth. "Shock is what finally validates psychiatrists and makes them look and feel like real doctors." Case histories are presented of seven persons subjected to shock. A clear, forceful statement of the antishock point of view.

Harper, Robert A. *The New Psychotherapies.* Englewood Cliffs, NJ: Prentice-Hall, 1975. 178 pp. $10.95; $3.45 (paper).
An academic and somewhat outmoded discussion of family, group, and sex therapy.

Herrink, Richie. *The Psychotherapy Handbook.* New York: Meridian, 1980. 752 pp. $9.95 (paper).
This guide to more than 250 different therapies in use today is a handy and concise reference to the ever-growing number of varieties of psychotherapy. Encyclopedic in scope, it features definitions, history, techniques, applications, and bibliographies for each therapy. Each chapter is written by either the originator of or a leading authority for that particular therapy. From the well-known to the obscure, from the mainstream to the controversial, each therapy is treated equally and allotted the same amount of space. Recommended.

Janot, Arthur. *Primal Man: The New Consciousness.* New York: Crowell, 1976. 532 pp. $10.
The author of the *Primal Scream* describes his new concept of consciousness and his belief that consciousness is liberated through the liberation of pain. Primal Man is relaxed because there are no longer deep buried pains constantly activating him and afflicting him with a variety of symptoms. Janot believes that Primal Therapy is the only real system of psychotherapy. For sophisticated lay readers.

Jencks, Beata. *Your Body–Biofeedback at Its Best.* Chicago: Nelson-Hall, 1978. 304 pp. $13.95; $7.95 (paper).
Demonstrates how to develop and use minds and bodies to accomplish the results for which mechanical biofeedback machines are designed.

Lewinsohn, Peter M., and others. *Control Your Depression.* Self-Management Series. Englewood Cliffs, NJ: Prentice-Hall, 1979. 354 pp. $14.95; $6.95 (paper); London: Prenctice-Hall £10.90; £5.05 (paper).
Four clinical psychologists discuss the nature, characteristics, and consequences of depression and suggest strategies for improvement. After outlining a nine-step self-change plan, the authors provide specific guidelines by which an individual can evaluate his or her own unique set of problems. The strategies involve learning to relax, engaging in pleasant activities, developing

and using social skills, controlling thoughts and thinking constructively, coping through self-instruction and coaching techniques. Also covered are methods of stress management and personality change. The work includes numerous charts and worksheets, as well as suggestions for further reading. Extremely practical and attuned to emotional wellness through personal action. Recommended.

Rathus, Spencer A., and Nevid, Jeffrey S. *BT: Behavior Therapy.* New York: NAL, 1978. 314 pp. $2.25 (paper).
Behavior therapists view problems such as anxiety and fears, nonassertiveness, sexual dysfunction, and lack of control as learned behavior and therefore capable of being unlearned. BT therapies are described for achieving relaxation, weight reduction, smoking cessation, sexual fulfillment, assertiveness, and dealing with anxiety.

Szasz, Thomas. *The Myth of Psychotherapy: Mental Healing as Religion, Rhetoric and Repression.* New York: Anchor, 1978. 236 pp. $8.95; $2.95 (paper).
Szasz believes that what is called psychotherapy is actually religion, or rhetoric, or repression, or a combination of all three. He denies the existence of psychotherapy in that "it is only a name we use for people speaking and listening to each other." This book is an extension of Szasz's rejection of the medical model of mental illness: "Medical disease stands in the same relation to mental disease as literal meaning stands to metaphorical meaning." Controversial.

Crisis Control

Calhoun, Lawrence G., Selby, James W., and King, H. Elizabeth. *Dealing with Crisis.* Englewood Cliffs, NJ: Prentice-Hall, 1976. 275 pp. $11.95; $4.95 (paper).
Encyclopedic compilation of information on critical human problems —adolescence, marital discord, abortion, divorce, rape, death and dying, sexual discord, suicide, aging. Useful.

Kliman, Ann S. *Crisis: Psychological First Aid for Recovery and Growth.* New York: Holt, 1978. 208 pp. $8.95.
A clinical psychologist describes the theory of therapeutic crisis intervention and its applications in recognizing, communicating about, and coping with the loss and trauma of death, injury, biological deficit, illness, divorce, rape, incest and suicide. Theoretical discussion is well illustrated by case history material.

Sutherland, N. S. *Breakdown.* New York: Stein & Day, 1977. 276 pp. $10; New York: NAL. $1.95 (paper).
Practical advice on how to cope with a "nervous breakdown." The author

describes how to seek competent therapy and mentions encounter groups and psychoanalysis among therapies to avoid.

Schizophrenia

Arieti, Silvano. *Understanding and Helping the Schizophrenic: A Guide for Family and Friends.* New York: Basic, 239 pp. $10.95.
An excellent discussion of the signs, symptoms, causes, and course of the illness, which afflicts more than three mlllion Americans. Arieti describes in simple language the thought patterns and unreal thinking of the schizophrenic. He provides valuable suggestions on how to relate to the patient and how to help. Recommended.

Bernheim, Kayla, and Levine, Richard. *Schizophrenia: Symptoms, Causes, and Treatments.* New York: Norton, 1979. 256 pp. $14.95.
Two clinical psychologists have produced a comprehensive, readable book to appeal to patients and their families and also to mental health technicians and allied health personnel. Topics discussed include the nature of schizophrenic thought, models of madness (the medical model, etc.), causes of schizophrenia (biochemical, neurological, physiological, and other factors), treatment, role of the family in treatment and recovery, hospitalization, and a look toward the future. Interesting and informative. Recommended.

O'Brien, Patrick. *The Disordered Mind: What We Know about Schizophrenia.* Englewoods Cliffs, NJ: Prentice-Hall, 1978. 304 pp. $9.95; $4.95 (paper); London: Prentice-Hall. £7.25; £3.60 (paper).
For sophisticated persons wishing to explore present-day thinking on schizophrenia, O'Brien has produced the ideal book. The coverage is broad, detailed, and reassuring. The extensive coverage includes a discussion of forty misconceptions of schizophrenia, problems in the diagnosis of schizophrenia, characteristics of schizophrenic thinking, what schizophrenia is not, types of schizophrenic disorders, prognosis for recovery, theories of schizophrenia and competing hypotheses, treatment modalities, and hospitalization. This is an excellent state-of-the-art review, well-substantiated by notes and references. Highly recommended.

PAMPHLETS

Blue Cross Association, 840 N. Lake Shore Dr., Chicago, IL 60611.
   Stress, 1974. 96 pp.

Mental Health Association, 1800 N. Kent St., Arlington, VA 22209.
Typical titles are:
   Civil Rights of Mental Patients.

Dealing with the Crisis of Suicide.
Facts about Mental Illness.
Family Life and Sex Education.
Health Insurance for Mental Illness.
Helping the Mental Patient at Home.
High Cost of Mental Illness.
Homosexuality and Mental Illness.
How to Deal with Mental Problems.
How to Deal with Your Tensions.
Marijuana.
Mental Illness Can Be Prevented.
New Directions for Community Mental Health.
Some Things You Should Know about Mental Illness.
What Every Child Needs for Good Mental Health.

National Clearinghouse for Mental Health Information, 5600 Fishers La., Rockville, MD 20857.

Caring about Kids: Dyslexia, 1978, NIH Pubn. No. (ADM) 78-616.
Caring about Kids: Helping the Hyperactive Child, NIH Pubn. No. (ADM) 78-561.
Caring about Kids: Stimulating Baby Senses, 1977, NIH Pubn. No. (ADM) 77-481.
Causes, Detection and Treatment of Childhood Depression, NIH Pubn. No. (ADM) 78-612.
Citizens' Guide to Community Mental Health Centers Amendments of 1975, 1977, NIH Pubn. No. (ADM) 77-397.
Consumer's Guide to Mental Health Services, 1975, NIH Pubn. No. (ADM) 75-214.
Conversations between Heart and Brain, 1978, NIH Pubn. No. (ADM) 78-708.
Dealing with the Crisis of Suicide, NIH Pubn. No. (OM) 2750.
Facts about College Mental Health, 1977, NIH Pubn. No. (ADM) 77-72.
Facts about Group Therapy, 1974, NIH Pubn. No. (ADM) 74-87.
Guide to Mental Health Education Materials, 1977, NIH Pubn. No. (ADM) 77-35.
It's Good to Know about Mental Health, 1977, NIH Pubn. No. (ADM) 77-67.
Learning about Depressive Illnesses, 1977, NIH Pubn. No. (ADM) 77-288.
Lithium in the Treatment of Mood Disorders, 1977, NIH Pubn. No. (ADM) 77-73.
Mental Health Matters: Behavior Modification, 1977, NIH Pubn. No. (ADM) 77-460.
Mental Health Matters: Child Mental Health, 1978, NIH Pubn. No. (ADM) 78-598.
Mental Health Matters: Depression, 1978, NIH Pubn. No. (ADM) 78-601.
Plain Talk about Dealing with the Angry Child, 1979, NIH Pubn. No. (ADM) 79-781.
Plain Talk about Feelings of Guilt, NIH Pubn. No. (ADM) 78-580.
Plain Talk about Stress, 1978, NIH Pubn. No. (ADM) 78-502.

Plain Talk about the Art of Relaxation, 1978, NIH Pubn. No. (ADM) 78-632.
Teaching Mothers Mothering, 1978, NIH Pubn. No. (ADM) 78-520.
When Your Child First Goes Off to School, 1973, NIH Pubn. No. (ADM)
    73-9045.
Yours, Mine and Ours, 1978, NIH Pubn. No. (ADM) 78-676.

Public Affairs Committee, Inc., 381 Park Ave., New York, NY 10016.
The following titles are related to mental health:

Behavior Modification, No. 540.
Dealing with the Crisis of Suicide, No. 406A.
A Death in the Family, No. 542.
Depression: Causes and Treatment, No. 488.
Helping Children Face Crises, No. 541.
How to Cope with Crises, No. 464.
How to Discipline Your Children, No. 154.
Male "Menopause": Crises in the Middle Years, No. 526.
Mental Health Is a Family Affair, No. 155.
Parents and Teenagers, No. 490.
Schizophrenia, No. 460.
Sensitivity Training and Encounter Groups, No. 474.
Serious Mental Illness in Children, No. 352.
Tensions—And How to Master Them, No. 305.
Understanding Stress, No. 538.
What Can You Do about Quarreling? No. 369.
What Should Parents Expect from Children? No. 154.
When Mental Illness Strikes Your Family, No. 172.
You and Your Adopted Child, No. 274.

AUDIOVISUAL PRODUCERS AND DISTRIBUTORS

Robert J. Brady Co.
A Prentice-Hall Company
Bowie, MD 20715
Death and dying; suicide and crisis
    intervention; reactive depression;
    relaxation; stress.

Concept Media
Box 19542
Irvine, CA 92714
Stress.

McGraw-Hill Films
110 15 St.
Del Mar, CA 92014

Abnormal behavior; transactional
    analysis; therapy.

Mendota Mental Health Institute
301 Troy Dr.
Madison, WI 53704
Treatment of children.

Omnia Corporation
1301 E. 79 St.
Suite 210
Minneapolis, MN 55420
Impotence.

Soundwords, Inc.
56-11 217 St.
Bayside, NY 11364
Understanding psychotherapy;
  psychosomatic disorders;
  understanding phobias; suicide;
  depression; mental problems.

Teach'em Inc.
Department 3-C
625 N. Michigan Ave.
Chicago, IL 60611
Depression; anorexia nervosa;
  anxiety, psychoneuroses;
  schizophrenia.

Trainex Corporation
Box 116
Garden Grove, CA 92642
Aggression; depression; anxiety; guilt;
  stress; suicide; the psychiatrist in
  society.

Walt Disney Educational Media
500 S. Buena St.
Burbank, CA 91521
Stress.

RESOURCE ORGANIZATIONS

**American Academy of Child
  Psychiatry**
1424 16 St. N.W.
Washington, DC 20036

American Mental Health Foundation
2 E. 86 St.
New York, NY 10028

**American Orthopsychiatric
  Association**
1775 Broadway
New York, NY 10019

American Psychiatric Association
1700 18 St. N.W.
Washington, DC 20009

American Psychological Association
1200 17 St. N.W.
Washington, DC 20036

**Group for the Advancement of
  Psychiatry**
419 Park Ave. S.
New York, NY 10016

Hogg Foundation for Mental Health
University of Texas
Austin, TX 78712

Mental Health Association
1800 N. Kent St.
Arlington, VA 22209

Mental Health Materials Center
419 Park Ave. S.
New York, NY 10016

**National Clearinghouse for Mental
  Health Information**
5600 Fishers La.
Rockville, MD 29852

**National Society for Autistic
  Children**
1234 Massachusetts Ave. N.W.
Washington, DC 20005

Network Against Psychiatric Assault
558 Capp St.
San Francisco, CA 94110

Neurotics Anonymous International Liaison
1341 G St. N.W.
Washington, DC 20005

Recovery Inc: The Association of Nervous and Former Mental Patients
116 S. Michigan Ave.
Chicago, IL 60603

Schizophrenics Anonymous International
Box 913
Saskatoon, Saskatchewan, Canada

Chapter 16

Alcoholism and Drug Abuse

BOOKS

Alcoholism

Allen, Chaney. *I'm Black and I'm Sober.* Minneapolis: CompCare, 1978. 279 pp. $6.95 (paper).
Allen demonstrates how Alcoholics Anonymous (AA) has worked a wonder in her life and includes practical aids to help others. Her list of "reality statements" points out the differences between "thinking drunk" and "thinking sober." Her Soul Chart illustrates stages in alcoholism and recovery. The author is well known for her work in alcoholism in minority groups.

Chafetz, Morris. *Why Drinking Can Be Good for You.* New York: Stein & Day, 1976. 191 pp. $8.95.
The author is a previous director of the National Institute on Alcohol Abuse and Alcoholism. Chafetz describes the situations in which modern medical practice considers alcohol to be beneficial—a useful adjunct to the essential human experience of socialization. Topics discussed include physical effects of alcohol; the hangover; alcohol and health; problems of young people; alcohol on the job; drinking and driving; alcohol and other drugs; diagnosis, treatment, and prevention of alcoholism. Clear, sensible, and practical advice in a highly readable form. Recommended.

Curlee-Salisbury, Joan. *When the Woman You Love Is an Alcoholic.* St. Meinrad, IN: Abbey, 1979. 96 pp. $1.95 (paper).
This book is written for the family and friends of alcoholic women who are bewildered by the seemingly contradictory dictates of love in a highly confusing situation. Topics of discussion are who is an alcoholic, the problem of

denial, when there are children, when she wants help, road to recovery, and special problems. Organizations and further readings are included as part of a section on where to look for help.

Fajardo, Roque. *Help Your Alcoholic Before He or She Hits Bottom: A Tested Technique for Leading Alcoholics into Treatment.* New York: Crown, 1976. 182 pp. $7.95.
Explores the myth that an alcoholic cannot be helped unless he or she wants help. Fajardo provides a manual for anyone who wants to help an alcoholic on the road to recovery.

Hornik, Edith. *The Drinking Woman.* Chicago: Follett, 1978. 191 pp. $8.95.
According to Hornick, drinking for a woman is a very different experience than it is for a man. She reinforces that point with reports of recent research and with interviews with recovering women. Hornick talks about traditional and modern attitudes toward women drinkers, self-image, hidden drinking, stresses and "stressors," family relationships, the unhealthy marriage, the alcoholic husband (who wants a drinking buddy), the man who keeps his wife out of treatment, women and Alcoholics Anonymous, the special problems of minority or elderly women. A comprehensive book about women and alcohol.

Kimball, Bonnie-Jean. *Alcoholic Woman's Mad, Mad World of Denial and Mind Games.* Center City, MN: Hazelden Foundation, 1978. 69 pp. $3.50 (paper).
Denial of the illness of alcoholism is a characteristic symptom in both sexes. The author describes how it is subtly different for women. She presents a touching, sensitive, and often humorous portrayal of the lonely, frightening world of the alcoholic woman.

McCabe, Thomas R. *Victims No More.* Center City, MN: Hazelden Foundation, 1978. 103 pp. $3.95.
The stress of internal tension that problem drinking generates within a particular family unit can cause the family to become nonfunctional. In this book, written for the spouse and children of a problem drinker, the author describes how the family can intervene and work together during the treatment process. McCabe offers advice on choosing a treatment facility and sympathetically describes some of the problems the family may encounter after treatment.

Mehl, Duane. *You and the Alcoholic in Your Home.* Minneapolis: Augsburg, 1979. 141 pp. $3.95 (paper).
Factors involved in the development and maintenance of drug and alcohol dependence—money, sex, social drinking patterns, and prescription drug availability—are discussed. The author describes in nontechnical language the drugs popular among today's youth. Treatment programs for the alcoholic are explored as well as companion groups for members of an alcoholic's family. The importance of Alcoholics Anonymous is emphasized.

Miller, William R., and Munoz, Ricardo. *How to Control Your Drinking*. Englewood Cliffs, NJ: Prentice-Hall, 1976. 246 pp. OP.
Designed specifically for persons who would like to cut down on drinking and not give up alcohol completely. Rejects the traditional, abstinence-oriented ideology of problem drinking. Details techniques for increasing self-control with things to do before drinking, things to do while drinking, and things to do instead of drinking. The emphasis is on self-help and how to relax, cope with depression, maintain a positive self-concept, and deal with situational factors. A most supportive and helpful book.

Nero, Jack. *Drink Like a Lady, Cry Like a Man: The Love Story of a Man and His Recovering Alcoholic Wife*. Minneapolis: CompCare, 1977. 285 pp. $6.95.
With wry humor that thinly veils his pain, Nero watches his wife change from the "life of the party" to an unreasonable, depressed alcoholic. And he makes her drinking *his* Number 1 problem. His earnest, but bumbling, attempts to "fix" her include supervising her "cutting down," psychiatry and a hospital for the emotionally disturbed, and a "controlled" vacation. Only after she chooses to go to a residential treatment center—and he begins to deal with his own mirror-alcoholic sickness in an Al-Anon group—do they recover.

Seixas, Judith. *Living with a Parent Who Drinks Too Much*. New York: Greenwillow, 1979. 116 pp. $6.95.
This book is to help children of alcoholics understand what is happening to them and to their parents. The message, clearly and directly conveyed to the child of an alcoholic parent, is that he or she is not alone; that there are many children far and near who live with a parent who drinks too much. The author describes how other children have effectively dealt with similar problems and feelings, and suggests ways in which life can be made more bearable and productive. Help can be obtained from Alateen, a group dedicated to helping children cope with problems of alcoholism in the family.

Weiner, Jack B. *Drinking*. New York: Norton, 1976. 241 pp. $8.95.
Weiner has skillfully created a representative portrait of the alcoholic today from interviews with a cross section of American alcoholics—nurses, bankers, secretaries, derelicts, nuns, homemakers, artists, and athletes. Dick Van Dyke claims on the book jacket, "Jack's book says it all. If everyone in America read it, there would no longer be a need to feel ashamed to ask for help."

Winters, Ariel. *Alternatives for the Problem Drinker: AA is Not the Only Way*. New York: Sterling, 1978. 160 pp. $8.95.
A good discussion of the many facets of the drinking problem. The impact of the Rand Report (1976), suggesting that some alcoholics could safely return to social drinking, is discussed in detail. Many persons consider Alcoholics Anonymous (AA) to be antijoy, puritanical, and punitive, reinforcing a sick dependency. Only 5 percent of the total ten million estimated alcoholics are

AA members. Winters discusses new trends in treatment, the nutritional approach, behavior modification, treatment centers and techniques for solitary self-help.

Juvenile Alcoholism

Addeo, Edmond G., and Addeo, Jovita Reichling. *Why Our Children Drink.* Englewood Cliffs, NJ: Prentice-Hall, 1975. 191 pp. OP.
A journalist and a nurse review the problem of teenage drinking in an attempt to foster responsible decision making about alcohol use. They consider the scope of the problem and the effect of lowering the legal age, and comment on several adolescent drinkers. After identifying four major influences on teenage drinking, the authors discuss alcohol education, the role of mass media, and the hard facts about alcohol. Includes suggestions for developing healthy attitudes and helping young people deal appropriately with drinking. Lists supportive organizations and literature. Dispassionate and realistic.

Alibrandi, Tom. *Young Alcoholics.* Minneapolis: CompCare, 1978. $5.50 (paper).
Alibrandi presents personal histories of young alcoholics, plus information on treatment, and helpful advice on how to recognize and cope with the problem. Based on a study conducted in Orange County, California.

Cross, Wilbur. *Kids and Booze: What You Must Know to Help Them.* New York: Dutton, 1979. 180 pp. $10.95; $5.95 (paper).
A nontechnical discussion that avoids theory and statistics. Instead, the author addresses many questions that concern parents and community members: What can be done to help the teenage problem drinker; how do you know if your child is a problem drinker; why do young people drink; how do you teach young people to make sensible decisions about drinking; how do parents' drinking habits influence their children; what role do the churches play in alcohol education. Excellent, practical advice accompanied by a listing of agencies concerned with alcoholism and suggestions for further reading. Recommended.

Englebardt, Stanley L. *Kids and Alcohol, The Deadliest Drug.* New York: Lothrop, 1975. 64 pp. $5.25. (Grades 5 and up).
This instructive work on juvenile drinking discusses the growing abuse of alcohol by youngsters; the chemical action of alcohol; health effects; the making of a problem drinker; determining factors; the recognition, prevention, and treatment of alcoholism. Especially valuable is Englebardt's nine-point "formula for avoiding alcoholism." References. Far superior to similar books.

Forrai, Maria S., and Anders, Rebecca. *A Look at Alcoholism.* Lerner Awareness Series. Minneapolis: Lerner, 1977. 36 pp. $4.95. (Grades 3–6).

Introducing youngsters to the subject of alcohol, the authors describe its healthy use as well as the many disastrous consequences of its abuse. Despite too many pictures of adult derelicts, Forrai and Anders nevertheless provide a message about alcohol and children, about how they inherit their parents' problems and how they can find help.

Haskins, Jim. *Teen-Age Alcoholism.* New York: Hawthorn, 1976. 156 pp. $6.95; $2.95 (paper).
In this book for adolescents the author presents a historical view of alcoholism, the social roots and causes of teenage drinking, and its physical and mental effects. Haskins also identifies four different types of alcoholism and various therapeutic approaches to the problem. Appendixes include a state-by-state directory of the National Council on Alcoholism and sources of further information. An adequate, historical overview; offers little on preventive measures.

Hyde, Margaret O. *Know about Alcohol.* New York: McGraw-Hill, 1978. 80 pp. $6.95 (Grades 4–6).
Introducing future drinkers to the positive and negative aspects of alcohol, the author covers such concerns as handling peer pressure, acquiring safe drinking habits, and choosing to abstain. Provides personal testimonies, a question-and-answer section, and recommended services and literature. A balanced, reassuring presentation.

Langone, John. *Bombed, Buzzed, Smashed or Sober: A Book about Alcohol.* Boston: Little, 1978. $7.95; New York: Avon, 1979. 157 pp. $1.50 (paper).
For everyone, but especially for junior and senior high school students, this book is most informative and lucid. Answers important questions such as: Do beer and wine have a slower effect than liquor? Is alcoholism an inherited disease? Will black coffee really sober you up? Good, basic, and relevant information to enable young persons to make intelligent decisions.

Lee, Essie E. *Alcohol—Proof of What?* New York: Messner, 1976. 192 pp. $7.29. (Grades 7 and up).
Directed at teenagers, this work by an educator and physical therapist reviews the history of alcohol; depicts an autopsy; dispels myths; and discusses such topics as alcohol and safety, adolescent drinking, and Alcoholics Anonymous for teens. Lee also provides an alcohol quiz and a directory for additional information. A straightforward, compelling work. Highly recommended.

Marshall, Shelly. *Young, Sober and Free.* Center City, MN: Hazelden Foundation, 1978. 137 pp. $4.95.
Marshall and her young collaborators relate for young persons the personal experiences of those who have lived through alcohol addiction. The emphasis is on the primary tools of recovery.

Snyder, Anne. *Kids and Drinking.* Minneapolis: CompCare, 1977. $2.50 (paper).
First-person stories are based on the experience of children the author has known in her work with young alcohol abusers. Sara, Kathy, and Tommy describe how they began drinking at ages nine, seven, and eight respectively, and how their drinking and their lives became out of control. Not intended as a scare book or a moralizer; the message is presented clearly and calmly to show that no one is too young to become an alcoholic.

Drug Abuse

Ausubel, David P. *What Every Well-Informed Person Should Know about Drug Addiction.* Chicago: Nelson-Hall, 1980. 161 pp. $8.95.
An excellent discussion of the drug problem and of the social and psychological characteristics of opiate addiction. The author believes that drug addiction is primarily a personality disorder and that a personality weakness predisposes some people toward addiction. Ausubel considers that that too large a share of research energies has been focused on the chemical, pharmacological, neurophysiological, and psychopharmacological aspects of addiction at the expense of concern for psychological factors. Although the book emphasizes opiate addiction, it does include materials on marijuana, cocaine, lysergic acid diethylamide (LSD), and barbiturates. Recommended.

Cohen, Sidney. *The Drug Dilemma,* 2nd ed. New York: McGraw-Hill, 1975. 103 pp. $9.50; $6.95 (paper); London: McGraw-Hill. £6.70; £4.45 (paper).
The author focuses attention primarily on the pharmacological and behavioral effects of LSD, marijuana, amphetamines, cocaine and other stimulants, narcotics, sedatives and tranquilizers, anesthetics and alcohol.

Forrai, Maria S., and Anders, Rebecca. *A Look at Drug Abuse.* Minneapolis: Lerner, 1977. 36 pp. $4.95.
Several photographs and a sparse text characterize this work for children about such drugs as alcohol, heroin, marijuana, nicotine, and caffeine. Although the authors describe many consequences of drug abuse and several types of therapy, the coverage is rather superficial.

Young, Lawrence A., and others. *Recreational Drugs.* New York: Berkley, 1979. 216 pp. $2.50 (paper); London: Collier Macmillan. £4.50 (paper).
A layman's guide to Quaaludes, snow, pot, catnip, angel dust, speed, lettuce opium, amies, downers, LSD, alcohol, ginseng, mescal beans. Chemical composition, effects, dosages, dangers, warning signals, and side effects of 88 recreational drugs are provided. A list of common names refers readers to the correct chemical name for each drug. An informative book that provides the basis for a rational, intelligent, and informed approach to the drug problem.

Smoking

Ducharme, Diane, Angel-Levy, Penny, and Mitz, Rick. *The Cigarette Papers: Snip the Strings to Your Habit.* Minneapolis: CompCare, 1979. $5.95 (paper).
Written by three former tobacco addicts who cumulatively burned up about 1,533,000 cigarettes, $34,492, and an occasional item of clothing during their approximately 30 total years of smoking. The book recognizes that people start smoking and quit smoking in different ways for varying reasons—and with varying amounts of pain. All three authors had slightly different experiences and do not always agree. What all three do agree on is that all smokers need a personalized program to successfully unhook from those tobacco-filled cylinders that act as crutches, tranquilizers, aphrodisiacs, and friends.

Harris, Roger Williams. *How To Keep On Smoking and Live.* New York: St. Martin's, 1978. 191 pp. $8.95; $3.95 (paper).
A unique book on the smoking problem, filled with both well and little-known facts about the habit and its various consequences. While providing an intriguing alternative to quitting, the author manages to lace his text with antismoking messages that are almost subliminal in their effect. In addition to his "second-best smoking plan," Harris includes a section on quitting and one entitled "Most Everything You Never Wanted to Know about Cigarettes and Didn't Know Who to Ask." Filled with humor and psychologically effective pictures and cartoons, the work has been applauded by several authorities on cancer. Appended are a bibliography and tables on the tar and nicotine content of American and Canadian cigarettes.

Madison, Arnold. *Smoking and You.* New York: Messner, 1975. 64 pp. $6.29. (Grade 4 and up).
With arresting photographs and diagrams, this work discusses the history of smoking, the tobacco industry today, chemical products of a lighted cigarette, and the surgeon general's reports. Madison graphically details the effects of smoking on the lungs, heart, and other organs. Glossary. A frightening collection of facts. Recommended.

Sonnett, Sherry. *Smoking.* A First Book. New York: Watts, 1977. 64 pp. $4.90. London: Watts. £2.25. (Grades 4–6).
Beginning with a detailed history of smoking, this book instructs young people about its consequences. Included are its effect on the lungs, heart, and other organs, and the risk of fires. The last chapter addresses the problem of children smoking. An impressive book, with striking illustrations.

PAMPHLETS

Al-Anon Family Group Headquarters, Box 182, Madison Square Sta., New York, NY 10010.

A very large number of pamphlets are available at nominal prices on many topics. Titles include:

Adult Children of Alcoholics.
Al-Anon: A Resource.
Al-Anon: Family Treatment Tools in Alcoholism.
Al-Anon and Alateen Groups at Work.
Al-Anon Fact File.
Al-Anon Interviews.
Al-Anon Is for Men.
Al-Anon, You and the Alcoholic.
Al-Anon's Twelve Concepts of Service.
Al-Anon's World Service Office.
Alcoholism, the Family Disease.
Allies for Al-Anon in Helping the Family.
Blueprint for Progress: Al-Anon's Fourth Step Inventory.
Double Winners.
Facts about Alateen.
Freedom from Despair.
A Guide for Sponsors of Alateen Groups.
Homeward Bound.
How Can I Help My Children?
It's a Teenaged Affair.
Jane's Husband Drank Too Much!
Living with Sobriety, Another Beginning.
Lois' Story.
My Wife Drinks Too Much.
Operation Alateen.
A Pebble in the Pond.
Purpose of the Al-Anon Group and Suggestions for Those Who Need Help.
So You Love an Alcoholic.
Sponsorship—What It's All About.
A Teacher Finds Guidance in Al-Anon.
This Is Al-Anon.
3 Views of Al-Anon.
To the Mother and Father of an Alcoholic.
Twelve Steps and Twelve Traditions for Alateen.
The Twelve Steps and Twelve Traditions of the Al-Anon Groups.
Understanding Ourselves and Alcoholism.
What Do You Do about the Alcoholic's Drinking?
What Is Al-Anon Anonymous?
What's "Drunk" Mama?
What's Next? Asks the Husband of the Alcoholic.
Youth and the Alcoholic Parent.

Alcoholics Anonymous World Services, Inc., Box 459, Grand Central Sta., New York, NY 10017.

A very large number of pamphlets are available at nominal prices on many topics. Titles include:

A.A. and the Alcoholic Employee.
A.A. and the Armed Services.
A.A. and the Medical Profession.
A.A. Fact File.
A.A. for the Woman.
The A.A. Group.
A.A. in Prisons.
A.A. in Treatment Centers.
The A.A. Member (formerly *A Community Resource*).
The A.A. Member and Drug Abuse.
A.A. Tradition: How it Developed.
A.A.'s Legacy of Service.
Alcoholics Anonymous in Your Community.
A Brief Guide to Alcoholics Anonymous.
Co-founder of Alcoholics Anonymous.
Do You Think You're Different?
44 Questions and Answers about the A.A. Program.
How A.A. Members Cooperate with Other Community Efforts to Help Alcoholics.
How It Works.
If You Are a Professional.
Inside A.A.
Is A.A. for You?
Is There an Alcoholic in Your Life?
It Happened to Alice!
The Jack Alexander Article.
Las Doce Tradiciones (Spanish).
The Last Talks of A.A.'s Co-founders.
Let's Be Friendly with our Friends.
A Letter to a Woman Alcoholic.
Los Doce Pasos (Spanish).
A Member's Eye View of Alcoholics Anonymous.
Memo to an Inmate Who May Be an Alcoholic.
Questions and Answers on Sponsorship.
Speaking at Non-A.A. Meetings.
This is A.A.
Three Talks to Medical Societies by Bill W.
Too Young?
Twelve Steps and Twelve Traditions (card).
The Twelve Traditions (illustrated).
Understanding Anonymity.
What Happened to Joe and His Drinking Problem.
Young People and AA.
Your A.A. General Service Office.

Blue Cross Association, 840 N. Lake Shore Dr., Chicago, IL 60611.

Alcoholism, 34 pp.
Drug Abuse: The Chemical Copout, 44 pp.

Do It Now Foundation, Box 5115, Phoenix, AZ 85010.

Alcohol: How It Can Affect Your Health, Nutrition, and the Vitamins in Your Body.
Alcohol, Drug & Apathy Abuse.
Alcohol/Drug Combinations.
All about Cocaine.
All about Downer Drugs.
AMYL/BUTYL Nitrite & Nitrous Oxide: A Report on Current Use of Two Popular Inhalants.
Aspirin: Uses and Abuses.
Barbiturates: Current Use, Patterns & Problems.
Barbiturates: Important Facts for Your Survival.
Comprehensive Drug Knowledge Test.
Drug I.Q. Test.
Drug Wipeout and Megavitamin Therapy.
Everything You've Always Wanted to Know about Chromosome Damage.
Facts about Angel Dust.
Facts for Needle Freaks.
Fetal Alcohol Syndrome.
Garbage: A Report on Street Ripoffs.
Gunk: All about Drugs & Pollution.
Junk: Getting Yourself Together.
Junk and You: Why People Use Heroin, and Why They Don't.
LSD: A Closer Look at Tripping.
LSD and the Market Place: From the Lab to the Street.
Marijuana: Unbiased Facts about the Killer Weed.
Medical Uses of Cannabis.
New Facts about Marijuana.
PCP, From Street Ripoff to Drug of Choice.
Quaaludes & Sopers (and Other Methaqualone Drugs).
Smack: The Strongest You Can Buy without a Prescription.
Smoking, Drinking & Pregnancy.
Sniffing: Good Smells & Bad Smells.
Speed and Whites: The Same Thing Sometimes.
Speedy Stuff & Coke: The Chemical Eye-Openers.
Tobacco Abuse.
True Facts about Sniffing.
Valium and Librium: The Pharmaceutical War against Anxiety.

Drug Enforcement Administration, Department of Justice, Washington, DC 20537.

Drugs of Abuse, 1978, 33 pp.

Hazelden Foundation, Box 176, Center City, MN 55012.
In addition to distribution and sale of many Alcoholics Anonymous and
Al-Anon pamphlets, the Hazelden Foundation has a number of other pam-
phlets available, such as:

Alcoholism and the Family.
Common Sense Re-education of an Abnormal Drinker.
Don't Tell Me I'm Not An Alcoholic.
Drugs—Use, Misuse, Abuse.
A Guide for the Family of an Alcoholic.
Guide for the Family of the Drug Abuser.
Help for the Marriage Partner of an Alcoholic.
I Had to Stop Because I Couldn't Quit.
If You Drink . . . What You Should Know and Do.
A Letter to Our Alcoholic Dad.
A Look at Relapse.
My Wife Thought I Could If I Would.
Reaching Out to the Alcoholic and the Family.
Recovery of Chemically Dependent Families.
Surrender Versus Compliance in Therapy.
Teen Drug Use: What Parents Can Do.
Thinking about Drinking.
The Woman Alcoholic and Her Total Recovery Program.

Health Communications Inc., 7541 Biscayne Blvd., Miami, FL 33138.

A Guide of Drug Information—Do You Know the Facts about Drugs?
The Female Alcoholic.
Young Drinkers: Teenagers and Alcohol.

National Clearinghouse for Drug Abuse Information, Box 1635, Rockville,
MD 20857.

Can Drug Abuse Be Prevented in the Black Community? 1977, DHEW Publica-
tion No. (ADM) 77-493.
Catching On: Parents, Peers and Pot.
Drug Abuse Facts: Hallucinogens.
Drug Abuse Facts: Marijuana.
Drug Abuse Facts: Narcotics.
Drug Abuse Facts: Sedatives.
Drug Abuse Facts: Stimulants.
Drug Abuse Prevention for Your Family.
A Family Response to the Drug Problem: Handbook.
For Parents Only: What You Need to Know about Marijuana.
Got a Minute?
Growing Up In America: A Background to Contemporary Drug Abuse.
Let's Talk About Drug Abuse: Some Questions and Answers, 1979, DHEW Publi-
cation No. (ADM) 78-706.

Parents, the Real Teachers.
This Side Up.
A Woman's Choice: Deciding about Drugs.

National Council on Alcoholism, 733 Third Ave., New York, NY 10017.

Alcohol: Pleasures and Problems.
Alcohol and the Adolescent.
Alcohol Beverages: Social Use—or Sick Abuse?
Pastoral Counselling and the Alcoholic.

National Highway Traffic Safety Administration, Department of Transportation, Washington, DC 20590.

How to Keep the Life of the Party Alive.
How to Talk to Your Teenager about Drinking and Driving.

National Institute on Alcohol Abuse and Alcoholism, 5600 Fishers La., Parklawn Bldg., Rockville, MD 20857.

Alcohol Abuse and Women: A Guide to Getting Help, 1979, DHEW Pubn. No.
    (ADM) 79-358, 25 pp.
Drinking Etiquette, 1979, DHEW Pubn. No. (ADM) 79-305, 13 pp.
The Drinking Question: Honest Answers to Questions Teenagers Ask about Drinking, 1979, DHEW Pubn. No. (ADM) 79-286. 28 pp.
Q/A Alcohol. Some Questions and Answers, 1979 DHEW Pubn. No. 79-312. 14
    pp.
Someone Close Drinks Too Much, 1979, DHEW Pubn. No. (ADM) 79-23. 15 pp.
The Unseen Crisis. Blacks and Alcohol, 1978, DHEW Pubn. No. (ADM) 78-478.
    15 pp.

Public Affairs Committee, Inc., 381 Park Ave. S., New York, NY 10016.

Alcoholism—A Sickness That Can Be Beaten, No. 547.
Cigarettes—America's No. 1 Health Problem, No. 439A.
Drinking on the Job, No. 544.
Drug Abuse and Your Child, No. 448.
Drugs—Use, Misuse, Abuse: Guidance for Families, No. 515.
How to Help the Alcoholic, No. 452.
Marijuana: Current Perspectives, No. 539.
The New Alcoholics: Teenagers, No. 499.
What You Should Know about Drug Abuse, No. 550.
The Woman Alcoholic, No. 529.
You and Your Alcoholic Parent, No. 500.

STASH, 118 S. Bedford St., Madison, WI 53703

Analysis of the LSD Flashback.

Drugs of Abuse: An Introduction to Their Actions and Potential Hazards.
Downers: The CNS Depressant Drugs.
Introduction to Amphetamine Abuse.
MDA: A Different Psychedelic.
Mescaline and Peyote: A Literature Review.
Methadone: The Drug and Its Use in the Treatment of Addiction.
PCP: The New Delusionogen.
Psilocybin and Psilocin: The Magic Mushrooms.
Who Took the Drugs?

AUDIOVISUAL PRODUCERS AND DISTRIBUTORS

Aims Instructional Media Services
Box 1010
Hollywood, CA 90028
Effects of alcohol and drugs on the
body.

American Medical Association Film
Library
535 N. Dearborn St.
Chicago, IL 60610
Drugs and the nervous system;
narcotics; alcoholism as a mental
health problem; teenage drinking.

Robert J. Brady Co.
A Prentice-Hall Company
Bowie, MD 20715
Cause of alcoholism; role of the
family; drugs and abuse.

Churchill Films
622 N. Robertson Blvd.
Los Angeles, CA 90069
Drugs and the nervous system.

Encyclopaedia Brittanica
Educational Corporation
425 N. Michigan Ave.
Chicago, IL 60611
Drug abuse, rehabilitation, heroin
addiction.

FMS Productions, Inc.
1040 N. Las Palmas Ave.
Los Angeles, CA 90038

Filmline Educational Services
1467 Tamarind Ave.
Hollywood, CA 90028
Alcohol recovery.

Guidance Associates, Inc.
Communications Pk.
Box 300
White Plains, NY 10602
Alcohol, a social problem; alcohol and
teenagers.

Hanna Barbera Productions
Educational Div.
3400 Cahuenga Blvd.
Hollywood, CA 90028
The drug scene.

Hazelden Foundation
Box 176
Center City, MN 55012
Drug abuse and prevention;
rehabilitation; alcohol abuse,
dependency, and prevention.

Johnson Institute
10700 Olson Memorial Hwy.
Minneapolis, MN 55441
Alcohol invervention.

Journal Films
930 Pitner Ave.
Evanston, IL 60202
Narcotics.

Lilly Film Library
Eli Lilly & Co.
Box 100 B
Indianapolis, IN 46206
Students look at drugs.

MTI Teleprograms, Inc.
4825 N. Scott St.
Suite 23
Schiller Park, IL 60176
Rehabilitation from drug abuse.

McGraw Hill Films
110 15 St.
Del Mar, CA 92014
Teenage drinking; heroin addiction.

Modern Talking Picture Service
2323 New Hyde Park Rd.
New Hyde Park, NY 11040
Drinking and driving.

National Association of Counties
 Research Foundation
1735 New York Ave. N.W.
Washington, DC 20006

National Drug Abuse Materials
 Distribution Center
Box 398
McLean, VA 22101
Drug abuse.

National Publications
Box 4116
Omaha, NE 68104

Parents' Magazine Films
Distributed by PMF Films, Inc.
Box 1000
Elmsford, NY 10523
Psychedelics; narcotics; stimulants;
    sedatives.

Paulist Communications
17575 Pacific Coast Hwy.
Box 1057
Pacific Palisades, CA 90272

Pyramid Films
Box 1048
Santa Monica, CA 90406
Physiological and behavioral effects of
    alcohol.

Soundwords, Inc.
56-11 217 St.
Bayside, NY 11364
Narcotic addiction; uppers and
    downers; marijuana and psychedelic
    drugs.

Southerby Productions
1709 E. 28 St.
Long Beach, CA 90806
Alcoholism and youth; alcoholism in
    high school.

Spenco Medical Corporation
Box 8113
Waco, TX 76710
Drug abuse and alcoholism posters,
    models, games, and audio-
    cassettes.

RESOURCE ORGANIZATIONS

Addiction Research Foundation
33 Russell St.
Toronto, Ontario

Al-Anon Family Group Headquarters
Box 182, Madison Square Sta.
New York, NY 10010

Alateen
Box 182
Madison Square Sta.
New York, NY 10010

**Alcohol and Drug Problems
Association of America**
1101 15 St. N.W.
Washington, DC 20005

**Alcohol, Drug Abuse and Mental
Health Administration**
Office of Communications and Public
Affairs
5600 Fishers La.
Rockville, MD 20857

**Alcoholics Anonymous World
Services, Inc.**
Box 459
Grand Central Sta.
New York, NY 10017

Center for Alcohol Studies
Rutgers Univ.
New Brunswick, NJ 08903

Center for Multicultural Awareness
2924 Columbia Pike
Arlington, VA 22204

Do It Now Foundation
Box 5115
Phoenix, AZ 85010

Drug Abuse Council, Inc.
1828 L St. N.W.
Washington, DC 20036

**Drug Enforcement Administration
(DEA)**
1405 I St. N.W.
Washington, DC 20537

Hazelden Foundation
Box 176
Center City, MN 55012

Iowa Drug Abuse Information Center
Cedar Rapids Public Library
428 Third Ave. S.E.
Cedar Rapids, IA 52401

Nar-Anon Family Group
Box 2562
Palos Verdes, CA 90274

Narcotics Anonymous
Box 622
Sun Valley, CA 91352

Narcotics Education, Inc.
6830 Laurel St. N.W.
Washington, DC 20012

**National Clearinghouse for Alcohol
Information**
Box 2345
Rockville, MD 20852

**National Clearinghouse for Drug
Abuse Information**
Box 1635
Rockville, MD 20857

**National Coordinating Council on
Drug Education**
1526 18 St. N.W.
Washington, DC 20036

National Council on Alcoholism
733 Third Ave.
New York, NY 10017

National Council on Drug Abuse
9 S. Michigan Ave.
Chicago, IL 60603

**National Institute on Alcohol Abuse
and Alcoholism**
5600 Fishers La.
Rockville, MD 20857

Pyramid Project
39 Quail Ct.
Suite 201
Walnut Creek, CA 94596

Veterans Administration
Alcohol and Dependency Service
810 Vermont Ave. N.W.
Washington, DC 20420

**Wisconsin Substance Abuse
  Clearinghouse**
420 N. Lake
Madison, WI 53706

Women for Sobriety Inc.
Box 618
Quakertown, PA 18951

Chapter 17

Other Health Problems and Concerns

BOOKS

Asthma and Allergies

See also Asthma and Allergies in Chapter 9, Children's Health.

Frazier, Claude A. *Psychosomatic Aspects of Allergy.* New York: Van Nostrand Reinhold, 1977. 257 pp. OP.
A lucid discussion of psychosomatic and emotional components of allergy. Frazier describes how prolonged emotional stress alters physical conditions and either becomes a factor in the cause of disease or aggravates underlying health problems. Stress is shown to be a factor in asthma, allergic rhinitis, skin disturbances, and gastrointestinal disease. Frazier indicates how to control the physical aspects of disease and how to keep a home allergen-free. Recommended.

Golos, Natalie, and Bolbitz, Frances Golos. *Coping with Your Allergies.* New York: Simon & Schuster, 1979. 351 pp. $11.95.
This book is written as a practical guide for the prevention and alleviation of allergies. It explains how to cope with sensitivities and the overload of pollutants in modern life. The authors advocate clinical ecology, which studies the individual's reaction to the environment. The book is particularly useful in its discussion of allergenic substances present in home furnishings, clothing and fabrics, cosmetics, and insecticides, and those encountered in traveling. The advice for nontoxic living is sensible and practical, but the soundness of the dietary information and the cookbook for the allergic person is debatable. Nonconventional, but useful.

Lane, Donald J., and Storr, Anthony. *Asthma: The Facts*. New York: Oxford Univ. Pr., 1979. 163 pp. $11.95.
A lucid compendium of useful information on the causes of asthma attacks; symptoms; effects of age, inheritance, and occupation; and treatment techniques such as bronchodilators and steroids. A final chapter presents information on self-help and some words of advice.

Mackarness, Richard. *Eating Dangerously: The Hazards of Allergies*. New York: Harcourt, 1976. 164 pp. $6.95.
The author, a British physician, presents evidence as to the wide prevalence of food allergies and shows how to recognize and avoid illness. MacKarness advocates a Stone Age–type diet, rich in animal fat and protein and practically free of sugar, cereals, and processed carbohydrates.

Back Pain

Linde, Shirley M. *How to Beat a Bad Back: Hundreds of Things to Achieve a Pain-Free Back*. New York: Rawson, Wade, 1979. 328 pp. $12.95; $6.95 (paper).
On any given day, 6.5 million people are in bed because of back pain. It is estimated that four out of every five people in the United States can expect to experience back trouble at some time in their lives. Bad backs are the number one claim on disability insurance policies and the second most frequent cause of absenteeism from work. Linde outlines techniques to tone muscles, improve posture, stretch ligaments, relax nerves, increase flexibility, reduce pain, and increase function. Specific information is presented on lifting, posture, diet, how to drive a car to best avoid backache; the best ways to sleep; and how to work to give your back the most protection. She suggests that surgery be regarded as a last resort only after a thorough exercise program has been tried. Also presented is a guide on where to go for information and further help on specific back problems. Recommended.

Stoddard, Alan. *The Back—Relief from Pain—Patterns of Back Pain—How to Deal with and Avoid Them*. New York: Arco. 1979. 125 pp. $7.95; $4.95 (paper).
A practical guide, by an osteopath, to back pain and techniques to relieve it. Stoddard explains the causes of back pain and describes the basic patterns of pain. He describes appropriate exercises and posture and shows how to minimize risks in sports, swimming, sex, and gardening. Methods of treatment covered include manipulation massage, traction, collars and corsets, sclerosing injections, electrotherapy, hydrotherapy, drugs, and surgery. Informative, with superb photographs showing posture and exercises.

Birth Control and Family Planning

Shapiro, Howard I. *The Birth Control Book*. New York: St. Martin's, 1977. $10.
A gynecologist active in Planned Parenthood and the National Organization

of Women (NOW) provides an extremely detailed guide to birth control. After introductory material on the reproductive system, Shapiro discusses contraceptive pills; intrauterine devices; diaphragms, spermicides, and condoms; coitus interruptus and rhythm; postcoital contraception; abortion; vasectomy; tubal ligation; hysterectomy; and currently experimental methods. Appendixes include Planned Parenthood directory, glossary, and bibliography. Rather graphic in places, not recommended for the overly sensitive.

Shivanandan, Mary. *Natural Sex.* New York: Rawson, Wade, 1979. 274 pp. $11.95; $6.95 (paper).
This work explains the rationale and benefits of practicing natural family planning instead of artificial birth control. Deemed more reliable than traditional rhythm, the ovulation method and the symptothermal methods depend on subtle changes in cervical mucus, basal body temperature, and other mid-cycle signs. According to the author, these methods can also increase body awareness and deepen the relationship between sexual partners. Appendixes include annotated list of natural family-planning organizations. Despite the need for further study, the work is intriguing.

Tucker, Tarvez. *Birth Control.* New Canaan, CT: Tobey, 1975. 158 pp. $2.95 (paper).
An excellent review of contraceptive methods, this work covers male and female anatomy and sexual function; the gynecological examination; choosing a doctor; birth control with oral contraceptives; intrauterine devices; diaphragms, and condoms; vaginal contraceptives; coitus interruptus, rhythm, and sterilization. Topics include the way in which a particular method works, its effectiveness, instructions for use, different designs and brands, cautions and side effects. Appended is a national directory of women's centers, health-care clinics, and referral services.

Wylie, Evan M. *All about Voluntary Sterilization.* New York: Berkley, 1977. 210 pp. $1.75 (paper).
This guide explains the procedures and results of vasectomy, tubal ligation, and laparoscopic tubal sterilization; discusses cost considerations, psychological effects, and vasectomy reversals; and compares sterilization with other birth control methods. Appended material includes recovery timetables for men and women, clinics and hospitals performing vasectomies and sterilizations by laparoscopy, and statements from various medical organizations. An unscholarly presentation.

Cosmetic Surgery

See also Surgery and the Consumer in Chapter 8, Wellness, Physical Fitness, and Self-Health Care.

Dicker, Ralph, and Syracuse, Victor. *Consultation with a Plastic Surgeon.* Chicago: Nelson-Hall, 1975. 273 pp. $10.95; New York: Warner. $2.50 (paper).
Answers to most of the common questions about plastic surgery are provided by two plastic surgeons.

Rosenthal, Sylvia. *Cosmetic Surgery: A Consumer's Guide.* New York: Lippincott, 1977. 250 pp. $10.95.
A comprehensive guide to cosmetic or aesthetic surgery that answers most questions: how to find and choose a plastic surgeon, what to ask during a consultation, what to expect from surgery, risks and complications, fees. Extensive coverage is given to face lifts; cosmetic correction of the eyelids, nose, jaw, chin, lips; hair transplants; augmentation, reduction, and reconstruction of the breasts; body contouring and skin improvement. The excellent text deserves better than the poor illustrations and photographs provided.

Digestive Tract Disorders

Galton, Lawrence. *Save Your Stomach.* New York: Crown, 1977. 287 pp. $8.95; New York: BJ Publg. Grp. $2.25 (paper).
A lay guide, by a medical journalist, to gastroenterology, diseases and conditions of the stomach and intestines. Popular topics covered include gastroenteritis, anal itching, constipation, diarrhea, diverticular disease, gallstones, irritable colon, liver disease, pancreatitis, peptic ulcer, ulcerative colitis, and regional enteritis. The effects of antacids, antibacterials, anticholinergics, and antiemetics are explained but no trade or generic names of drugs are provided. Useful.

Nugent, Nancy. *How to Get Along with Your Stomach: A Complete Guide to the Prevention and Treatment of Stomach Distress.* Boston: Little, 1978. 271 pp. $8.95.
A highly readable description of many popular medical topics: hiatal hernia, heartburn, esophagitis, obesity, dyspepsia, gastritis, hyperacidity, nausea, morning sickness, peptic ulcers, constipation, and ulcerative colitis. In each instance, the nature of the disorder, symptoms, and treatment are discussed, accompanied by references for further reading. Informative presentation of the essentials of the digestive system and the important role that stress plays. Recommended.

Holt, Robert Lawrence. *Hemorrhoids: The Problem, Personal Treatments, Medical Treatment.* Oceanside, CA: California Health Pubns., 1977. 195 pp. OP.
To those who suffer from them, there is nothing amusing about hemorrhoids. The author explains clearly how and why hemorrhoids develop. Preventive measures recommended include increased intake of fiber, improved diet, use

of good toilet habits, and exercise. Suppositories, ointments, and laxatives are not recommended: "The use of commercial preparations is a poor substitute for an intelligent diet and improved toilet habits." For those conditions not amenable to home treatment, Holt recommends cryohemorrhoidectomy, a technique of eliminating hemorrhoids by a freezing process. The author claims that cryorectal surgery is a reliable and valuable alternative to excision for the removal of hemorrhoids in many cases. An interesting book that will doubtless be of great value to many persons afflicted with hemorrhoids. Recommended.

Epilepsy

See also Epilepsy under Other Health Problems and Concerns in Chapter 9, Children's Health.

Sands, Harry, and Minters, Frances C. *The Epilepsy Fact Book.* Philadelphia: Scribner's, 1979. 116 pp. $7.95.
Sponsored by the Epilespy Foundation of America, this work discusses the nature of the disorder, its possible causes, types of seizures, diagnostic and treatment methods. Also covered are the various problems of living with epilepsy and sources of help. There is a separate chapter on epileptic children. Includes sections with facts and figures, glossary, and bibliography. Designed specifically for lay readers; straightforward and comprehensive.

Genetics

Hendin, David, and Marks, Joan. *The Genetic Connection: How to Protect Your Family against Hereditary Disease.* New York: Morrow, 1978. 251 pp. $8.95.
The joint effort of a medical writer and a specialist in genetic counseling, this work discusses the problem of inherited disease, describes several specific defects, and explains the role of genetic counseling and such prenatal tests as amniocentesis (sampling of amniotic fluid from the uterus). Also covered are the alternatives of aborting a defective child or caring for one that is brought to term. Lists of resources, treatment centers, and literature are appended.

Milunsky, Aubrey. *Know Your Genes.* Boston: Houghton, 1977. 335 pp. $9.95; New York: Avon. $1.95 (paper); London: Houghton, £6.00.
A Harvard pediatrician and geneticist thoroughly discusses genes and chromosomes, birth defects and genetic counseling, prenatal diagnosis, heredity and specific diseases, determining the sex of a baby, multiple births, and test-tube babies and other ethical problems. Also covered are infections, X rays, and drugs that cause birth defects; amniocentesis; artificial insemination. Appendixes include a list of biochemical diseases that can be diagnosed prenatally. Highly informative and readable.

Nyhan, William L. *The Heredity Factor: Genes, Chromosomes, and You.* New York: Grosset & Dunlap, 1976. 320 pp. OP.
An eminent geneticist provides an extensive guide to genetic disorders and their prevention through such means as genetic counseling and prenatal diagnosis. Includes numerous case histories, pertinent questions, a chart of genetic diseases, a glossary, and selected readings. Somewhat technical, but readable and authoritative.

Headache

Rose, F. Clifford. *Migraine: The Facts.* New York: Oxford Univ. Pr., 1979. 100 pp. $10.95.
A well-written book for migraine sufferers and their families, as well as for nurses, doctors, and other health professionals who encounter migraine. Chapters cover "triggers" such as food and birth control pills; the effects of factors such as stress; the various types of migraine; the relationship between migraine and the environment; and the reasons for the feeling of elation or exhaustion that sometimes follow an attack. A good discussion of diagnosis, prevention, and treatment with clear illustrations and drawings. Recommended.

Saper, Joel R., and Magee, Kenneth R. *Freedom from Headaches: A Personal Guide for Understanding and Treating Headache, Face and Neck Pain.* New York: Simon & Schuster, 1979. 222 pp. $8.95.
A clear explanation by two neurologists of the pain associated with headaches and the various types: migraine, tension, cluster, sinus, and psychogenic. Also discussed are headaches as symptoms of other medical conditions such as infection and meningitis; headaches and food; and how to select a doctor and what to expect from him or her. Will answer most questions asked by the layperson.

Speer, Frederic. *Migraine.* Chicago: Nelson-Hall, 1977. 160 pp. $9.95; $5.95 (paper).
A useful book for migraine sufferers, families, and friends with specific recommendations for control and relief.

Hearing Impairment

See also Hearing and Vision in Chapter 11, Health of the Elderly.

Helleberg, Marilyn M. *Your Hearing Loss: How to Break the Sound Barrier.* Chicago: Nelson-Hall, 1979. 257 pp. $12.95.
A valuable guide for those with various degrees and types of hearing impairment. Using a question-and-answer format, Helleberg covers basic types of

hearing loss, causes and symptoms, self-help techniques for auditory training and lipreading, hearing-aid selection and adjustments, vocational rehabilitation, social and psychological problems relating to hearing loss, medical and surgical treatments, organizations serving the hearing handicapped, and suggestions for family and friends. Informative, practical, and useful. Recommended.

Human Sexuality

Barlow, David. *Sexually Transmitted Diseases: The Facts.* New York: Oxford Univ. Pr., 1979. 140 pp. $8.95.
The author is Consultant Physician, Department of Genitourinary Medicine, St. Thomas's Hospital, London. Dr. Barlow has succinctly digested most, if not all, of what the average person would ever want to know about syphilis, gonorrhea, chancroid, trichomoniasis (a form of vaginitis), candidiasis (a fungus disease), scabies, pubic lice, herpes genitalis, genital warts, and so on. He claims that Great Britain and Ireland are "the only countries in the world to have made a separate medical specialty out of the study, diagnosis and treatment of the sexually transmitted diseases, and this is reflected in a lower incidence of infection and a generally higher standard of patient care and clinic facilities than is found elsewhere." Perhaps, after all, the British invented the slogan "Clean Living is the Only Safeguard." The book is informative and lucidly written and contains excellent color photographs, diagrams, and a glossary. Cartoons interject a very necessary sense of humor. Highly recommended.

Rowan, Robert L. and Gillette, Paul G. *Gay Health Guide.* Boston: Little, 1978. 239 pp. $9.95.
A comprehensive guide to health problems common to homosexually active men and women that offers both clinical information and preventive advice. Written by a psychologist and a urologist, the handbook defines and examines the medical problems related principally to homosexuality in terms of prevention, causes, effects, and methods of treatment. For problems that merit medical attention, the guide includes advice on how to find physicians who are understanding of the health problems of gays, and ways of evaluating a doctor's ability to treat venereal disease. Additional chapters discuss problems in sexual performance, emotional problems related to homosexuality, ambisexuality and "going straight," transvestism and homosexual activity in marriage, and questions and answers about health problems that commonly cause difficulties for gays.

Secondi, John J. *For People Who Make Love: A Doctor's Guide to Sexual Health.* New York: Taplinger Publishing, 1975. 191 pp. $7.95.
This work offers detailed information about the symptoms, diagnosis, and treatment of sexually related disorders. Among these are trichomoniasis,

moniliasis, hemophilus vaginalis, crab lice, viral hepatitis, mononucleosis, herpes simplex, venereal warts, and chancroid. Dr. Secondi devotes extensive space to both gonorrhea and syphilis, describing symptoms, complications, syphilitic stages, effects on fetuses and newborns, diagnosis, treatment, and preventive measures. There is also a question-and-answer section, advice on getting help, recommended treatment schedules for gonorrhea and syphilis, glossary and bibliography. Sensitive and thorough.

Woods, Nancy Fugate, and Woods, James S. *Human Sexuality in Health and Illness.* St. Louis: Mosby, 1979. 232 pp. $9.95 (paper); London: Mosby. £5.75.
Aimed at professionals, this work by a professor of nursing and a research pharmacologist has some value for lay readers also. Topics include sexual patterns and cycles; sexuality during pregnancy; abortion; sexual assault; the sexual effects of drugs, illness, handicaps, and procedures like mastectomy and hysterectomy. A scholarly, rather detached study.

Infertility

Decker, Albert, and Loebl, Suzanne. *Why Can't We Have a Baby?* New York: Dial Pr., 1976. 245 pp. $7.95; New York: Warner. $2.50 (paper).
The authors attempt to describe the problem of infertility and what can be done as a remedy. A great deal of information is presented on the causes of infertility, male and female reproductive organs, tests, fertility drugs, surgical procedures, miscarriage, and artificial insemination. In addition, 50 frequently asked questions are answered, and a glossary is supplied. The writing, however, lacks sparkle and the illustrations are sparse and of poor quality.

Harrison, Mary. *Infertility: A Couple's Guide to Its Causes and Treatments.* Boston: Houghton, 1979. 204 pp. $7.95; $3.95 (paper); London: Houghton. £4.75.
Written from the patient's point of view, this work discusses normal conception; the possible causes of infertility and habitual miscarriage; recognizing the problem and seeking help; basic diagnostic tests for both men and women and special tests; the emotional burden of infertility; various treatments; the effects of birth control measures; medical innovations. Appended are summaries of diagnostic workups, organizational addresses, anatomical illustrations, notes, bibliography, and glossary. In part a journal of Harrison's own experiences and impressions, the work is written with both authority and compassion.

Kaufman, Sherwin A. *You Can Have a Baby: New Hope for the Childless, Including Facts about Test Tube Births and Other New Techniques.* New York: Elsevier/Nelson, 1978. 206 pp. $8.95.
An obstetrician surveys the causes and treatments of infertility. He describes the tests conducted to determine the type of infertility and possible remedies.

Culdoscopy and laparoscopy permit the physician to make a visual examination of the uterus, ovaries, and fallopian tubes. Also described is the successful birth of the Steptoe "test-tube" baby. Included are sections on reproductive biology and a glossary. A thorough, articulate presentation, compassionate but realistic.

Menning, Barbara Eck. *Infertility: A Guide for the Childless Couple.* Englewood Cliffs, NJ: Prentice-Hall, 1977. 178 pp. $9.95; $3.45 (paper); London: Prentice-Hall. £6.95; £2.40 (paper).
The founder of a support organization for infertile people discusses various causes, tests, and treatments of infertility in both men and women; myths; prevention of the problem; selecting a doctor; patients' rights; miscarriage and stillbirth; the cultural and psychological aspects of infertility; adjusting to an incurable problem; alternatives such as adoption, artificial insemination, and childfree living. Includes glossary, bibliography, and list of resources. A broad overview of the problem, with touching anecdotes that highlight its emotional effects.

Philipp, Elliot. *Overcoming Childlessness: Its Causes and What To Do about Them.* New York: Taplinger, 1975. 186 pp. $8.50.
The head of an infertility clinic discusses the conditions necessary for conception, problem evaluation, and treatments. Dr. Philipp strongly recommends that a *team* of specialists performs the evaluation. He describes the questions that will be asked of the couple, as well as the examination and possible tests. Also discussed are improving male fertility without surgery, artificial insemination, surgical procedures for men and women, psychology, the maintenance of an existing pregnancy, delivery, genetics, and chromosomes. Includes address of the American Fertility Society. Informative, but not well organized.

Stangel, John J. *Fertility and Conception: An Essential Guide for Childless Couples.* New York: Paddington, 1979. 223 pp. $8.95.
A specialist in problems of fertility discusses the anatomy and processes of reproduction, causes of both male and female infertility and of miscarriage, treatments and possible solutions in the future. Includes glossary, statistics, suggestions for further information. With detailed explanations of both disorders and procedures, Stangel does much to dispel myths and reassure couples about conception. Most current; superior to similar works.

Kidney Disease

Glabman, Sheldon, and Freese, Arthur S. *Your Kidneys, Their Care and Their Cure.* New York: Dutton, 1976. 185 pp. OP.
An excellent, informative summary of pertinent information on the warning signals of kidney disease, urinary-tract infections, kidney stones, prostate

problems, nephritis and nephrosis, pregnancy and kidney disease, systemic diseases and the kidneys (hypertension, diabetes, gout, etc.), kidney failure, dialysis, artificial kidneys and transplants. Answers most of the questions the layperson may pose.

Multiple Sclerosis

Forsythe, Elizabeth. *Living with Multiple Sclerosis.* Salem, NH: Faber, (dist. by Merrimack Bk. Serv.), 1979. 144 pp. $11.95; $6.95 (paper); London: Faber. £4.95; £2.50 (paper).
A personal narrative by a British doctor and journalist who describes in flawless prose her own reactions to the diagnosis and subsequent progress of her illness. Although a physician, she knew very little about multiple sclerosis. The book is full of sound common sense and practical advice. Attention is paid to diet, treatment, exercise, rest, psychological effects, and the capacity to work. Chapters relating to social services, voluntary societies, and how to select a doctor reflect the current situation in the United Kingdom and are not relevant to the American scene. Nevertheless, the book is useful for those with multiple sclerosis and their families. Recommended.

Mathews, Bryan. *Multiple Sclerosis: The Facts.* New York: Oxford Univ. Pr., 1978. 103 pp. $8.95.
A professor of clinical neurology at Oxford University has presented the essential facts relating to what multiple sclerosis is, early symptoms, the course of the disease, diagnosis, causes, treatment, and practical management. It will be most helpful to those who need to know—patients, families, friends, and health professionals. Unfortunately, Dr. Mathews has lost sight of the level of understanding of a lay audience, viz: "Professor Field has now developed a simpler test, avoiding the somewhat remote intervention of guinea pigs, in which red blood cells from the subject are exposed in an electric field and the effect of the PUFA's linoleic and arachidonic acid on their mobility is measured." A good summary of current knowledge but beyond the reach of persons without highly specialized training. Useful, however, for reference.

Ginther, John R. *But You Look So Well.* Chicago: Nelson-Hall, 1978. 160 pp. $10.95.
While not a killer, multiple sclerosis (MS) is a crippler with a range of symptoms so complex that early and proper diagnosis is often missed. This book is a personal, in-depth examination of multiple sclerosis by a university professor and a victim whose family, at his doctor's insistence, kept the true diagnosis of his disease from him for ten years. It describes, in lay terms, the scientific, emotional, and practical problems involved, and offers advice and hope for victims and their families.

Skin Care

Feinberg, Herbert S. *All about Hair.* New York: Simon & Schuster, 1979. 182
pp. $10.
A consumer's guide to causes of hair loss, dandruff, and hair restoration. A
good description with illustrations is provided to explain hairpieces, hair
weaving, hair implanting, and hair transplants. The discussion is informative
and lucid. The book is also valuable as to methods for controlling dandruff
and in the selection of appropriate shampoos and conditioners, which are
listed by brand name. Recommended.

Flandermeyer, Kenneth L. *Clear Skin: A Step-by-Step Program to Stop Pimples,
Blackheads, Acne.* Boston: Little, 1979. 211 pp. $8.95; $5.95 (paper).
Eighty-six percent of all adolescents have some degree of acne by the age of
seventeen; forty-three percent of those who consult a doctor are over twenty
and a third of American females between twenty and fifty have acne. Fact is
separated from fiction in explaining the causes of acne. Acne is not caused by
unfulfilled sexual desires, chocolate, greasy foods or colas; moisturizers and
makeup, pressure on the skin, certain drugs such as cortisone, and stress may
cause or aggravate acne. The home treatment recommended involves the use
of desquamating or exfoliating agents, or, more popularly, drying-peeling
(DP) agents. Guidance is provided on assessing the severity of one's acne and
the selection and purchase of DP agents, washing, and application of agents
such as benzoyle peroxide. Most persons will prefer to obtain the assistance of
a physician to confirm diagnosis and to obtain an individualized treatment
plan.

Goldstein, Norman. *The Skin you Live In: How to Recognize and Prevent Skin
Problems and Keep Your Skin Youthful and Attractive.* New York: Hart, 1978.
205 pp. $10.95; $5.95 (paper).
A concise guide to topics of widespread concern: acne, warts, psoriasis, sunburn, moles, skin discolorations, insect bites, burns, rashes, poison ivy, hives,
scabies, and fungi. Summary information is given on how to protect oneself
from the sun, home care of hair and nails, and how to spot serious skin trouble.
Great emphasis is placed on self–skin care and on how to attain a healthy,
youthful, attractive skin. Little detail is provided, however, of treatment
modalities and what to expect from a dermatologist. It is more an explanation
of self–skin care than a simplified guide to present-day dermatology.

PAMPHLETS

American College of Obstetricians and Gynecologists, One E. Wacker Dr.,
Chicago, IL 60601.
Causes and Treatments for Genetic Disorders.

Important Facts about Venereal Diseases.
Infertility: Causes and Treatments.

American Medical Association, 535 N. Dearborn St., Chicago, IL 60610.
A large number of high-quality pamphlets are available at minimal cost.
Typical titles include:

Aesthetic-Cosmetic Surgery . . . What it Can and Cannot Do, OP 208.
Aging Skin, OP 333.
Allergic Contact Rashes, OP 239.
Allergies, OP 007.
Anesthesiology, OP 066.
Appendicitis, OP 358.
Arthritis, OP 053.
Athelete's Foot, OP 349.
Atopic Eczema or Atopic Dermatitis, OP 379.
Birth Control, OP 155.
Cancer: Facts You Should Know, OP 046.
Common Sense about Moles, OP 178.
Constipation, OP 142.
Dandruff, OP 029.
Dermatologist Talks about Warts, OP 334.
Diseases of the Colon and Rectum, OP 367.
Gallbladder Disease, OP 350.
Hair You Can Do Without, OP 396.
Hay Fever and Its Complications, OP 301.
Infertility, OP 172.
Kidney Disease, OP 118.
Peptic Ulcer, OP 236.
Poison Plant Rashes, OP 025.
Psoriasis: The Scaling Disease, OP 116.
Sexually Transmitted Diseases, OP 383.
Something Can Be Done about Acne, OP 035.
Sun and Your Skin, OP 319.
What to Do When Hearing Fades, OP 028.

Bureau of Community Health Services, Health Services Administration, 5600
Fishers La., Rockville, MD 20857.

The Extra Advantages of Family Planning, 1979, DHEW Pub. No. (HSA)
79-5658, 9 pp.
Family Planning and Health, 1979, DHEW Pub. No. (HSA) 79-5657, 10 pp.
The Man Who Cares, 1979 DHEW Pub. No. (HSA) 79-5651, 9 pp.
Planning Your Future Includes Family Planning, 1975, DHEW Pub. No. (HSA)
75-16014, 9 pp.

National Clearinghouse for Family Planning Information, Box 2225, Rockville, MD 20852.

Among the materials available for distribution are:

a series of six patient education pamphlets on encouraging the practice of family planning by specific target groups.
a grid presentation of contraceptive methods.
a community involvement pamphlet on teenage pregnancy.
a series of four self-instructional booklets on contraception, sterilization, and the pelvic examination.
informed consent for sterilization pamphlets.
motivation posters for target audiences.
a Spanish-language flip-chart and Spanish translations of selected other publications.

Office of Communications, National Institutes of Health, Bethesda, MD 20014.

Acne, DHEW Pub. No. (NIH) 79-188.
Asthma, NIH Pub. No. 79-525.
Digestive Diseases: Recent Research Advances, Future Opportunities and Needs, DHEW Pub. No. (NIH) 76-1073.
Dust Allergy, DHEW Pub. No. (NIH) 75-490.
Epilepsy, DHEW Pub. No. (NIH) 77-156 (also in Spanish).
Food Allergy, DHEW Pub. No. (NIH) 75-533.
Headache, DHEW Pub. No. (NIH) 76-158.
Hearing Loss, DHEW Pub. No. (NIH) 78-157.
Kidney Disease and Artificial Kidneys, DHEW Pub. No. (NIH) 73-376.
Multiple Sclerosis, DHEW Pub. No. (NIH) 79-75.
Questions and Answers about Allergies, DHEW Pub. No. (NIH) 78-189.
Sexually Transmitted Diseases, DHEW Pub. No. (NIH) 78-909.
What are the Facts about Genetic Disease? DHEW Pub. No. (NIH) 77-370.

Public Affairs Committee, Inc., 381 Park Ave. S., New York, NY 10016.

Family Planning: Today's Choices, No. 513.
Voluntary Sterilization, No. 507.
Why Can't You Have a Baby? No. 309.

RESOURCE ORGANIZATIONS

American Academy of Allergy
611 Wells St.
Milwaukee, WI 53202

Asthma and Allergy Foundation of America
801 Second Ave.
New York, NY 10017

Epilepsy Foundation of America
1828 L St. N.W.
Washington, DC 20036

Muscular Dystrophy Association
810 Seventh Ave.
New York, NY 10019

**National Association of Patients on
  Hemodialysis and Transplantation**
505 Northern Blvd.
Great Neck, NY 11021

National Kidney Foundation
2 Park Ave.
New York, NY 10016

National Migraine Foundation
5214 N. Western Ave.
Chicago, IL 60625

National Multiple Sclerosis Society
205 E. 42 St.
New York, NY 10017

National Psoriasis Foundation
6415 Southwest Canyon Ct.
Portland, OR 97221

Appendix 1

Organizational Guide to Pamphlet Suppliers

This guide includes all suppliers of pamphlet and booklet materials listed in the Pamphlets sections of Chapters 8 through 17 (Part III). Entries are arranged by type of organization and are alphabetical by name within each category. There are six major types of pamphlet-producing organizations: commercial firms, government agencies and clearinghouses, insurance companies, pharmaceutical companies, professional associations and societies, and voluntary health organizations. Consult the subject index to locate specific pamphlet suppliers in the text.

COMMERCIAL FIRMS

Arandel Publishing Co.
141 Linden St.
Wellesley, MA 02187

Becton, Dickinson & Co.
Consumer Product Div.
Rutherford, NJ 07070

Robert J. Brady Co.
A Prentice-Hall Company
Bowie, MD 20715

Channing L. Bete, Inc.
45 Federal St.
Greenfield, MA 01301

Health Communications, Inc.
7541 Biscayne Blvd.
Miami, FL 33138

Medical Datamation
Southeast and Harrison
Bellevue, OH 44811

Physician's Art Service, Inc.
Patient Information Library
343-B Serramonte Plaza Office Ctr.
Daly City, CA 94015

Pritchett and Hull Associates
2996 Grandview Ave. N.E.
Atlanta, GA 30305

Public Affairs Committee, Inc.
381 Park Ave. S.
New York, NY 10016

UpFront, Inc.
Box 330589
Coconut Grove, FL 33133

GOVERNMENT AGENCIES AND CLEARINGHOUSES

**Administration for Children, Youth
and Families**
Office of Human Development
Services
200 Independence Ave. S.W.
Washington, DC 20201

**Alcohol, Drug Abuse, and Mental
Health Administration**
5600 Fishers La.
Parklawn Bldg.
Rockville, MD 20857

Arthritis Information Clearinghouse
Box 34427
Bethesda, MD 20034

**Bureau of Community Health
Services**
Health Services Administration
5600 Fishers La.
Rockville, MD 20857

Bureau of Health Planning
Health Resources Administration
3700 East-West Hwy.
Hyattesville, MD 20782

Cancer Information Clearinghouse
Office of Cancer Communications
National Cancer Institute
7910 Woodmont Ave.,
Suite 1320
Bethesda, MD 20014

Center for Disease Control
Bureau of Health Education
1600 Clifton Rd. N.E.
Atlanta, GA 30333

Clearinghouse on the Handicapped
Office for Handicapped Individuals
200 Independence Ave. S.W.
Washington, DC 20201

Consumer Information Center
Pueblo, CO 81009

**Consumer Product Safety
Commission**
5401 Westbard Ave.
Bethesda, MD 20207

Diabetes and Arthritis Program
Division of Chronic Diseases
Department of Health and Human
Services
200 Independence Ave. S.W.
Washington, DC 20201

Drug Enforcement Administration
Department of Justice
Washington, DC 20537

**John E. Fogarty International
Center for the Advanced Study in
the Health Sciences**
9000 Rockville Pike
Bethesda, MD 20014

Food and Drug Administration
Office of Consumer Inquiries
5600 Fishers La.
Parklawn Bldg.
Rockville, MD 20857

Food and Nutrition Service
Department of Agriculture
500 12 St. S.W.
Washington, DC 20250

Health Resources Administration
3700 East-West Hwy.
Hyattsville, MD 20782

Health Services Administration
5600 Fishers La.
Parklawn Bldg.
Rockville, MD 20857

**High Blood Pressure Information
Center**
National Heart, Lung and Blood
Institute
National Institutes of Health
7910 Woodmont Ave.
Bethesda, MD 20014

**National Clearinghouse for Alcohol
Information**
Box 2345
Rockville, MD 20852

**National Clearinghouse for Drug
Abuse Information**
Box 1635
Rockville, MD 20857

**National Clearinghouse for Family
Planning Information**
Box 2225
Rockville, MD 20852

**The National Clearinghouse for
Mental Health Information**
National Institute of Mental Health
5600 Fishers La.
Rockville, MD 20852

**National Clearinghouse for
Smoking and Health**
Office on Smoking and Health
5600 Fishers La.
Rockville, MD 20857

National Clearinghouse on Aging
Administration on Aging
330 Independence Ave. S.W.
Washington, DC 20201

**National Diabetes Information
Clearinghouse**
805 15th St. N.W.
Suite 500
Washington, DC 20005

National Eye Institute
National Institutes of Health
Bldg. 31
Bethesda, MD 20014

**National Health Information
Clearinghouse**
InterAmerica Research Associates,
Inc.
1555 Wilson Blvd.
Suite 600
Rosslyn, VA 22209

**National Health Planning
Information Center**
Prince Georges Plaza Branch
Box 1600
Hyattsville, MD 20788

**National Health Standards and
Quality Information
Clearinghouse**
6110 Executive Blvd.
Suite 250
Rockville, MD 20852

**National Heart, Lung and Blood
Institute**
9000 Rockville Pike
Bldg. 31, Room 5A-03
Bethesda, MD 20014

**National High Blood Pressure
Education Program**
See High Blood Pressure
Information Center

**National Highway Traffic Safety
Administration**
U.S. Department of Transportation
Washington, DC 20590

**National Institute of Allergy and
Infectious Diseases**
9000 Rockville Pike
Bethesda, MD 20014

**National Institute of Arthritis,
Metabolism and Digestive
Diseases**
National Institutes of Health
9000 Rockville Pike
Bethesda, MD 20205

**National Institute of Child Health
and Human Development**
9000 Rockville Pike
Bethesda, MD 20205

National Institute of Mental Health
5600 Fishers La.
Rockville, MD 20857

**National Institute of Neurological
and Communicative Disorders &
Stroke**
National Institutes of Health
Bethesda, MD 20014

National Institute on Aging
9000 Rockville Pike
Bldg. 31
Bethesda, MD 20250

**National Institute on Alcohol Abuse
and Alcoholism**
5600 Fishers La.
Parklawn Bldg.
Rockville, MD 20857

National Institute on Drug Abuse
5600 Fishers La.
Parklawn Bldg.
Rockville, MD 20857

National Institutes of Health
9000 Rockville Pike
Publications Bldg. 31
Bethesda, MD 20014

**Occupational Safety and Health
Administration**
Department of Labor
200 Constitution Ave. N.W.
Washington, DC 20210

Office of Cancer Communications
National Cancer Institute
Bethesda, MD 20014

Office of Communications
National Institutes of Health
Bethesda, MD 20014

Office of Consumer Affairs
Department of Health and Human
Services
330 Independence Ave. S.W.
Washington, DC 20201

Office of Nursing Home Affairs
Public Health Service
5600 Fishers La.
Rockville, MD 20857

**President's Committee on Mental
Retardation**
Rehabilitation Services
Administration
3300 C St. S.W.
Mary E. Switzer Bldg.
Washington, DC 20201

Public Health Service
Health Services Administration
5600 Fishers La.
Parklawn Bldg.
Rockville, MD 20857

Social Security Administration
6401 Security Blvd.
Altmeyer Bldg.
Baltimore, MD 21235

INSURANCE COMPANIES

Aetna Life and Casualty
Public Relations Department
151 Farmington Ave.
Hartford, CT 06115

Blue Cross and Blue Shield of Central New York
433 S. Warren St.
Box 4809
Syracuse, NY 13221

Blue Cross Association
840 N. Lake Shore Dr.
Chicago, IL 60611

Connecticut General Life Insurance Company
Hartford, CT 06152

Health Insurance Institute
1850 K St. N.W.
Washington, DC 20006

Kemper Insurance Companies
Communications and Public Affairs
Long Grove, IL 60049

Liberty Mutual Insurance Company
Public Relations Department
175 Berkeley St.
Boston, MA 02117

Metropolitan Life Insurance Company
Health and Safety Education Division
One Madison Ave.
New York, NY 10010

Prudential Insurance Company of America
Public Relations Department
Box 36
Newark, NJ 07101

PHARMACEUTICAL COMPANIES

Abbott Laboratories
Abbot Park, D-383
North Chicago, IL 60064

Ames Co.
Division of Miles Laboratories, Inc.
1127 Myrtle St.
Elkhart, IN 46514

Ayerst Laboratories
685 Third Ave.
New York, NY 10017

CIBA-Geigy Co.
Medical Education Division
550 Morris Ave.
Summit, NJ 07901

C. B. Fleet Co.
4615 Murray Pl.
Lynchburg, VA 24506

Hollister, Inc.
211 E. Chicago Ave.
Chicago, IL 60611

Johnson and Johnson
Educational Services
Patient Care Division
501 George St.
New Brunswick, NJ 08903

Kimberly Clark Corporation
Neenah, WI 54956

Lederle Laboratories
Public Affairs Department
Pearl River, NY 10965

Eli Lilly and Co.
Box 618
Indianapolis, IN 46206

Mead Johnson
Public Relations Department
Evansville, IN 44721

Merck, Sharp and Dohme
Public Relations Department
West Point, PA 19486

Organon
Advertising Department
West Orange, NJ 08869

Ortho Pharmaceutical Corporation
Professional Services Department
Rte. 202
Raritan, NJ 08869

Parke Davis and Co.
Joseph Campau Ave.
Detroit, MI 48232

Personal Products Co.
Milltown, NJ 08850

Pfizer, Inc.
235 E. 42 St.
New York, NY 10017

A. H. Robins
Public Affairs Department
1407 Cummings Dr.
Richmond, VA 23220

Ross Laboratories
Education Services Department
Columbus, OH 43216

Sandoz
Rte. 10
East Hanover, NJ 07936

G. D. Searle
Public Relations
Box 1045
Skokie, IL 60676

Smith, Kline and French Laboratories
1500 Spring Garden St.
Philadelphia, PA 19101

E. R. Squibb & Sons, Inc.
Box 4000
Princeton, NJ 08540

Syntex Laboratories
3401 Hillview Ave.
Palo Alto, CA 94304

Tampax, Inc.
Box 7001
Lake Success, NY 11042

Upjohn
Public Relations Department
7000 Portage Rd.
Kalamazoo, MI 49001

Warner Chilcott Laboratories
201 Tabor Rd.
Morris Plains, NJ 07950

Winthrop Laboratories
90 Park Ave.
New York, NY 10016

PROFESSIONAL ASSOCIATIONS AND SOCIETIES

American Academy of Pediatrics
Box 1034
Evanston, IL 60204

**American Association of Retired
Persons/National Retired Teachers
Association**
1909 K St. N.W.
Washington, DC 20049

**American College of Obstetricians
and Gynecologists**
One E. Wacker Dr.
Chicago, IL 60601

**American Dental Association Bureau
of Health Education and
Audiovisual Services**
211 E. Chicago Ave.
Chicago, IL 60611

American Dietetic Association
430 N. Michigan Ave.
Chicago, IL 60611

American Health Care Association
1200 15 St. N.W.
Washington, DC 20005

American Hospital Association
Center for Health Promotion
840 N. Lake Shore Dr.
Chicago, IL 60611

American Medical Association
535 N. Dearborn St.
Chicago, IL 60610

American Osteopathic Association
212 E. Ohio St.
Chicago, IL 60611

American Podiatry Association
20 Chevy Chase Circle N.W.
Washington, DC 20015

**American Society for
Psychoprophylaxis in Obstetrics**
1523 L St. N.W.
Washington, DC 20005

**American Society of Dentistry for
Children**
211 E. Chicago Ave.
Chicago, IL 60611

**American Society of Hospital
Pharmacists**
4630 Montgomery Ave.
Washington, DC 20014

**National Council for
Homemaker-Home Health Aide
Services, Inc.**
65 Irving Pl.
New York, NY 10003

National Dairy Council
6300 W. River Rd.
Rosemont, IL 60018

The Nutrition Foundation, Inc.
888 17 St. N.W.
Washington, DC 20006

**Pharmaceutical Manufacturers
Association**
1155 15 St. N.W.
Washington, DC 20005

Society for Nutrition Education
2140 Shattuck Ave.
Suite 1110
Berkeley, CA 94704

VOLUNTARY HEALTH ORGANIZATIONS

Al-Anon Family Group Headquarters
Madison Square Sta.
Box 182
New York, NY 10010

Alcoholics Anonymous World Services, Inc.
Grand Central Sta.
Box 459
New York, NY 10017

Allergy Foundation of America
801 Second Ave.
New York, NY 10017

American Cancer Society
777 Third Ave.
New York, NY 10017

American Cleft Palate Educational Foundation
University of Pittsburgh
331 Salk Hall
Pittsburgh, PA 15261

American Diabetes Association, Inc.
600 Fifth Ave.
New York, NY 10020

American Foundation for the Blind, Inc.
15 W. 16 St.
New York, NY 10011

American Heart Association
7320 Greenville Ave.
Dallas, TX 75231

American Lung Association
1740 Broadway
New York, NY 10010

American National Red Cross
17 and D Sts. N.W.
Washington, DC 20006

American Parkinson's Disease Association
147 E. 50 St.
New York, NY 10022

Arthritis Foundation
3400 Peachtree Rd. N.E.
Atlanta, GA 30326

Asthma and Allergy Foundation of America
801 Second Ave.
New York, NY 10017

Better Vision Institute
230 Park Ave.
New York, NY 10017

C/SEC, Inc. (Cesarean/Support, Education and Concern)
15 Maynard Rd.
Dedham, MA 02026

C-Section Experience
Box 65
Glencoe, IL 60022

Canadian Diabetic Association
1491 Yonge St.
Toronto, Ontario M4T-125
Canada

Cesarean Birth Council International
Box 4331
Mountain View, CA 94040

Citizens for Better Care
960 E. Jefferson Ave.
Detroit, MI 48207

Concerned Relatives of Nursing Home Patients
3137 Fairmount Blvd.
Cleveland Heights, OH 44118

Cystic Fibrosis Foundation
6000 Executive Blvd.
Suite 309
Rockville, MD 20852

DES Action
Box 1977
Plainview, NY 11803

Diabetes Association of Greater Cleveland
2022 Lee Rd.
Cleveland Heights, OH 44118

Diabetes Education Center
4959 Excelsior Blvd.
Minneapolis, MN 55416

Do It Now Foundation
Institute for Chemical Survival
Box 5115
Phoenix, AZ 85010

Epilepsy Foundation of America
1828 L St. N.W.
Washington, DC 20036

Hazelden Foundation
Box 176
Center City, MN 55012

HealthRight
Women's Health Forum
41 Union Sq.
Rm. 106
New York, NY 10003

Hospice, Inc.
765 Prospect St.
New Haven, CT 06511

Joslin Clinic
Joslin Diabetes Foundation, Inc.
One Joslin Pl.
Boston, MA 02215

Juvenile Diabetes Foundation
23 E. 26 St.
New York, NY 10010

La Leche League International, Inc.
9616 Minneapolis Ave.
Franklin Park, IL 60131

Leukemia Society of America
211 E. 43 St.
New York, NY 10017

Maternity Center Association
48 E. 92 St.
New York, NY 10028

Medic Alert Foundation
Box 1009
Turlock, CA 95380

Mental Health Association
1800 N. Kent St.
Arlington, VA 22209

Metropolitan Medical Center
Diabetes Education
900 S. Eighth St.
Minneapolis, MN 55404

Muscular Dystrophy Association
810 Seventh Ave.
New York, NY 10019

Myasthenia Gravis Foundation
6230 Park Ave.
New York, NY 10017

National Alliance of Senior Citizens, Inc.
Box 40031
Washington, DC 20016

National Association of Patients on Hemodialysis and Transplantation, Inc.
505 Northern Blvd.
Great Neck, NY 10021

National Council on Alcoholism
733 Third Ave.
Suite 1405
New York, NY 10017

The National Council on the Aging
1828 L St. N.W.
Washington, DC 20036

**National Foundation for Ileitis and
Colitis**
295 Madison Ave.
New York, NY 10017

**National Foundation—
March of Dimes**
Box 2000
White Plains, NY 10620

National Hemophilia Foundation
25 W. 39 St.
New York, NY 10018

National Kidney Foundation
116 E. 27 St.
New York, NY 10016

National Psoriasis Foundation
6415 S.W. Canyon Ct.
Portland, OR 97221

**National Society for the Prevention
of Blindness, Inc.**
79 Madison Ave.
New York, NY 10016

**National Sudden Infant Death
Syndrome Foundation**
310 S. Michigan Ave.
Chicago, IL 60604

**National Tay-Sachs and Allied
Diseases Association, Inc.**
122 E. 42 St.
Suite 3705
New York, NY 10017

National Women's Health Network
2025 I St. N.W.
Suite 105
Washington, DC 20006

Nutrition in the Life Cycle
Box 24770
Los Angeles, CA 90024

Overeaters Anonymous
World Service Office
2190 190 St.
Torrance, CA 90504

Parkinson's Disease Foundation
640 W. 168 St.
New York, NY 10032

**Sex Information and Education
Council of the United States
(SIECUS)**
84 Fifth Ave.
New York, NY 10011

Sight Center
1909 E. 101 St.
Cleveland, OH 44106

**STASH (Student's Association for
the Study of Hallucinogens)**
118 S. Bedford St.
Madison, WI 53703

United Cerebral Palsy Association
66 E. 34 St.
New York, NY 10016

United Ostomy Association
1111 Wilshire Blvd.
Los Angeles, CA 90017

Appendix 2

Directory of Audiovisual Producers and Distributors

This directory lists all sources of audiovisual materials included in the Audiovisual Producers and Distributors sections of Chapters 8 through 16 (Part III). Entries are arranged alphabetically by name. Consult the subject index to locate specific producers and distributors in the text.

Abbott Laboratories
Abbott Park, D-383
North Chicago, IL 60064

Aims Instructional Media Services
Box 1010
Hollywood, CA 90028

American Cancer Society
777 Third Ave.
New York, NY 10017

American College of Obstetricians and Gynecologists
Film Service
Box 299
Wheaton, IL 60187

American Dental Association
211 E. Chicago Ave.
Chicago, IL 60611

American Heart Association Film Library
8615 Directors' Row
Dallas, TX 75247

American Hospital Association
840 N. Lake Shore Dr.
Chicago, IL 60611

American Learning Systems
1106 Jeanette Ave.
Columbus, GA 31906

American Lung Association
1740 Broadway
New York, NY 10019

American Medical Association Film Library
535 N. Dearborn St.
Chicago, IL 60610

American Podiatry Association
20 Chevy Chase Circle N.W.
Washington, DC 20015

Ames Co.
Division of Miles Laboratories, Inc.
1127 Myrtle St.
Elkhart, IN 46514

**M. D. Anderson Hospital and
Tumor Institute**
Dept. of Medical Communication
Houston, TX 77030

Arthritis Foundation Film Library
3400 Peachtree Rd. NE
Atlanta, GA 30326

Association Films
866 Third Ave.
New York, NY 10022

A T & T—Long Lines
Medical Department
Room 2B 200
Bedminster, NJ 07921

Baptist Medical Center—Montclair
800 Montclair Rd.
Birmingham, AL 35213

**Becton, Dickinson & Co. Consumer
Products**
Consumer Products Division
Rutherford, NJ 07070

Benchmark Films
145 Scarborough Rd.
Briarcliff Manor, NY 10510

Robert J. Brady Co.
A Prentice-Hall Company
Bowie, MD 20715

Cancer Care
One Park Ave.
New York, NY 10016

**Cancer Center of University
Hospitals At-Home
Rehabilitation Center**
2074 Abington Rd.
Cleveland, OH 44106

**The Canadian Diabetic Association,
Inc.**
1491 Yonge St.
Toronto, Ontario M4T 1Z5
Canada

Churchill Films
662 N. Robertson Blvd.
Los Angeles, CA 90069

Communications in Learning, Inc.
2929 Main St.
Buffalo, NY 14214

Concept Media
Box 19542
Irvine, CA 92714

**Core Communications in Health,
Inc.**
919 Third Ave.
New York, NY 10022

CRM Educational Films
110 15 St.
Del Mar, CA 92014

Department of Human Resources
Bureau of Health Services
275 E. Main St.
Frankfort, KY 40601

Diabetes Education Center
4959 Excelsior Blvd.
Minneapolis, MN 55416

Walt Disney Educational Media
500 S. Buena St.
Burbank, CA 91521

Educational Activities, Inc.
1937 Grand Ave.
Baldwin, NY 11510

**Encyclopaedia Britannica
Educational Corporation**
425 N. Michigan Ave.
Chicago, IL 60611

Filmline Educational Services
1467 Tamarind Ave.
Hollywood, CA 90028

FMS Productions, Inc.
1040 N. Las Palmas Ave.
Los Angeles, CA 90038

Focus International, Inc.
One E. 53 St.
New York, NY 10022

Guidance Associates, Inc.
Communications Park
Box 300
White Plains, NY 10602

Hanna Barbara Productions
Educational Division
3400 Cahuenga Blvd.
Hollywood, CA 90028

Hazelden Foundation
Box 176
Center City, MN 55012

Health Film Library
Box 309
Madison, WI 53701

Hear Center
301 E. Del Mar Blvd.
Pasadena, CA 91101

Hollister, Inc.
211 E. Chicago Ave.
Chicago, IL 60611

**International Association of Cancer
Victims and Friends**
434 S. San Vincente Blvd.
Los Angeles, CA 90048

International Films Bureau, Inc.
332 S. Michigan Ave.
Chicago, IL 60604

International Union against Cancer
3, rue de Conseil General
CH-1205 Geneva, Switzerland

Jeppersen Sanderson
8025 E. 40 Ave.
Denver, CO 80207

Johnson Institute
10700 Olson Memorial Hwy.
Minneapolis, MN 55441

Journal Films
930 Pitner Ave.
Evanston, IL 60202

Juvenile Diabetes Foundation
23 E. 26 St.
New York, NY 10010

La Leche League International, Inc.
9616 Minneapolis Ave.
Franklin Park, IL 60131

Leukemia Society of America
211 E. 43 St.
New York, NY 10017

Lilly Film Library
Eli Lilly & Co.
Box 100 B
Indianapolis, IN 46206

McGraw-Hill Films
110 15 St.
Del Mar, CA 92014

Medcom
1633 Broadway
New York, NY 10019

Medfact, Inc.
1112 Andrew Ave. N.E.
Massillon, OH 44646

Medi-Cine Sales Corporation
8201 Pendleton Pike
Indianapolis, IN 46226

Mendota Mental Health Institute
301 Troy Dr.
Madison, WI 53704

Milner-Fenwick, Inc.
2125 Green Spring Dr.
Timonium, MD 21093

Modern Talking Picture Service
2323 New Hyde Park Rd.
New Hyde Park, NY 11040

Monoject
Division of Sherwood
Medical Dept.
1831 Clive St.
St. Louis, MO 63103

MTI Teleprograms, Inc.
4825 N. Scott St.
Suite 23
Schiller Park, IL 60176

National Association for Human Development
1750 Pennsylvania Ave. N.W.
Washington, DC 20006

National Association of Counties Research Foundation
1735 New York Ave. N.W.
Washington, DC 20006

National Audiovisual Center
General Services Administration
National Archives and Records Service
Washington, DC 20409

National Council for Homemaker-Home Health Aide Services, Inc.
67 Irving Pl.
New York, NY 10003

National Council on the Aging
1828 L St. N.W.
Washington, DC 20036

National Dairy Council
50 S. Parker
Indianapolis, IN 46201

National Drug Abuse Materials Distribution Center
Box 398
McLean, VA 22101

National Foundation/March of Dimes
Box 2000
White Plains, NY 10602

National Health Films
Box 13973
Sta. K
Atlanta, GA 30324

National Health Systems
Box 1501
Ann Arbor, MI 48106

National Pharmaceutical Council
1030 15 St. N.W.
Washington, DC 20005

National Publications
Box 4116
Omaha, NE 68104

National Society for the Prevention
of Blindness, Inc.
79 Madison Ave.
New York, NY 10016

Omnia Corporation
1301 E. 79 St.
Suite 210
Minneapolis, MN 55420

Paramount Communications
5151 Marathon St.
Hollywood, CA 90038

Parents' Magazines Films
Distributed by PMF Films Inc.
Box 1000
Elmsford, NY 10523

Paulist Communications
17575 Pacific Coast Hwy.
Box 1057
Pacific Palisades, CA 90272

Perennial Education, Inc.
477 Roger Williams
Box 855, Ravinia
Highland Park, IL 60035

Pfizer Laboratories
Divison of Pfizer, Inc.
Film Library
267 W. 25 St.
New York, NY 10001

Pharmaceutical Manufacturers
Association
1155 15 St. N.W.
Washington, D.C. 20005

Phoenix Films
470 Park Ave. S.
New York, NY 10016

Pritchett and Hull Associates, Inc.
2122 Faulkner Rd. N.E.
Atlanta, GA 30324

Professional Research, Inc.
12960 Coral Tree Pl.
Los Angeles, CA 90066

Pyramid Films
Box 1048
Santa Monica, CA 90406

Ross Laboratories
625 Cleveland Ave.
Columbus, OH 43216

St. Louis Park Medical Research
Foundation
5000 W. 39 St.
St. Louis Park, MN 55416

St. Mary's Hospital Medical Center
Community Relations Department
707 S. Mills St.
Madison, WI 53715

Schering Corporation
Professional Services
Galloping Hill Rd.
Kenilworth, NJ 07033

Single Concept Films
2 Terrain Dr.
Rochester, NY 14618

Sister Kenny Institute
27 St. at Chicago Ave.
Minneapolis, MN 55407

Society for Nutrition Education
2140 Shattuck Ave.
Berkeley, CA 94704

Soundwords, Inc.
56-11 217 St.
Bayside, NY 11364

Southerby Productions
1709 E. 28 St.
Long Beach, CA 90806

Spenco Medical Corporation
Box 8113
Waco, TX 76710

Sterling Educational Films
241 E. 34 St.
New York, NY 10016

Teach'em, Inc.
Department 3-C
625 N. Michigan Ave.
Chicago, IL 60611

Time-Life Films
Multimedia Division
100 Eisenhower Dr.
Box 644
Paramus, NJ 07652

Train-Aide Educational Systems
1015 Grandview
Glendale, CA 91201

Trainex Corporation
Box 116
Garden Grove, CA 92642

TV Film Library
475 Riverside Dr.
Room 860
New York, NY 10027

United Ostomy Association
1111 Wilshire Blvd.
Los Angeles, CA 90017

University of British Columbia
P.A. Woodward Instructional
 Resource Ctr.
Room 105
Vancouver, British Columbia
 V6T 1W5

**University of Kansas Medical
 Center**
Education Resource Center
College of Health Sciences
Rainbow Blvd. at 39th
Kansas City, KS 66103

Upjohn
Professional Film Library
7000 Portage Rd.
Kalamazoo, MI 49001

**Vision Multimedia Communication,
 Inc.**
Box 8527
Orlando, FL 32806

West Glen Communications, Inc.
565 Fifth Ave.
New York, NY 10017

Wexler Film Productions
801 N. Seward St.
Los Angeles, CA 90028

Wyeth Film Library
Box 8299
Philadelphia, PA 19101

Xerox Films
245 Long Hill Rd.
Middletown, CT 06457

Appendix 3

Directory of Publishers

This directory provides current addresses for American and British publishers of in-print books annotated in the *Source Guide*. Also listed are publishers of bibliographies and other publications whose addresses are not included in the bibliographic information of the text entries. Publishers are alphabetized by their key word or words, which are the same words used in the annotations (e.g., Bowker = R. R. Bowker Co.). Between the time the main text of this book was prepared and the directory was compiled, a number of publishers changed their names, affiliations, or addresses. Thus, cross-references are provided in the directory to refer readers to publishers' new names or parent companies, and addresses have been updated.

Abbey Press
St. Meinrad, IN 47577

Abelard-Schuman Ltd.
10 E. 53 St.
New York, NY 10022

Academy Publications
Box 5224
Sherman Oaks, CA 91413

Addison-Wesley Publishing Co. Inc.
Jacob Way
Reading, MA 01867

Addison-Wesley Publishers Ltd. (U.K.)
West End House
11 Hills Place
London W1R 2LR

Alcohol, Drug Abuse, and Mental Health Administration
5600 Fishers Lane
Rockville, MD 20857

Alcoholics Anonymous World Services Inc.
Box 459
Grand Central Station
New York, NY 10017

**Al-Anon Family Group
  Headquarters**
Box 182
Madison Square Station
New York, NY 10010

**The Alexander Graham Bell
  Association for the Deaf**
3417 Volta Place N.W.
Washington, DC 20007

**George Allen & Unwin Publishers
  Ltd. (U.K.)**
40 Museum St.
London WC1A 1LU

American Cancer Society
777 Third Ave.
New York, NY 10017

**American College of Obstetricians
  and Gynecologists**
One East Wacker Dr.
Chicago, IL 60601

American Diabetes Association
600 Fifth Ave.
New York, NY 10020

American Hospital Association
840 N. Lake Shore Dr.
Chicago, IL 60611

American Media
790 Hampshire Rd., Suite H
Westlake Village, CA 91361

American Medical Association
535 N. Dearborn St.
Chicago, IL 60610

**American Pharmaceutical
  Association**
2215 Constitution Ave. N.W.
Washington, DC 20037

**American Society for Health
  Manpower Education and
  Training**
840 N. Lake Shore Dr.
Chicago, IL 60611

**American Society of Hospital
  Pharmacists**
4630 Montgomery Ave.
Washington, DC 20014

Anchor Books
see Doubleday

Anderson World Inc.
1400 Stierlin Rd.
Mountain View, CA 94043

Andover Publishing Group
c/o Brick House Publishing Co.
3 Main St.
Andover, MA 01810

Andrews & McMeel Inc.
4400 Johnson Dr.
Fairway, KS 66205

Anthelion Press Inc.
Box 614
Corte Madera, CA 94925

Apple Press
5536 S.E. Harlow
Milwaukie, OR 97222

Arbor House Publishing Co.
235 E. 45 St.
New York, NY 10017

Arco Publishing Inc.
219 Park Ave. S.
New York, NY 10003

Arlington House Publishers
333 Post Rd. W.
Westport, CT 06880

Arrow Books Ltd. (U.K.)
see Hutchinson Publishing Group
Ltd.

Arrow Publishing Co. Inc.
Box 115, 1238 Chestnut St.
Newton Upper Falls, MA 02164

**Arthritis Information
Clearinghouse**
Box 34427
Bethesda, MD 20034

Aspen Systems Corp.
20010 Century Blvd.
Germantown, MD 20767

Association Press
c/o Follett Publishing Co.
1010 W. Washington Blvd.
Chicago, IL 60607

Atheneum Publishers
597 Fifth Ave.
New York, NY 10017

Augsburg Publishing House
426 S. Fifth St.
Minneapolis, MN 55415

Avon Books
959 Eighth Ave.
New York, NY 10019

BBC Publications (U.K.)
35 Marylebone High St.
London W1M 4AA

BJ Publishing Group
200 Madison Ave.
New York, NY 10016

Baker Book House
Box 6287
Grand Rapids, MI 49506

Ballantine Books Inc.
201 E. 50 St.
New York, NY 10022

Bantam Books Inc.
666 Fifth Ave.
New York, NY 10103

Bantam Books Ltd. (U.K.)
Century House
61-63 Uxbridge Rd.
Ealing, London W5 5SA

A. S. Barnes & Co. Inc.
11175 Flintkote Ave., Suite C
San Diego, CA 92121

Barron's Educational Series Inc.
113 Crossways Park Dr.
Woodbury, NY 11797

Basic Books Inc., Publishers
10 E. 53 St.
New York, NY 10022

Basic Books Inc. (U.K.)
see Harper & Row Ltd.

Beacon Press Inc.
25 Beacon St.
Boston, MA 02108

Beacon Press (U.K.)
c/o Harper & Row Ltd.
28 Tavistock St.
London WC2E 7PN

Berkley Publishing Corp.
200 Madison Ave.
New York, NY 10016

Bi World Industries
Box 62
Provo, UT 84601

Biomedical Communications
472 Park Ave. S.
New York, NY 10016

A. C. Black Publishers Ltd. (U.K.)
35 Bedford Row
London WC1R 4JH

Bobbs-Merrill Co. Inc.
Box 558, 4300 W. 62 St.
Indianapolis, IN 46206

The Book Publishing Co.
156 Drakes Lane
Summertown, TN 38483

Boston Public Library
Box 286, 666 Boylston St.
Boston, MA 02117

R. R. Bowker Co.
1180 Avenue of the Americas
New York, NY 10036

R. R. Bowker Co. (U.K.)
Box 5, Epping
Essex CM16 4BU
England

Brooks/Cole Publishing Co.
555 Abrego St.
Monterey, CA 93940

Brunner-Mazel Inc.
19 Union Square W.
New York, NY 10003

Bull Publishing Co.
Box 208
Palo Alto, CA 94302

Bureau of Community Health Services
Health Services Administration
5600 Fishers Lane
Rockville, MD 20857

California Ethnic Services Task Force
c/o Alameda County Library
224 W. Winton Ave.
Hayward, CA 94544

California Health Publications
Box 963, 347 Mermaid
Laguna Beach, CA 92652

California State Library
Box 2037
Sacramento, CA 95809

Canada Books International (U.K.)
One Bedford Rd.
Finchley
London N2 9DB

Cancer Information Clearinghouse
Office of Cancer Communications
National Cancer Institute
7910 Woodmont Ave., Suite 1320
Bethesda, MD 20014

Jonathan Cape Ltd. (U.K.)
30 Bedford Square
London WC1B 3EL

Celestial Arts Publishing Co.
231 Adrian Rd.
Millbrae, CA 94030

Center for Disease Control
Bureau of Health Education
1600 Clinton Rd. N.E.
Atlanta, GA 30333

Center for Health Promotion
see American Hospital Association

Chicago Nutrition Association
550 S. Fourth Ave.
Des Plains, IL 60016

Child's World
1556 Weatherstone Lane
Elgin, IL 60120

The Children's Hospital of Vanderbilt University
Nashville, TN 37232

Chilton Book Co.
Chilton Way
Radnor, PA 19089

Christoper Publishing House
53 Billings Rd.
North Quincy, MA 02171

Churchill Livingstone Inc.
19 W. 44 St., Suite 301
New York, NY 10036

Churchill Livingstone (U.K.)
23 Ravelston Terrace
Edinburgh EH4 3TL,
Scotland

Cleveland Area Metropolitan Library System (CAMLS)
1101 Euclid Ave.
Cleveland, OH 44106

Collier Macmillan Ltd. (U.K.)
Stockley Close
Stockley Rd.
West Drayton,
Middlesex UB7 9BE,
England

William Collins Sons & Co. Ltd. (U.K.)
14 St. James's Place
London SW1A 1PS

Columbia University Press
562 W. 113 St.
New York, NY 10025

Community Health Information Network (CHIN)
c/o Mount Auburn Hospital
330 Mount Auburn St.
Cambridge, MA 02238

CompCare Publications
2415 Annapolis Lane
Minneapolis, MN 55441

Congressional Quarterly Inc.
1414 22 St. N.W.
Washington, DC 22037

Consumer Guide Publications International Ltd.
3841 W. Oakton St.
Skokie, IL 60076

Consumer Health Information Program and Services/Salud y Bienestar (CHIPS)
c/o Carson Regional Library
(Los Angeles County Public Library System)
151 E. Carson St.
Carson, CA 90745

Consumer Information Center
Pueblo, CO 81009

Consumers Union
256 Washington St.
Mount Vernon, NY 10550

Contemporary Books Inc.
180 N. Michigan Ave.
Chicago, IL 60601

Corgi Books Ltd. (U.K.)
Century House
61-63 Uxbridge Rd.
Ealing, London W5 5SA

Cornell University Press
124 Roberts Place
Ithaca, NY 14850

Corwin Books
One Century Plaza
2029 Century Park E.
Los Angeles, CA 90067

Coward, McCann & Geoghegan Inc.
200 Madison Ave.
New York, NY 10016

Thomas Y. Crowell Co., Publishers
10 E. 53 St. CRO
New, York, NY 10022

Crown Publishers Inc.
One Park Ave.
New York, NY 10016

F. A. Davis Co.
1915 Arch St.
Philadelphia, PA 19103

John Day Co. Inc.
c/o Harper & Row, Publishers
10 E. 53 St.
New York, NY 10022

Delacorte Press
c/o Dell Publishing Co.
One Dag Hammarskjold Plaza
245 E. 47 St.
New York, NY 10017

Dell Publishing Co.
One Dag Hammarskjold Plaza
245 E. 47 St.
New York, NY 10017

Andre Deutsch Ltd. (U.K.)
105 Great Russell St.
London WC1B 3LJ

Devin-Adair Co. Inc.
143 Sound Beach Ave.
Old Greenwich, CT 06870

Diabetes Association of Greater Cleveland
2022 Lee Rd.
Cleveland Heights, OH 44118

Dial Press
One Dag Hammarskjold Plaza
245 E. 47 St.
New York, NY 10017

Dodd, Mead & Co.
79 Madison Ave.
New York, NY 10016

Dolphin
see Doubleday

Dorison House Publishers Inc.
802 Park Square Bldg.
Boston, MA 02116

Doubleday & Co. Inc.
245 Park Ave.
New York, NY 10167

Douglas-West Publishers Inc.
7060 Hollywood Blvd.
Los Angeles, CA 90028

Dow Jones Books
Box 300
Princeton, NJ 08540

Duke University Press
Box 6697, College Station
Durham, NC 27708

E. P. Dutton
2 Park Ave.
New York, NY 10016

Eccles Health Sciences Library
University of Utah
Salt Lake City, UT 84112

Wm. B. Eerdmans Publishing Co.
255 Jefferson Ave. S.E.
Grand Rapids, MI 49503

Elsevier/Nelson Books
2 Park Ave.
New York, NY 10016

Paul S. Eriksson, Publisher
Battell Bldg.
Middlebury, VT 05753

Esselte Video Inc.
see Nord Media Inc.

M. Evans & Co. Inc.
216 E. 49 St.
New York, NY 10017

Faber & Faber
99 Main St.
Salem, NH 03079

Faber & Faber Ltd. (U.K.)
3 Queen Square
London WC1N 3AU

Farrar, Straus & Giroux Inc.
19 Union Square W.
New York, NY 10003

Fawcett Book Group
1515 Broadway
New York, NY 10036

**John E. Fogarty International
Center for Advanced Study in the
Health Sciences**
National Institutes of Health
9000 Rockville Pike
Bethesda, MD 20014

Follett Publishing Co.
1010 W. Washington Blvd.
Chicago, IL 60607

Fontana Books (U.K.)
see William Collins

**Food and Nutrition Information
and Educational Materials Center**
National Agricultural Library
Rm. 304
Beltsville, MD 20705

Fount Paperbacks (U.K.)
see William Collins

Four Winds Press
c/o Scholastic Book Services
50 W. 44 St.
New York, NY 10036

Free Press
see Macmillan

W. H. Freeman & Co., Publishers
660 Market St.
San Francisco, CA 94104

Funk & Wagnalls Inc.
c/o Harper & Row, Publishers
10 E. 53 St.
New York, NY 10022

Gale Research Co.
Book Tower
Detroit, MI 48226

General Mills Inc.
Minneapolis, MN 55427

Glide Publications
330 Ellis St.
San Francisco, CA 94102

Victor Gollancz Ltd. (U.K.)
14 Henrietta St.
Covent Garden
London WC2E 8QJ

Great Ocean Publishers
738 S. 22 St.
Arlington, VA 22202

Warren H. Green Inc.
8356 Olive Blvd.
St. Louis, MO 63132

Greenwillow Books
105 Madison Ave.
New York, NY 10016

Greenwood Press Inc.
88 Post Rd. W.
Westport, CT 06881

Greenwood Press (U.K.)
3 Henrietta St.
London WC2E 8LT

Grosset & Dunlap Inc.
51 Madison Ave.
New York, NY 10010

Grove Press Inc.
196 W. Houston St.
New York, NY 10014

Grune & Stratton Inc.
111 Fifth Ave.
New York, NY 10003

Grune & Stratton (U.K.)
c/o Academic Press
24-28 Oval Rd.
Camden Town
London NW1 7DX

Habitex (Les Editions de l'Homme)
955 rue Amherst
Montreal, PQ H2L 3K4, Canada

Robert Hale Ltd. (U.K.)
Clerkenwell House
Clerkenwell Green
London EC1R OHT

G. K. Hall & Co.
70 Lincoln St.
Boston, MA 02111

Halsted Press
c/o John Wiley & Sons Inc.
605 Third Ave.
New York, NY 10016

Halsted Press (U.K.)
c/o John Wiley & Sons Ltd.
Baffins Lane
Chichester, W. Sussex P019 1UD,
England

Harcourt Brace Jovanovich Inc.
757 Third Ave.
New York, NY 10017

Harmony Books
see Crown

Harper & Row, Publishers Inc.
10 E. 53 St.
New York, NY 10022

Harper & Row Ltd. (U.K.)
28 Tavistock St.
London WC2E 7PN

Hart Associates
12 E. 12 St.
New York, NY 10003

Hart-Davis, MacGibbon Ltd. (U.K.)
c/o Granada Publishing Ltd.
Box 9, 29 Frogmore
St. Albans, Hertfordshire AL2 2NF,
England

Harvard University Press
79 Garden St.
Cambridge, MA 02138

Harvester Press Ltd. (U.K.)
2 Stanford Terrace
Hassocks, E. Sussex BN6 8QK,
England

Hawthorn Books
see Dutton

Hayes Publishing Co. Inc.
6304 Hamilton Ave.
Cincinnati, OH 45224

Hazelden Foundation
Box 176
Center City, MN 55012

Health Care Financing
Administration
330 C St. S.W.
Washington, DC 20201

Health Insurance Institute
1850 K St. N.W.
Washington, DC 20006

Health Plus Publishers
Box 22001
Phoenix, AZ 85028

Health Resources Administration
3700 East-West Highway
Hyattsville, MD 20786

Health Sciences Publishing Corp.
451 Greenwich St.
New York, NY 10013

Health Services Administration
5600 Fishers Lane
Rockville, MD 20857

Health Services and Mental Health
Administration
see Health Services Administration

Health Services Communications
Association (HESCA)
Education Committee
Box 1207
Milledgeville, GA 31061

Hearst Books
224 W. 57 St.
New York, NY 10019

William Heinemann Ltd. (U.K.)
15-16 Queen St.
London W1X 8BE

William Heinemann Medical Books
Ltd. (U.K.)
23 Bedford Square
London WC1

High Blood Pressure Information
Center
National Heart, Lung and Blood
Institute
120/80 National Institutes of Health
Bethesda, MD 20014

Highly Specialized Promotions
391 Atlantic Ave.
Brooklyn, NY 11217

Hippocrene Books Inc.
171 Madison Ave.
New York, NY 10016

Hodder & Stoughton Ltd. (U.K.)
47 Bedford Square
London WC1B 3DP

Holt, Rinehart & Winston Inc.
383 Madison Ave.
New York, NY 10017

Holt-Saunders Ltd. (U.K.)
One St. Anne's Rd.
Eastbourne, E. Sussex BN21 3UN,
England

Houghton Mifflin Co.
2 Park St.
Boston, MA 02107

Houghton Mifflin Publishers Ltd.
(U.K.)
41-45 Beak St.
London W1R 3LE

Human Sciences Press Inc.
72 Fifth Ave.
New York, NY 10011

Hunter House Inc.
748 E. Bonita Ave., Suite 105
Pomona, CA 91767

Hutchinson Publishing Group Ltd. (U.K.)
3 Fitzroy Square
London W1P 6JD

Alan Hutchinson Publishing Ltd. (U.K.)
2 Logan Mews
London W8 6QP

I.B.E.G. Ltd. (U.K.)
2-4 Brook St.
London W1Y 1AA

Information Canada
c/o Canadian Government
Canadian Government Publishing
   Centre, Supply and Services
   Canada
Hull, PQ K1A OS9, Canada

International Book Distribution Ltd. (U.K.)
66 Wood Lane End
Hemel Hempstead,
Hertfordshire HP2 4RG,
England

International Universities Press Inc.
315 Fifth Ave.
New York, NY 10016

Joint Information Services of the American Psychiatric Association & the National Association for Mental Health
1700-18 St. N.W.
Washington, DC 20009

Judson Press
Valley Forge, PA 19481

Keats Publishing Inc.
Box 876, 36 Grove St.
New Canaan, CT 06840

Keats Publishing Inc. (U.K.)
c/o Thorsons Publishers Ltd.
Denington Estate
Wellingborough,
Northamptonshire NN8 2RQ,
England

Kellogg Foundation
400 North Ave.
Battle Creek, MI 49016

Kentucky-Ohio-Michigan Regional Medical Library Network
Health Information Library
   Program
Shiffman Medical Library
Wayne State University
Detroit, MI 48201

Alfred A. Knopf Inc.
see Random House

Kogan Page Ltd. (U.K.)
120 Pentonville Rd.
London N1 9JN

LSP Books Ltd. (U.K.)
8 Farncombe St.
Farncombe, Godalming
Surrey GU7 3AY
England

Allen Lane (U.K.)
17 Grosvenor Gardens
London SW1W 0BD

Lange Medical Publications
Drawer L
Los Altos, CA 94022

Lea & Febiger
600 S. Washington Square
Philadelphia, PA 19106

Lea & Febiger (U.K.)
c/o Henry Kimpton Ltd.
7 Leighton Place
Leighton Rd.
London NW5 2QL

Lerner Publications Co.
241 First Ave. N.
Minneapolis, MN 55401

Les Femmes Publishing
231 Adrian Rd.
Millbrae, CA 94030

Libraries Unlimited Inc.
Box 263
Littleton, CO 80160

J. B. Lippincott Co.
E. Washington Square
Philadelphia, PA 19105

Little, Brown & Co.
34 Beacon St.
Boston, MA 02106

Lorenz Press Inc.
501 E. Third St.
Dayton, OH 45401

Lothrop, Lee & Shepard Books
105 Madison Ave.
New York, NY 10016

Robert B. Luce Inc.
6919 Radnor Rd.
Bethesda, MD 20034

METRO
see New York Metropolitan
Reference and Research Library
Agency

MTP Press Ltd. (U.K.)
Falcon House
Cable St.
Lancaster LA1 1PE,
England

McGraw-Hill Book Co.
1221 Avenue of the Americas
New York, NY 10020

McGraw-Hill Book Co. Ltd. (U.K.)
McGraw-Hill House
Shoppenhangers Rd.
Maidenhead,
Berkshire SL6 2QL,
England

David McKay Co. Inc.
2 Park Ave.
New York, NY 10016

Macmillan Publishing Co. Inc.
866 Third Ave.
New York, NY 10022

Richard Marek Publishers
200 Madison Ave.
New York, NY 10016

Marquis Who's Who Inc.
200 E. Ohio St.
Chicago, IL 60611

Massachusetts Medical Society
10 Shattuck St.
Boston, MA 02115

**Medical & Technical Publishing
Co. Ltd. (U.K.)**
see MTP Press

**Medical Economics Co. Book
Division**
680 Kinderkamack Rd.
Oradell, NJ 07649

Merck & Co. Inc.
Box 2000
Rahway, NJ 07065

Meridian Books
see New American Library

Merrimack Book Service Inc.
99 Main St.
Salem, NH 03079

Julian Messner
see Simon & Schuster

Metropolitan Life Insurance Company
Health and Safety Education Division
One Madison Ave.
New York, NY 10010

Monarch Press
see Simon & Schuster

Moore Publishing Co.
Box 3036
W. Durham Station
Durham, NC 27705

William Morrow & Co. Inc.
105 Madison Ave.
New York, NY 10016

C. V. Mosby Co.
11830 Westline Industrial Dr.
St. Louis, MO 63141

C. V. Mosby Co. (U.K.)
Year Book Medical Publishers Ltd.
Barnard's Inn, Holborn
London EC1N 2JA

Mss. Information Corp.
Box 985
Edison, NJ 08817

John Murray Publishers Ltd.
50 Albemarle St.
London W1X 4BD

NAL
see New American Library

National Association for Mental Health
1800 N. Kent. St.
Rosslyn, VA 22209

National Association of Parents & Professionals for Safe Alternative in Childbirth
Box 267
Marble Hill, MO 63764

National Audiovisual Center
National Archives and Records Service
General Services Administration
Washington, DC 20409

National Cancer Institute
Office of Cancer Communications
7910 Woodmont Ave., Suite 1320
Bethesda, MD 20014

National Chamber Foundation
1615 H St. N.W.
Washington, DC 20062

National Clearinghouse for Alcohol Information
Box 2345
Rockville, MD 20852

National Clearinghouse for Drug Abuse Information
Box 1635
Rockville, MD 20850

National Clearinghouse for Family Planning Information
Box 2225
Rockville, MD 20852

National Clearinghouse for Mental Health Information
5600 Fishers Lane
Rockville, MD 20857

National Council on Aging
1828 L. St. N.W.
Washington, DC 20036

National Dairy Council
6300 W. River Rd.
Rosemont, IL 60018

**National Diabetes Information
  Clearinghouse**
805 15 St. N.W., Suite 500
Washington, DC 20005

**National Heart, Lung and Blood
  Institute**
9000 Rockville Pike
Bethesda, MD 20014

National Institute on Drug Abuse
5600 Fishers Lane
Rockville, MD 20857

National Institute of Mental Health
5600 Fishers Lane
Rockville, MD 20857

National Institutes of Health
9000 Rockville Pike
Bethesda, MD 20205

National League for Nursing Inc.
10 Columbus Circle
New York, NY 10019

National Library of Medicine
8600 Rockville Pike
Bethesda, MD 20014

**National Nutrition Education
  Clearinghouse**
2140 Shattuck Ave.
Berkeley, CA 94704

National Women's Health Network
2025 I St. N.W., Suite 105
Washington, DC 20006

Thomas Nelson Inc.
Box 946
405 Seventh Ave. S.
Nashville, TN 37203

Nelson-Hall Publishers
111 N. Canal St.
Chicago, IL 60606

New American Library Inc.
1633 Broadway
New York, NY 10019

**New York Metropolitan Reference
  and Research Library Agency
  (METRO)**
33 W. 42 St.
New York, NY 10036

**New York University Medical
  Center**
Patient Education Center
560 First Ave.
New York, NY 10016

Nord Media
127 E. 56 St.
New York, NY 10019

Northwestern University
Program on Women
619 Emerson St.
Evanston, IL 60201

W. W. Norton & Co. Inc.
500 Fifth Ave.
New York, NY 10036

The Nutrition Foundation Inc.
888 17 St. N.W.
Washington, DC 20006

Oaklawn Press Inc.
283 S. Lake Ave., Suite 200
Pasadena, CA 91101

Okpaku Communications
444 Central Park W.
New York, NY 10025

101 Productions
834 Mission St.
San Francisco, CA 94103

Open Books Publishing Ltd. (U.K.)
11 Goodwin's Court
London WC2N 4LB

Oryx Press
2214 N. Central at Encanto
Phoenix, AZ 85004

Oxford University Press Inc.
200 Madison Ave.
New York, NY 10016

Oxford University Press (U.K.)
Ely House
37 Dover St.
London W1X 4AH

Pacific Mutual Life Insurance Company
700 Newport Center Dr.
Newport Beach, CA 92663

Pacific Southwest Regional Medical Library Service
Biomedical Library
University of California at Los Angeles
Los Angeles, CA 90024

Paddington Press Ltd.
95 Madison Ave.
New York, NY 10016

Paddington Press Ltd. (U.K.)
21 Bentinck St.
London W1M 5RL

Pan Books Ltd. (U.K.)
Cavaye Place
London SW10 9PG

Pantheon Books
see Random House

Parker Publishing Co.
see Prentice-Hall

Paulist Press
1865 Broadway
New York, NY 10023

Penguin Books Inc.
625 Madison Ave.
New York, NY 10022

Penguin Books Ltd. (U.K.)
Bath Rd., Harmondsworth
Middlesex UB7 0DA,
England

Pergamon Press Inc.
Maxwell House
Fairview Park
Elmsford, NY 10523

Pergamon Press Ltd. (U.K.)
Headington Hill Hall
Oxford OX3 0BW,
England

Perrier—Great Waters of France
595 Madison Ave.
New York, NY 10022

Pharmaceutical Manufacturers Association
1155 15 St. N.W.
Washington, DC 20005

Pierian Press
Box 1808
Ann Arbor, MI 48106

Pinnacle Books Inc.
One Century Plaza
2029 Century Park E.
Los Angeles, CA 90067

Plenum Publishing Corp.
233 Spring St.
New York, NY 10013

Pocket Books Inc.
1230 Avenue of the Americas
New York, NY 10020

Popular Library Inc.
1515 Broadway
New York, NY 10036

Praeger Publishers
521 Fifth Ave.
New York, NY 10017

Prentice-Hall Inc.
Englewood Cliffs, NJ 07632

Prentice-Hall International Inc. (U.K.)
66 Wood Lane End
Hemel Hempstead
Hertfordshire HP2 4RG,
England

Princeton University Press
41 William St.
Princeton, NJ 08540

George Prior Associated Publishers Ltd. (U.K.)
37-41 Bedford Row
London WC1R 4JH

Prodist
see Neale Watson

Proteus Publishing Ltd. (U.K.)
Bremar House
27 Sale Place
London W2 1PT

Pruett Publishing Co.
3235 Prairie Ave.
Boulder, CO 80301

Public Citizen Health Research Group
2000 P St. N.W.
Washington, DC 20036

Publications International Ltd.
3841 W. Oakton
Skokie, IL 60076

G. P. Putnam's Sons
200 Madison Ave.
New York, NY 10016

Quail Street Publishing Co. Inc.
22 Aries Court
Newport Beach, CA 92663

Raintree Publishers Inc.
205 W. Highland Ave.
Milwaukee, WI 53203

Random House Inc.
201 E. 50 St.
New York, NY 10022

Rawson, Wade Publishers Inc.
630 Third Ave.
New York, NY 10017

Reader's Digest Press
200 Park Ave.
New York, NY 10017

Regnery/Gateway Inc.
116 S. Michigan Ave.
Chicago, IL 60603

Re-runs Unlimited
4907 Cordell Ave.
Bethesda, MD 20014

Research Press
2612 N. Mattis Ave.
Champaign, IL 61820

Rider & Co. (U.K.)
see Hutchinson Publishing Group
Ltd.

Robinson Press Inc.
Box 25, 218 W. Mountain Ave.
Fort Collins, CO 80521

Rodale Press Inc.
33 E. Minor St.
Emmaus, PA 18049

J. I. Rodale & Co. Ltd. (U.K.)
Griffin Lane
Aylesbury, Buckinghampshire
HP19 3AS, England

Richards Rosen Press Inc.
29 E. 21 St.
New York, NY 10010

Routledge & Kegan Paul Ltd.
9 Park St.
Boston, MA 02108

Routledge & Kegan Paul Ltd. (U.K.)
39 Store St.
London WC1E 7DD

Ruben Publishing
Box 414
Avon, CT 06001

Running Press
38 S. 19 St.
Philadelphia, PA 19103

St. Martin's Press Inc.
175 Fifth Ave.
New York, NY 10010

Samaritan Health Service
Health Education Resource Center
1410 W. Third St.
Phoenix, AZ 85002

W. B. Saunders Co.
W. Washington Square
Philadelphia, PA 19105

W. B. Saunders Co. (U.K.)
see Holt-Saunders Ltd.

Schocken Books Inc.
200 Madison Ave.
New York, NY 10016

Charles Scribner's Sons
597 Fifth Ave.
New York, NY 10017

Seabury Press Inc.
815 Second Ave.
New York, NY 10017

Seaview Books
747 Third Ave.
New York, NY 10017

Sheldon Press (U.K.)
Holy Trinity Church
Marylebone Rd.
London NW1 4DU

Sierra Club Books
530 Bush St.
San Francisco, CA 94108

Signet Books
see New American Library

Simon & Schuster Inc.
1230 Avenue of the Americas
New York, NY 10020

Sister Kenny Institute
1800 Chicago Ave.
Minneapolis, MN 55404

Charles B. Slack Inc.
6900 Grove Rd.
Thorofare, NJ 08086

Society for Nutrition Education
2140 Shattuck Ave.
Berkeley, CA 94704

Souvenir Press Ltd. (U.K.)
43 Great Russell St.
London WC1B 3PA

Sphere Books Ltd. (U.K.)
30-32 Gray's Inn Rd.
London WC1X 8JL

Springer Publishing
200 Park Ave. S.
New York, NY 10003

Standard Publishing
8121 Hamilton Ave.
Cincinnati, OH 45231

Stanford University Press
Stanford, CA 94305

State University of New York Press
State University Plaza
Albany, NY 12246

Stein & Day Publishers
Scarborough House
Briarcliff Manor, NY 10510

Sterling Publishing Co. Inc.
2 Park Ave.
New York, NY 10016

George F. Stickley Co.
210 W. Washington Square
Philadelphia, PA 19106

Lyle Stuart Inc.
120 Enterprise Ave.
Secaucus, NJ 07094

Summit Books
see Simon & Schuster

Summit Books, Australia (U.K.)
c/o WHS Distributors
Euston St.
Freemen's Common
Aylestone Rd.
Leicester LE2 7SS,
England

Superintendent of Documents
Government Printing Office
Washington, DC 20402

Syracuse University Press
1011 E. Water St.
Syracuse, NY 13210

Taplinger Publishing Co. Inc.
200 Park Ave. S.
New York, NY 10003

J. P. Tarcher Inc.
9110 Sunset Blvd., Suite 212
Los Angeles, CA 90069

Teach'em Inc.
625 N. Michigan Ave.
Chicago, IL 60611

Teachers College Press
Columbia University
1234 Amsterdam Ave.
New York, NY 10027

Technomic Publishing Co. Inc.
265 Post Rd. W.
Westport, CT 06880

Ten Speed Press
Box 7123
Berkeley, CA 94707

Charles C. Thomas, Publisher
301-27 E. Lawrence Ave.
Springfield, IL 62717

Thorsons Publishers Ltd. (U.K.)
Denington Estate
Wellingborough
Northamptonshire NN8 2RQ,
England

Times Books
3 Park Ave.
New York, NY 10016

Tobey Publishing Co. Inc.
One Aldwyn Center
Villanova, PA 19085

Touchstone Press
Box 81
Beaverton, OR 97005

Triad Publishing Co. Inc.
Box 13096
University Station
Gainesville, FL 32604

Tulsa City-County Library System
400 Civic Center
Tulsa, OK 74103

Turnstone Books (U.K.)
37 Upper Addison Gardens
London W14 8AJ

**Two Continents Publishing Group
Inc.**
171 Madison Ave.
New York, NY 10016

U. S. Government Printing Office
see Superintendent of Documents

University of California Press
2223 Fulton St.
Berkeley, CA 94720

**University of Michigan Medical
School**
Michigan Diabetes Research and
Training Center

2715 Medical Science II
Ann Arbor, MI 48109

University of New Mexico Press
Alburquerque, NM 87131

University of Southern California
Andrus Gerontology Center
Publications Office
University Park, CA 90007

University of Wisconsin Press
114 N. Murray St.
Madison, WI 53715

University Park Press
233 E. Redwood St.
Baltimore, MD 21202

Van Nostrand Reinhold Co.
135 W. 50 St.
New York, NY 10020

**Van Nostrand Reinhold Co. Ltd.
  (U.K.)**
Molly Millar's Lane
Wokingham, Berkshire RG11 2PY,
England

Veterans Administration Hospital
Patient Education Resource Center
San Francisco, CA 94121

Viking Press
625 Madison Ave.
New York, NY 10022

Vintage College Books
see Random House

Henry Z. Walck Inc.
see David McKay

Walker & Co.
720 Fifth Ave.
New York, NY 10019

Frederick Warne & Co. Inc.
2 Park Ave.
New York, NY 10016

Warner Books Inc.
75 Rockefeller Plaza
New York, NY 10019

Neale Watson Academic Publications, Inc.
156 Fifth Ave.
New York, NY 10010

Franklin Watts Inc.
730 Fifth Ave.
New York, NY 10019

Franklin Watts Ltd. (U.K.)
8 Cork St.
London W1X 2HA

Wayne State University
Division of Library Science
Detroit, MI 48202

George Weidenfeld & Nicolson Ltd. (U.K.)
91 Clapham High St.
London SW4 9TA

Albert Whitman & Co.
560 W. Lake St.
Chicago, IL 60606

Wideview Books
747 Third Ave.
New York, NY 10017

Wildwood House Ltd. (U.K.)
One Prince of Wales Passage
117 Hampstead Rd.
London NW1 3EF

John Wiley & Sons Inc.
605 Third Ave.
New York, NY 10158

John Wiley & Sons Ltd. (U.K.)
Baffins Lane, Chichester
W. Sussex PO19 1UD,
England

Williams & Wilkins Co.
428 E. Preston St.
Baltimore, MD 21202

Winchester Press Inc.
Box 1260, 1421 S. Sheridan
Tulsa, OK 74101

World Publications
see Anderson World

John Wright & Sons Ltd. (U.K.)
42-44 Triangle W.
Bristol BS8 1EX,
England

Wyden Books
747 Third Ave.
New York, NY 10017

Year Book Medical Publishers Ltd. (U.K.)
Barnard's Inn
Holborn
London EC1N 2JA

Zondervan Corp.
1415 Lake Dr. S.E.
Grand Rapids, MI 49506

Author Index

Title Index

NOTE: Pamphlet titles listed in Part III (Chapters 8—17) are not indexed.

Subject Index